"This book brings together the sharpest minds in the psychoanalytic field of today and draws attention to an urgent question within psychoanalysis – how to improve standards of observation, conceptualization and communication of clinical material. The authors engage in in-depth discussions of the scientific status of psychoanalytic knowledge, moving from clinical inquiry to clinical research. A distinguishing feature of the book is the way it highlights how the establishment of various Clinical Working Parties has opened the analytic room and stimulated a productive dialogue between colleagues with different theoretical perspectives in which "arguments of authority" are replaced by a commitment to distinguish between observation and interpretation. This book is a unique contribution to the attempts to bridge the gap between clinicians and researchers, and to create a culture of scientific inquiry. It is of interest for a wide audience, university students, psychoanalytic candidates as well as teachers and practicing psychoanalysts."

Dr. Siri Erika Gullestad, PhD Psychoanalyst. Directed the Department of Psychology and the Clinic for Psychoanalytic Psychotherapy at the University of Oslo.

"It is absolutely fascinating what the systematic study of clinicians' thinking can teach us about patients and about the ways we can work with them most effectively. This book provides an excellent summary of the way in which conceptualisations and technique about patient groups and clinical situations can be refined and used to advance the science of clinical psychoanalysis.

The broad international perspectives will at the same time inform us about diversity of clinical approaches and, far more important, move towards generating a common language in what is now an unnecessarily fragmented field. This is a major contribution to a rapidly developing and crucial field in our discipline."

Prof. Peter Fonagy, Head of the Division of Psychology and Language Sciences at UCL; Chief Executive of the Anna Freud National Centre for Children and Families.

"For more than 100 years psychoanalysis has been seeking its place between the natural sciences and hermeneutics, denounced by some as mechanistic and by others as unscientific. This amazing book brings together a myriad of brilliant minds to shed light on this false choice, where precisely psychoanalysis is played out in its legitimacy as a discipline of the mind, in clinical research. The conversations it brings together have an additional merit: its editors come from the Southern Hemisphere. Those of us who work in these southern confines look at the school disputes being debated in the North with a certain skepticism, which allows us to look at the different perspectives from an advantageous point of view that facilitates integration. This is a book that every psychiatrist, psychologist, psychotherapist, and psychoanalyst who is passionate about borderline questions should study. Whoever reads it will not be disappointed."

Prof. Juan Pablo Jiménez, Director of the Chilean Millennium Institute for Research on Depression and Personality, MIDAP.

Clinical Research in Psychoanalysis

This book offers different theoretical approaches to what clinical research is. *Clinical Research in Psychoanalysis* is a unique contribution to the attempts to bridge the gap between clinicians and researchers and to create a culture of a more rigorous and systematic inquiry. It provides an innovative experience because for the first time different methods and perspectives were used to analyse one same clinical material. This was done by analysts from different working parties of the International Psychoanalytical Association (IPA), from a range of different schools of psychoanalytic thought. This allows the reader to have a vision of the different methods that are currently being used by some working parties of the IPA and to learn about the strengths of each one for certain situations and types of research. This book revaluates clinical research, intending to make links between the analysts working through the working parties and the different ways of thinking in clinical research. By covering key topics, such as how working parties can facilitate different types of research, the place of metaphor in psychoanalytic research and practice, and the future for psychoanalytic research, this text is a fruitful dialogue between different theoretical conceptions and between clinicians and researchers that will expand our perspectives on the evidence we find in clinical material and will broaden our views on the patient.

This book offers a unique and invaluable experience to psychologists and psychoanalysts who are trying to improve their clinical practice and bring research evidence into their psychoanalytic practice. It is an invaluable contribution to the psychoanalytic training of candidates, teachers, and students.

Marina Altmann de Litvan, PhD, is a child and adolescent psychoanalyst (IPA) and a training and supervising analyst of the Uruguayan Psychoanalytical Association and is Chair of the Clinical Research Subcommittee and former Chair of the Clinical Observation Committee of the IPA (2010–2017). She received the Mary Sigourney Award 2017.

Psychoanalytic Ideas and Applications Series
IPA Publications Committee

Recent titles in the Series include

Unpresented States and the Construction of Meaning: Clinical and Theoretical Contributions
edited by Howard B. Levine, Gail S. Reed and Dominique Scarfone

The Ethical Seduction of the Analytic Situation: The Feminine–MaternalOrigins of Responsibility for the Other
Viviane Chetrit-Vatine

Time for Change: Tracking Transformations in Psychoanalysis—The Three-Level Model
edited by Marina Altmann de Litvan

Hostile and Malignant Prejudice: Psychoanalytic Approaches
edited by Cyril Levitt

Freud and Culture
Eric Smadja

Play, Gender, Therapy: Selected Papers of Eleanor Galenson
edited by Nellie L. Thompson

Psychopathology of Work: Clinical Observations
edited by Christophe Dejours

Finding the Body in the Mind: Embodied Memories, Trauma, and Depression
Marianne Leuzinger-Bohleber

Clinical Research in Psychoanalysis

Theoretical Basis and Experiences through Working Parties

Edited by
Marina Altmann de Litvan

Routledge
Taylor & Francis Group
LONDON AND NEW YORK

First published 2022
by Routledge
2 Park Square, Milton Park, Abingdon, Oxon OX14 4RN

and by Routledge
605 Third Avenue, New York, NY 10158

Routledge is an imprint of the Taylor & Francis Group, an informa business

British Library Cataloguing-in-Publication Data
A catalogue record for this book is available from the British Library

Library of Congress Cataloging-in-Publication Data
Names: Altmann de Litvan, Marina, editor.
Title: Clinical research in psychoanalysis : theoretical basis and experiences through working parties / Marina Altmann de Litvan [editor].
Description: Abingdon, Oxon ; New York, NY : Routledge, 2021. |
Series: The international psychoanalytical association psychoanalytic ideas and applications series | Includes bibliographical references and index. |
Identifiers: LCCN 2021001427 (print) | LCCN 2021001428 (ebook) |
ISBN 9781032023175 (hbk) | ISBN 9780367760380 (pbk) |
ISBN 9781003182870 (ebk)
Subjects: LCSH: Psychoanalysis--Research. | Psychoanalytic interpretation.
Classification: LCC RC504 .C58 2021 (print) | LCC RC504 (ebook) |
DDC 616.89/17--dc23
LC record available at https://lccn.loc.gov/2021001427
LC ebook record available at https://lccn.loc.gov/2021001428

ISBN: 978-1-032-02317-5 (hbk)
ISBN: 978-0-367-76038-0 (pbk)
ISBN: 978-1-003-18287-0 (ebk)

DOI: 10.4324/9780000000002

Typeset in Palatino
by Taylor & Francis Books

Contents

Illustrations

Figures

Tables

Prologue

Mark Solms

Psychology, the science of the mind, has always been an embarrassment. Scientific methods are grounded in systematic empirical observation, where *empirical* means 'gathered by means of the senses'. The nub of the problem for us is the fact that the mind – the object of investigation in psychology – is a subject, not an object. This necessarily implies that it cannot be observed empirically, as empiricism is conventionally defined.

The extent of the embarrassment becomes apparent when we consider the fact that, if the mind is something subjective, you can only observe your own. This makes objective observation impossible. It also makes *systematic* observation impossible. How do you measure subjective phenomena? Measurement is essential for objective and systematic observation. In the absence of measurement, how do you control for 'observer bias', for example, especially when the thing you are observing is your own beloved self? In science, we always strive to exclude such distorting factors. How you *feel* about the thing you are studying is not only irrelevant but it positively interferes with systematic observation, and it is therefore excluded as far as possible in science. But how do you exclude subjectivity from the science of subjectivity?

Different schools of psychology have dealt with this problem in different ways. The most infamous of them was behaviourism. The behaviourists, who dominated psychological science for much of the 20th century, ruled subjective data out of science and insisted that we can only study the externally observable inputs and outputs of the mind: stimuli and responses. In effect, they excluded the psyche from psychology.

Psychoanalysis adopted the opposite approach: We took the view that the methods of science must be adapted to its objects of study, not the other way round. We accepted the unavoidable fact that the object of study in psychology is subjective and that it therefore can only be studied introspectively and, moreover, that our data will accordingly be heavily biased by subjective factors. The psychoanalytic method is grounded in these unavoidable facts about the nature of the mind – it positively embraces them – and it has made them the cornerstones of its theories.

This is the origin of foundational concepts in psychoanalysis such as 'resistance', 'censorship', and 'countertransference'. These facts also explain why feelings play such a central role in psychoanalytic observation, because feelings are the direct empirical equivalent of sensory data in the physical sciences.

Taking full account of the ubiquity of these complex factors in subjective observation, psychoanalysis has sought, for more than a century now, to discern the lawful organisation of what we might call the mind *in itself* – that is, the objective reality of the mind, which, perforce, lies behind subjective experience and explains it. Freud used the term *metapsychology* for this systematic endeavour to discern the *implicit* nature of the mind (where *meta* means 'beyond' and *psyche* means 'subjectivity').

The development of a technical vocabulary to achieve such a description of the apparatus of the mind poses special problems of its own. When we cannot point to an object and say, 'term *X* denotes that part over there, and term *Y* denotes that other part', we run the risk that our terms themselves replace the (invisible) things they are meant to denote. But in a science of the mind – the mind as opposed to behaviour – we cannot escape the necessity of a figurative terminology. As Freud wrote one hundred years ago:

> [We are] obliged to operate with the scientific terms, that is to say with the figurative language, peculiar to psychology (or, more precisely, to depth psychology). We could not otherwise describe the processes in question at all, and indeed we could not even become aware of them. The deficiencies in our description would probably vanish if we were already in a position to replace the psychological terms by physiological and chemical ones.
>
> (Freud, 1920/1955, p. 60)

In other words, the deficiencies in our description would vanish if our terms denoted externally observable things. But, unfortunately, they do not. Although it is possible (nowadays) *also* to discern the underlying structure and functions of the mind via their physiological and chemical manifestations, the fact remains that such phenomena do not constitute the mind *itself*; the mind will forever and always be something subjective.

The authors of the various chapters in this remarkable book take these historical facts and truisms as their starting point and then report on recent methodological developments, on a range of systematic research efforts embodying new ways of obtaining and coding the data of our subjective observational field. These developments, led by the authors themselves, working individually and in collaboration with one another (with the enthusiastic support of the International Psychoanalytical Association and its component organisations), attest to the ongoing vitality and fruitfulness of the psychoanalytic approach to the mind.

Being an academic mental scientist myself, I remember only too well the dark days of behaviourism, and I continue to endure the limitations of its successor school in psychology (cognitivism, which treats the mind as though it were no different from a computer). The book you are about to read, more than any other that I have read in recent years, demonstrates the enormous value of an alternative approach, the psychoanalytic one, which – for all its own faults – has the distinction of accepting that subjective experience must be the very foundation of any psychological science that deserves the name. Psychoanalysis is still a young science, so the authors of this book are pioneers, although they stand on the shoulders of giants. As Chair of the Research Committee of the IPA, the Clinical Research Subcommittee of which is chaired by Marina Altmann de Litvan, I am incredibly proud of what they have achieved – and are continuing to achieve.

But the authors of this book are not martyrs. They know, as every psychoanalyst does, how richly rewarding it is to immerse yourself in truly psychological research. As Freud wrote to Einstein, discussing the lack of scientific standing of psychoanalysis compared with physics: 'Admittedly, it is not altogether a matter of regret that one has opted for psychology. There is no greater, richer, more mysterious subject, worthy of every effort of the human intellect, than the life of the mind' (Freud, 1929/1995, p. 122).

16 May 2020

Notes

1 The exchanging and sharing of different models and different methods has many previous and remarkable experiences: (a) the 'Fact, Image, and Metaphor' colloquium, which took place in Colonia, Uruguay, in 1996; (b) a panel in the 2010 congress hosted by the Uruguayan Psychoanalytic Association, in which several methods were presented and shared. This activity meant an important contribution to the raising of awareness of the different models being used; (c) in 2013 in Prague the IPA Clinical Observation Committee had 18 groups working with the same clinical material using the same method (3-LM); (d) panels organised by William Glover and Bernard Reith: 'Expanding the Field: Clinical Working Parties Today' (Prague Congress 2013), 'Expanding the Field: Clinical Working Parties Today (II) Continuing the Dialogue' (Turin 2014, Boston 2015); (e) in July 2015, during the Boston Congress, the IPA Clinical Observation Committee organised a panel and a small discussion group called 'Metaphors and the Use of the Analyst as Tools to Improve Our Clinical Practise'; (f) continuing the work on this topic, at the 2019 IPA Congress held in London, two panels deepened the discussion: 'Transformation in female bodily experiences and bodily metaphors' (Altmann de Litvan, 2021; Fitzpatrick-Hanly, 2019; Fitzpatrick-Hanly, Leuzinger-Bohleber, & de León de Bernardi, 2021).

2 The board of the IPA reviewed research funding in 2012 and 2013. In a setting of falling revenues, there was concern about an excessive dependence on empirical outcome studies. In my view, there also was a retreat from a recognition of the need for expertise in respect of all kinds of research.

3 With the generous support of the IPA and the São Paulo Psychoanalytic Society.

References

Freud, S. (1955). Beyond the pleasure principle. In J. Strachey (Ed.), *The standard edition of the complete psychological works of Sigmund Freud* (Vol. XVIII). London, England: The Hogarth Press. (Original work published 1920)

Freud, S. (1995). Letter to Einstein. In I. Grubrich-Simitis, 'No greater, richer, more mysterious subject … than the life of the mind'. An early exchange of letters between Freud and Einstein. *The International Journal of Psychoanalysis*, 76(1), 115–122. (Original work published 1929)

Introduction

Marina Altmann de Litvan

This book is the fruit of the work of several analysts, the authors who contributed their articles and many others who generously shared their material, clinical work, ideas, and knowledge for the discussion of the cases and organised or participated in discussion groups, conferences, and panels.

Clinical research is a crucial issue for psychoanalysts because psychoanalytic knowledge has emerged mostly from the clinical setting. The psychoanalyst uses subjective data and a subjective instrument – the patient's free association and the analyst's evenly suspended attention – to make observations. As Hinshelwood (2013) stated, clinical knowledge cannot be abandoned without losing a large part of our framework to think about our work.

The purpose of this book is to enhance the dialogue among International Psychoanalytical Association (IPA) working parties (WPs), which work with clinical material from different standpoints and with different approaches. I, as the editor of this book, working with the colleagues of the Clinical Research Subcommittee, thought that our first step should be to reflect on what clinical research is for psychoanalysis. Thus, we invited different authorities on the subject, who have shared their different conceptions.

The book shows the confluence of the interest and work of different IPA committees. On the one hand, the work that was carried out by the Clinical Research Subcommittee, chaired by David Taylor (2010–2017), proposed a set of conferences around the world aiming to improve understanding of clinical research, departing form the working clinician and not from 'above', as Taylor points out in his prologue. On the other hand, in 2011 the IPA Clinical Observation Committee (which I chaired from 2010 to 2017) designed a model for group observation of clinical materials, called the Three-Level Model for Observing Patient Transformations (3-LM). Discussing different clinical materials with hundreds of analysts in different congresses and psychoanalytic societies, metaphors emerged as a relevant element to observe the patient's process. Previous work (Altmann de Litvan, 2021; de León de Bernardi & Altmann de Litvan, 2014) encouraged us to go deeper on this path.

We have introduced metaphor as a clinical tool, as a concept that is close to the clinical work of the analyst in order to work together and to promote a dialogue between working groups.

Our selection of metaphors as key to this observation was based on previous findings that were the result of working with clinical materials, in which we discovered that metaphors were useful to have access to and understand some of the key issues of the patient. We found that metaphors in both symbolic and subsymbolic forms create new modes of understanding. We arrived at the conclusion that the metaphorical processes and metaphors can acquire a relevant significance in the psychoanalytic experience, resulting in true access to the key unconscious problems of the patient. Having found that metaphors were key to the observation of clinical materials, we asked ourselves whether this view was shared by other working groups. This path led us to the idea of different WPs working with the same clinical material, each of them with their own methods.

To further explore these findings, we asked ourselves some questions. *How can a single clinical material be approached by different WPs or by WPs adopting different psychoanalytic research methods*? This was the question addressed at the conference titled 'The Different Phases of Clinical Research' (in 2016), organised by Liana Pinto Chaves, member of the Clinical Research Subcommittee, and Regina Fonseca, chair of the Scientific Committee of the São Paulo Society in Brazil. There, the same clinical material was analysed by the different IPA WPs.

In October 2017, we organised, along with the Uruguayan Psychoanalytic Association, the third conference, 'Working From the Clinic, Metaphor and Interpretation' (Altmann de Litvan, de León, & Uriarte). In that conference we wanted to observe how each of the WP's methodologies approached the same clinical material, which questions were addressed, and which results each WP sought.[1]

The proposed questions for the dialogue were the following.

How do the different groups discover and work on the metaphors? Do they come from the patient? From the analyst? From the group? Or are they co-created by the couple or the group? In what context of the analytic process do metaphors arise?

Although not all WPs prioritised the metaphor in the same way, we believe that the result of the work generated by these questions is remarkably interesting and valuable for the analysts.

A lot has been said about a conflict between two opposed cultures within psychoanalysis (Snow, 1959):

> One culture primarily interpretive, emphasising meaning and purposefulness in human behaviour and relying primarily on the traditional case study method or on qualitative methods and another culture relying primarily on methods from the physical, natural, and social sciences, which search for sequences of cause and effect and use probabilistic rather than individualistic models of data analysis and explanation. (Blatt, Corveleyn, & Luyten, 2006, p. 573)

These two cultures resulted in a clash, expressed, for example, in the debates between André Green, Peter Fonagy, Robert Wallerstein, and Robert Emde (Sandler, Sandler, & Davies, 2000).

But these different psychoanalytic cultures can interact at the clinical level, even when they differ in their understandings of the nature of clinical research. Additionally, their internal perspectives on what psychoanalysis and being a psychoanalyst mean are different, and these perspectives play a – rather unconscious – role in the choices psychoanalysts make while using the different methods and taking part in groups or WPs.

WPs are an effort to go beyond languages and the cognitive processing model of the different IPA geographical regions.

> Working parties and working groups (WP) are ongoing clinical research groups of experienced analysts that hold/sponsor workshops where individual cases are studied using defined methods combining free association, reflective elaboration, and structured research questions, comparing the cases and workshop proceedings to develop and test hypotheses relevant to its inquiry. (Glover & Reith, personal communication)

As Glover and Reith remind us, WPs originated in the European Psychoanalytic Federation and developed different models that show the diversity of traditions, theories, and languages in the European Psychoanalytic Federation to widen the net for listening to the unconscious. Later, the model was used in Latin and North America with variations and new initiatives such as Cassorla's 'microscopy of the session' and Zysman's 'unconscious theories in the psychoanalyst's mind'. To coordinate and encourage these efforts to move forward, the IPA has recently formed a Working Parties Committee, chaired by Dr. Ruggero Levy.

Glover and Reith emphasise that each working group has a question, a method, and a setting. The question varies for each group and addresses a key aspect of psychoanalysis. In most models, the methods progress from free association to reflective elaboration on the question, using semi-structured protocols that invite thinking about the case more systematically, beginning to categorise and formulate hypotheses for further investigation.

My personal focus as a psychoanalyst has always been, and still is, what is beneficial for the patient, within the psychoanalytic office but also outside analysis. Although I belong to the Río de la Plata psychoanalytic tradition, I have been constantly in contact with and interested in different approaches, from both Europe and the United States. The certainty that all views are valuable and that opening to new perspectives makes us better analysts and researchers has not only been part of my training and my practice but also my life philosophy.

When I decided, from my role as chair of the Clinical Research Subcommittee, to be the editor of this book, I saw the opportunity to offer the readers a volume showing what it is like to gather different minds and different approaches with one common aim: to understand the patient and the psychoanalytic process better.

This book is an invitation to explore the way in which a single clinical material can be approached by different WPs, as each of them adopts a different psychoanalytic research method and reflects upon this experience.

This might represent a new approach to single-case studies, which is different from either the empiric approach, as carried out by Kächele, Schachter, and Thomä (2009), and from the traditional psychoanalytical case study, as developed by Freud.

The methods that each WP presents are outside the session itself and in the context of an observation group integrated by analysts. The material seen by our colleagues invites us to find new forms of approaching it. We are not repeating identical situations but rather are promoting the possibility of a conceptual reproduction. WPs enable the creation of a space in which the clinical experience prevails and analysts find it possible to focus on their clinical observations regardless of their different theoretical frameworks (Nieto, Bernardi, Fernandez, Ginés, & Muller, 1982).

It is particularly valuable in the context of present debates for Hinshelwood (2013) to have placed his main emphasis on clinical practice as the primary context for the generation of knowledge. Hinshelwood's inference is that because single-case studies generate valid knowledge in the natural sciences, they should equally be expected to do so in psychoanalysis. The question then is how to design such a model of validation.

What is clinical research in psychoanalysis?

The scientific validity of clinical cases has often been questioned or criticised, from Popper (1959) to Grünbaum (1984). Widlöcher (1994) argued that even before wondering whether clinical cases can satisfactorily meet scientific criteria, one should ponder whether most of the cases reported have scientific goals at all. He emphasises that most clinical cases published serve to the advance of knowledge but do not aim to provide scientific proof. He defends the idea that clinical psychoanalytic cases aim at deepening knowledge relating to and resulting from psychoanalytic practice, and this practice follows different methodological rules from those followed in scientific research. Therefore, the advances made in practical knowledge relate more to a spirit of discovery than to scientific evidence.

Widlöcher (1994) stated that this does not mean that scientific studies cannot be conducted on facts explored by psychoanalysis, clinical cases, mental processes, or theoretical concepts. Case reports are probably not the best method to progress in scientific research. He considers that it remains to be seen whether the scientific findings have an impact on practice. He supports the idea that psychoanalysts do not have to seek scientific objectiveness in clinical case reports.

Psychoanalytic knowledge is originated in a kind of research that is different from the kind done in other sciences. Hinshelwood (2013) pointed out that the subjective nature of our data and our instrument to make observations raises suspicion, but we must remain confident that problems arising from subjectivity can be in fact resolved with careful thought, observation, and a logic designed specifically for research into the psychoanalysis of subjective data.

We can say that all analysts 'investigate' in the session, in the broad sense of the term (enquiry, exploration, *Untersuchung*), because we make use of a method that leads us into the discovery of the unconscious aspects of the material. In this way, the co-creation of 'dyadic truths', characteristic of any analysis and any analyst–patient couple, is produced (Jiménez, 2009). The central aim is the progress of the therapeutic process, and the advance of knowledge is the means to achieve this progress. This activity, as Liberman pointed out (Liberman, 1971), takes place with the patient during the session, and it is therefore also called 'online' research (Leuzinger-Bohleber, Kallenbach, & Schoett, 2016) or 'research on the couch' (Hinshelwood, 2013; Bernardi, Chapter 6, this book).

Thus, psychoanalysis is essentially a clinical discipline that is supported by its own method. Still, as Bernardi states, it can and should resort to a variety of other methodologies when the questions it seeks to answer so demands it (Bernardi, Chapter 6, this book).

However, because treatment and research are not identical, there is no assurance that 'the observation of the analyst and his theoretical conclusions drawn from observations are reliable' (Kächele, Schachter, & Thomä, 2009).

Some authors, like Marianne Leuzinger-Bohleber (Leuzinger-Bohleber & Fischmann, 2006), clearly distinguish clinical research (carried out with the psychoanalytic method in the session) from extraclinical research, which studies the analytic materials or other related issues by using the methodologies characteristic of rigorous scientific research. This distinction is valid if we are interested in discriminating the methods employed. If, on the other hand, we are interested in underscoring the result or purpose sought, it would be advisable to call the full set of procedures that provide us with evidence that is useful for the comprehension of a problem or a situation that is relevant to psychoanalysis 'research at the service of clinical work' (Bernardi, Chapter 6, this book).

As I have already mentioned, different authors emphasise different aspects, but they all agree that clinical research is done outside the analytical session, at a second moment. There are different ways of understanding what clinical and extraclinical research is. What is important is to assess which method is best suited to answer our questions.

The question about psychoanalytic research leads us to what we understand as a psychoanalytic fact. The characteristics of psychoanalytic clinical facts are that they are observable and communicable and that they have, at the same time, a fixed and a transformational aspect (Canestri, 2006; Quinodoz, 1994; Sandler & Sandler, 1994; Tuckett, 1994; Widlöcher, 1994).

The first task is to identify significant clinical facts; that is, to distinguish the 'selected facts' from the 'overvalued ideas' of the analyst (Britton & Steiner, 1994). The expression 'selected fact' – borrowed from Bion (1967), who took it, in turn, from Poincaré – refers to elements that make it possible to gather and attribute meaning to a set of data that, until then, seemed disconnected. It is important then for us to become sensitive to this kind of facts. In this book we are trying to observe specific psychoanalytic facts: metaphors.

Joseph Sandler and Anne Marie Sandler (1994) said that facts reflect the way in which we organise the data we received by our senses (analytical listening), and this organisation is highly selective. We shall further assume that such structures are developed from the beginning of life, on the basis of the individual's conscious or unconscious subjective experience, built on a substratum of given psychobiological dispositions and capacities. The private theories of psychoanalysis play a major role in the organisation of facts and their conceptualisation.

Clinical research offers a valuable occasion for the comparison and examination of the contribution of each perspective. What is analytical listening like for each group? The book aims to show the different approaches to clinical material. Do the differences make the results from one method incomparable to the results from the other? Because this could be questionable, in a clinical sense, as we are observing the same patient, we aim to know whether the outcome is comparable. And we must add whether the discussion is useful and enlightening for the analyst.

The book is based on the experiences of the ordinary analyst who works with the patient, who faces their loneliness and wonders about their patients. In general, there is a widespread concern to improve the listening of the analyst, refining their observations and improving their work. Many WPs place the mind of the analyst as central. We are not talking about process or outcome research.

In the analytic session, the psychoanalyst has at their disposal the means indicated by Freud: the patient's free association and the analyst's evenly suspended attention. As human beings, we have a natural sensitivity for apprehending unconscious emotional phenomena. This sensitivity, which human beings share with other mammals, is reformulated, but not suppressed, by language and finds expression in the representations of our internal world.

Research work moves one step forward when we manage to go deeper with the listening of the unconscious emotional aspects in a first step and then, in a second step, we revise in a critical and systematic form what has been observed, seeking higher validity and reliability.

By using this comprehension of what happens in the session as a starting point, we can propose different metapsychological models. As Freud claimed, oftentimes the more general and abstract constructions of a theory are the top of the building, not its foundation. The foundation, Freud insists (1914/1958), is observation, and it is observation that can corroborate or falsify our speculations. Metapsychology must be considered from this point of view (Bernardi, 2014). I agree with Bernardi (Chapter 6, this book) that psychoanalysis is not to be located 'between' science and hermeneutics: It belongs to both fields and should make use of the resources in both.

Clinical material is an important path to approach our knowledge of the experience of human suffering from a psychoanalytic perspective. In recent times, the development of clinical discussion groups with different perspectives or methodologies has promoted advancements in this field.

Why metaphors?

Freud frequently resorted to different kinds of metaphors to express theoretical concepts and models: the military metaphors, the energetic metaphors, and so forth. But he did not explore the psychic formation of the metaphor or its clinical meaning (Rizzuto, Chapter 10, this book; de León de Bernardi, Chapter 11, this book). He referred to metaphors only in his exploration of jokes and in *Totem and Taboo*. In *The Interpretation of Dreams* he speaks of metaphorical semitones, linking the metaphor to an associative chain that opens up meanings.

From a psychoanalytic perspective, metaphors are defined as

> an effect of a substitution of one signifier for another, a process in which the occulted signifier nevertheless remains in touch with the occulting signifier. It is crucial for the understanding of the structure of repression and its role in the formations of the unconscious, the symptom and the operation of the name-of-the-father: in repression an occluded signifier is forced into the unconscious, the symptom stands in for unconscious material which causes it and the name-of-the-father substitutes for the desire of the mother. It is also the dimension in which the interpretation aims at truth. (Skelton, 2006)

This definition gives an important role to language; the unconscious is structured by language. At the same time, there is another position, coming from developmental studies – especially those focusing on early infant–caregiver interactions. Research in this area has provided an empirical basis for distinguishing primary or root metaphors (i.e., metaphors that originate in preverbal bodily awareness), from metaphors that are more strongly shaped by experience (Modell, 1997). Developmental studies have also enhanced analysts' understandings of the ways in which variations in infant–caregiver mirroring (a metaphoric concept itself) shape subsequent personality dynamics (Stern et al., 1988).

In the analytic field, metaphors are understood as metaphoric processes. Katz (2013) stated that multiple metaphoric processes are always ongoing in an individual's life and they can merge, diverge, overlap, combine, contradict, and conflict with each other.

'A metaphoric process can be thought of as an unconscious trail, which includes and encodes emotional, procedural, dynamic, and other unconscious ingredients of experience. … They are the way in which humans communicate, verbally and non-verbally, intrapsychically and intervivos' (Katz, 2013, p. 15).

I would say there is an experiential level in the session; metaphor is the language of experience. Metaphor is an organising concept in psychoanalytic theory and technique. Every analyst does bring their own language, their own style, their own use of metaphor to the treatment.

In my experience, many times metaphor acquires its quality when advancing the analytical process. For example, the patient can say something at some point in treatment and, in that moment, it may not have a metaphorical sense. Later on during the analysis that expression may acquire a metaphoric meaning. Several metaphors can appear during the analytic process having emotional, cognitive, and visual content. Sometimes they are images or words with high emotional or cognitive content. Metaphorical language is not arbitrary and unmotivated, nor simply ornamental, but is embedded in and central to our entire idea-creating, thinking process, originally arising from our basic bodily (sensorimotor) developmental experiences.

Wurmser (2013) stated that the analyst's work has to be largely metaphorical and he quoted Arlow (1979), who spoke of the whole of psychoanalysis as a metaphorising odyssey. Metaphor has been moved by Lakoff and Johnson (1980) from mental product to mental process (Wallerstein, 2011)

In recent years, psychodynamic theorists have used research findings from outside psychoanalysis to explore the ways in which metaphors can enhance our understanding of a broad array of psychoanalytic concepts. The most widely discussed links involve neuropsychology, wherein research on brain structure and function has elucidated the biological underpinnings of unconscious mental processes, has helped trace the evolutionary roots of human behavioural predispositions, and has been used to examine the interplay of neuropsychological, social, and cultural influences on affective experience and emotional responding (e.g., Modell, 2005; Slipp, 2000).

Cognitive science has been a third area of emphasis, with cognitive research helping elucidate the role of the metaphor in contextualising memories and the process by which retrieval of schema-based memories inevitably results in some degree of distortion and reconstruction (Michels, 1994). These latter findings have been particularly relevant for understanding the long-term negative effects of early trauma and the obstacles to accessing and working through traumatic memories in psychoanalytic treatment (Katz, 2013).

Certain human experiences need metaphors and figures of speech in order to be expressed. They evoke the memories of nature or scenes from literature and from art that help us understand the meanings of those experiences. They are part of the interaction that arises in the analytic field between the analyst and the patient (see de León de Bernardi, Chapter 11, this book).

The metaphor does not always appear in beautiful and ordered packages that can be easily taken out of context for analysis. People use metaphorical language and participate in metaphorical thinking, in complex, often contradictory patterns that make simple conclusions about the ubiquity and structure of the metaphor difficult to elaborate.

The metaphor is creative, novel, and culturally sensitive and allows us to transcend the mundane while being rooted in generalised patterns of body experience that are common to all people (Gibbs, 2010). Metaphors in both verbal and nonverbal forms create new modes of understanding. It is fundamental for many aspects of thought but, nevertheless, special for creative language.

The metaphorical processes and metaphors can acquire a relevant significance in the psychoanalytic experience, resulting in true access keys to the unconscious problems of the patient. Different thinkers of psychoanalysis have given metaphor a central value in both metapsychological constructions and in psychoanalytic communication. Modell (2005) conceptualised metaphors as detectors of unconscious patterns and established a very firm connection between metaphors, bodily sensations, and feelings.

The affective experience, inexpressible sometimes, finds in the components of the metaphor an instrument capable of articulating in the word and, perhaps, in the imagination, in the meaning, and in the image, a way to articulate a dialogue, a connection with the analyst and perhaps sometimes with things that the patients themselves could not even name.

Metaphors have an important unconscious construction in finding meanings (Modell, 2005) that allow us to display or find the lines of force (pattern detectors) of the clinical material and therefore occupy a central role in the organisation and categorisation of emotional memory.

As mentioned above, in the work experience of the different groups, metaphors emerge as common elements. All groups chose metaphors to account for key aspects of the clinical material and the evolution of the patient. But are the metaphors considered equally by all groups? What are the differences?

As we have pointed out, metaphors are a very vast and complex concept that has been largely used in our psychoanalytic community but with different meanings and levels of abstraction. So, to some degree, focusing on metaphors has also meant a challenge, because the same clinical material was being observed by different WPs, following a research proposal.

Working in clinical observation groups with the 3-LM, several metaphors were observed, as well as their use by patient and analyst. But, different from the proposal of this book, the emergence of metaphors as elements to be observed originated not from a research proposal, as is the case in this book, but during the group experiences themselves, where time and time again metaphors rose as significant elements. Sometimes the importance of metaphors became explicit in an interpretation and sometimes it was not even conscious. However, groups observed this importance and usefulness of metaphors in interpretations as possible tools to understand the patient and the process better.

In turn, it has been highlighted how the observation made by different psychoanalysts of the transformations of metaphors in the analytic process contributes to the establishment of a common base for the exchange among them (Bernardi, 2017; Rizzuto, 2009, 2015).

Our work was guided by different questions: How do the different WPs discover and work on the metaphors? Do metaphors come from the patient or from the analyst or are they co-created by both? Do metaphors emerge in the group? In what context of the analytic process do metaphors arise? What can we learn from metaphors in the different clinical settings? Can we equate the changes that occur in metaphors throughout the analysis with changes in the patient's internal and external world? Do metaphors show changes in the way of mental processing, the structure, or the patient's conflicts? Does the symbolic content of the metaphors really change throughout the analysis?

What is the potential of metaphors in the development of the analytical process and what might be their limitations? Will we find an answer to these questions in this book? Probably we will not find one single answer to the questions but different ones, and we may even not find any answers to some of them. However, the exercise of looking for those answers being guided by the different approaches and methods of each WP, in groups of analysts of diverse origins, has resulted in a very rich clinical research exercise. Hopefully, it will inspire other analysts to continue looking for what is best for the patient and for the psychoanalytic process, not limiting their views to their own perspective or to the training received but opening up to new developments and new findings that may improve their own views.

It is my personal hope that psychoanalysts continue searching for dialogue among different schools of thought and that the group observation done by the different WP reaches as many analysts as possible, because it is of real value for our practice and, most of all, for our patients. I see this book as a contribution in that direction.

About the content of this book

Part I introduces us to psychoanalytical clinical practice and clinical research, framed in philosophical and scientific concepts. Authors develop their ideas about the challenge that different practices face for clinical practice and clinical research to be mutually enriching.

Part II presents different conceptual and methodological perspectives on psychoanalytical clinical research within distinct historical, societal, and institutional contexts. This part explains how we move from the clinical inquiry to clinical research and how extraclinical research is included. Experienced authors from different regions in psychoanalysis discuss different significant issues about this topic.

Part III discusses the role of metaphors in the psychoanalytic process, based on clinical examples. Key metaphors in the analytic process and the metaphorising process are presented as a facilitating path from concrete observation to symbolisation and conceptualisation. Metaphors, however, are seen as a complex element that cannot be understood entirely from the surface and demand deep reflection in the context of the analyst–patient relationship.

Part IV presents a detailed account of the history of the IPA WPs and their methods, focusing on answering the questions of whether these methods can be understood as research tools. Different authors present the methods of initiating psychoanalysis, comparative clinical methods, 3-LM, microscopy of the session, Faimberg's method 'listening to listening', and specificity of psychoanalysis. They explain, as well as other aspects, their aims, how they select clinical materials, the setting in which they work, and how they later reflect using the material gathered in the groups. Some of the methods use their findings as starting points to reflect and investigate.

Part V presents three different WPs – 3-LM, comparative clinical methods, and specificity – doing clinical research on the same clinical material and with the same setting. They present what they observed as clinical facts, metaphors, and interpretations.

The relevance of the first interviews in the analytic process is compared by the working group Initiating Psychoanalysis and the Three-Level Model for Observing Patient Transformations (3-LM).

In Part VI the reader will find a reflection upon the work presented in the whole book. The analysts who presented clinical material to be studied by the different working groups share their thoughts about the experience. A synthesis of the convergences and divergences between the different WPs is presented, followed by an analysis of the need for evidence in clinical research and of the role of metaphors as a research tool through three WPs.

References

Altmann de Litvan, M. (2021). Changes and no change in the representation of self and others through images and metaphors. In M. A.Fitzpatrick-Hanly, M. Altmann de Litvan, & R. Bernardi (Eds.), *Change through time in psychoanalysis: Transformations and interventions with the Three-Level Model*, Chapter 4, pp. 79–101. London, England: Routledge.

Arlow, J. A. (1979). Metaphor and the psychoanalytic situation. *The Psychoanalytic Quarterly*, 48(3), 363–385.

Bernardi, R. (2014). The assessment of changes: Diagnostic aspects. In M. Altmann de Litvan (Ed.), *Time for change: Tracking transformations in psychoanalysis – The Three-Level Model*. London, England: Karnac.

Bernardi, R. (2017). A common ground in clinical discussion groups: Intersubjective resonance and implicit operational theories. *The International Journal of Psychoanalysis*, 98(5), 1291–1309.

Bion, W. R. (1967). Notes on memory and desire. In R. Lang (Ed.), *Classics in psychoanalytic technique*. New York, NY, and London, England: Jason Aronson.

Blatt, S. J., Corveleyn, J., & Luyten, P. (2006). Minding the gap between positivism and hermeneutics in psychoanalytic research. *Journal of the American Psychoanalytic Association*, 54(2), 571–610.

Britton, R., & Steiner, J. (1994). Interpretation: Selected fact or overvalued idea? *The International Journal of Psychoanalysis*, 75, 1069–1078.

Canestri, J. (2006). Implicit understanding of clinical material beyond theory. In J. Canestri (Ed.), *Psychoanalysis: From practice to theory*. Chichester, England: John Wiley.

de León de Bernardi, B., & Altmann de Litvan, M. (2014). The Three-Level Model in psychoanalytic training. In M. Altmann de Litvan (Ed.), *Time for change: Tracking transformations in psychoanalysis – The Three-Level Model*. London, England: Karnac.

Fitzpatrick-Hanly, M. A. (2019). Panel report, IPA Congress 2019: Transformation in female bodily experiences and bodily metaphors. *The International Journal of Psychoanalysis*, 100(5), 1031–1033.

Fitzpatrick-Hanly, M. A., Leuzinger-Bohleber, M., & de León de Bernardi, B. (2021). Bodily metaphors as anchor points in facilitating change. In M. A. Fiztpatrick-Hanly, M. Altmann de Litvan, & R. Bernardi (Eds.), *Change through time in psychoanalysis: Transformations and interventions with the Three-Level Model*. London, England: Routledge.

Freud, S. (1958). Remembering, repeating and working-through (further recommendations on the technique of psycho-analysis II). In J. Strachey (Ed.), *The standard edition of the complete psychological works of Sigmund Freud* (Vol. XII). London, England: The Hogarth Press. (Original work published 1914)

Gibbs, R. (2010). The wonderful, chaotic, creative, heroic, challenging world of researching and applying metaphor: A celebration of the past and some peeks into the future. In G. Low, Z. Todd, A. Deignan, & L. Cameron (Eds.), *Researching and applying metaphor in the real world*. Amsterdam, the Netherlands: John Benjamins.

Grünbaum, A. (1984). *The foundations of psychoanalysis*. Berkeley: University of California Press.

Hinshelwood, R. D. (2013). *Research on the couch: Single-case studies, subjectivity and psychoanalytic knowledge*. London, England: Routledge.

Jiménez, J. P. (2009). Grasping psychoanalysts' practice in its own merits. *The International Journal of Psychoanalysis*, 90(2), 231–248.
Kächele, H., Schachter, J., & Thomä, H. (2009). *From psychoanalytic narrative to empirical single case research: Implications for psychoanalytic practice*. New York, NY, and London, England: Routledge.
Katz, S. M. (2013). Metaphoric processes. In S. M. Katz (Ed.), *Metaphor and fields: Common ground, common language, and the future of psychoanalysis*. New York, NY, and London, England: Routledge.
Lakoff, G., & Johnson, M. (1980). *Metaphors we live by*. Chicago, IL: The University of Chicago Press.
Leuzinger-Bohleber, M., & Fischmann, T. (2006). What is conceptual research in psychoanalysis? *The International Journal of Psychoanalysis*, 87(5), 1355–1386.
Leuzinger-Bohleber, M., Kallenbach, L., & Schoett, M. J. (2016). Pluralistic approaches to the study of process and outcome in psychoanalysis. The LAC depression study: A case in point. *Psychoanalytic Psychotherapy*, 30(1), 4–22.
Liberman, D. (1971). *Lingüística, interacción comunicativa y proceso psicoanalítico*. Buenos Aires, Argentina: Galerna/Nueva Visión.
Michels, R. (1994). Validation in the clinical process. *The International Journal of Psychoanalysis*, 75, 1133–1140.
Modell, A. H. (1997). Reflections on metaphor and affects. *Annual of Psychoanalysis*, 25, 219–233.
Modell, A. H. (2005). Emotional memory, metaphor, and meaning. *Psychoanalytic Inquiry*, 25(4), 555–568.
Nieto, M., Bernardi, R., Fernandez, A., Ginés, M. A., & Muller, L. (1982). El futuro del psicoanálisis en Latinoamérica. Presentation at the XIV Congreso Psicoanalítico de América Latina. *Revista Uruguaya de Psicoanálisis*, 50, 1–18.
Popper, K. R. (1959). *The logic of scientific discovery*. London, England: Hutchinson.
Quinodoz, J. M. (1994). Clinical facts or psychoanalytic clinical facts. *The International Journal of Psychoanalysis*, 75, 963–976.
Rizzuto, A. M. (2009). Metaphoric process and metaphor: The dialectics of shared analytic experience. *Psychoanalytic Inquiry*, 29(1), 18–29.
Rizzuto, A. M. (2015). *Freud and the spoken word: Speech as a key to the unconscious*. London, England: Routledge.
Sandler, J., & Sandler, A. M. (1994). Comments on the conceptualisation of clinical facts in psychoanalysis. *The International Journal of Psychoanalysis*, 75, 995–1010.
Sandler, J., Sandler, A. M., & Davies, R. (Eds.). (2000). *Clinical and observational psychoanalytic research: Roots of a controversy*. London, England: Routledge.
Skelton, R. M. (Ed.). (2006). *The Edinburgh international encyclopaedia of psychoanalysis*. Edinburgh, Scotland: Edinburgh University Press. Retrieved from http://www.pep-web.org/document.php?id=zbk.069.0001m#yp0003165995600
Slipp, S. (2000). Introduction to neuroscience and psychoanalysis. *Journal of the American Academy of Psychoanalysis*, 28(2), 191–201.
Snow, C. P. (1959). *The two cultures*. Cambridge, England: Cambridge University Press.
Stern, D., Bruschweiler-Stern, N., Harrison, A., Lyons-Ruth, K., Morgan, A., Nahum, J., & Tronick, E. (1988). The process of therapeutic change involving implicit knowledge: Some implications of developmental observations for adult psychotherapy. *Infant Mental Health Journal*, 19(3), 300–308.

Tuckett, D. (1994). The conceptualisation and communication of clinical facts in psychoanalysis. *The International Journal of Psychoanalysis*, 75(5–6), 865–870.
Wallerstein, R. (2011). Metaphor in psychoanalysis: Bane or blessing? *Psychoanalytic Inquiry*, 31, 90–106.
Widlöcher, D. (1994). A case is not a fact. *The International Journal of Psychoanalysis*, 75, 1233–1244.
Wurmser, L. (2013). Metaphor and conflict. In S. M. Katz (Ed.), *Metaphor and fields: Common ground, common language, and the future of psychoanalysis*. New York, NY, and London, England: Routledge.

Note on the IPA's Committee for Clinical Research in Psychoanalysis

David Taylor

One of Charles Hanly's first initiatives when he became International Psychoanalytical Association (IPA) president in 2009 was to propose a group that looked out for psychoanalytic clinical research, which he thought had been neglected by the IPA. As both a philosopher and a psychoanalyst, Hanly could argue compellingly that the future of psychoanalysis depended primarily on its capacity to distinguish what is factual and substantial within itself from what is vacuous. Only secondarily does it depend on its ability to generate new ideas about the human psyche or on a willingness to expose them to empirical forms of research. This remains the case.

This, then, was why the Clinical Research Subcommittee (CRSCo) came into being: a child of that decade-ago context; a legacy that has lasted of an effort to redirect the IPA's research activities by means of a wholesale administrative reorganisation. Peter Fonagy was then the chair of the IPA's International Research Board. He and Hanly invited me to be the CRSCo's first chair.

I accepted on condition that the CRSCo's *raison d'être* would be psychoanalytic research per se. That meant supporting the use of the psychoanalytic method to make discoveries using standards of truth or falsehood that are appropriate to the study of the human subject. There are no instruments or forms. It would not genuflect, neither to supposedly more empirical scientific methods nor to pseudo-profound ideas that seem so attractive to some fellow practitioners even while having little or no readily discernible basis in psychic reality. What phenomena exactly psychoanalysis thinks are essential to the study of the human subject, and what criteria of truth or falsehood apply, were tactfully left unstated.

The CRSCo had forerunners. These included a collection of IPA-funded groups devoted to conceptual research and others to clinical observation. Several members of a dissolved IPA Conceptual Research Committee became a nucleus for the new CRSCo. These were Anna Ursula Dreher (Frankfurt, Germany), Susanna Fischbein (Buenos Aires, Argentina), Clara López-Moreno (Buenos Aires, Argentina), and Norbert Freedman (New York, United States). Within the next year, they were joined by Liana Pinto Chaves (São Paulo,

Brazil), Donald Moss (New York, United States), and, a little while later, Rudi Vermote (Leuven, Belgium), Kay Long, (New Haven, Connecticut, United States), and Mitchell Wilson (San Francisco, California, United States). Each one brought intelligence, independence of position, readiness to work together (perhaps a little variable), rigour, expertise in differing special areas, and knowledge. They also brought networks in their countries and regions.

The CRSCo quickly became an active, productive working group with its own identity and programme. This was achieved by meeting six times per year, largely via audio link. The technology often failed. As well as managing their own multiplicity of tongues, members coped with frequent losses of audio connection and the intrusion of noises sounding like electronic plumbing in deep underwater ocean trenches.

It is invidious to single out individuals for special mention, but Norbert Freedman should be an exception: a New York psychoanalyst blind from his youth, a refugee from Nazi Germany. As he did, the CRSCo depended on listening to words and sensing feelings. Psychoanalytic sessions also depend on these capacities. Norbert was an adept. Sadly, a few years into the life of the CRSCo, he died at age 88 following a fall while he was going about his still-active life. All felt it a privilege to have worked with him.

Out of such experiences, the CRSCo created what was to become a lasting sense of its purpose. Certain refractory problems presented themselves repeatedly. To consider them, the CRSCo proposed designated clinical research panels at successive IPA congresses.

For example, everyone thinks they know good psychoanalytic clinical research when they see it, but if asked to formulate criteria these are tentative and unconvincing. Therefore, in 2011, in a Mexico City congress panel, members of the CRSCo examined three papers to spell out what were their epistemological strengths and weaknesses (see Chaves, 2012).

We wanted to eschew using customary explanations such as 'unconscious functioning' to describe an important characteristic of psychoanalytic findings, namely, how they go beyond what we customarily say – or think – about ourselves. The method chosen for Prague in 2013 was to examine the grounds on which the analyst imputes motives, actions, and phantasies to the analysand when neither the analyst nor the analysand has any direct knowledge of them (Chaves & Taylor, 2013). In Boston in 2015, simultaneous states of knowing and not-knowing were examined (Bronstein, 2015).

Other questions considered included the optimal relationship between clinical and formal research methods; empirical and platonic (metaphysical or metapsychological) ways of thinking; psychoanalysis as rooted in biological science; and psychoanalysis as hermeneutics. There were different positions on these matters, but by and large a sympathetic tolerance developed among the members of the committee: a tolerance that underpinned the CRSCo's confidence in its ability to put clinical knowledge firmly alongside the findings of empirical science in several Sandler conferences. Their programmes were co-organised with Marianne Leuzinger-Bohleber, vice-chair of the International Research Board, and Peter Fonagy. Both often attended CRSCo meetings (see, for example, Fonagy, Kächele, Leuzinger-Bohleber, & Taylor, 2012).

The regular contacts between CRSCo members also led to an appreciation of the effects on what counts as knowledge of the different traditions, languages, and geographical regions. This appreciation led the CRSCo to propose a rolling programme of working conferences in different parts of the world to improve understanding of clinical research, starting from the working clinician upwards rather than a model from 'above'.

The first of these was organised by William Glover and Donald Moss in the United States and was held in San Francisco in October 2013. It was titled, 'Says Who? Evidence, Fact, and Belief in Clinical Psychoanalysis'. In his thoughtful account, Donald Moss noted some reluctance among psychoanalysts when together in a setting enquiring into 'evidence' to make statements about phantasies or internal structures or object relations. It seemed they felt less anxious when referring to aspects of analyst–analysand interaction they deemed observable; imputing internal mental processes by venturing outside the protection of a reality shared by the group involved a distinct anxiety, or fear.

Charles Hanly's term ended in 2013. He was succeeded by Stefano Bolognini. Peter Fonagy resigned. Mark Solms became chair of the IRB.[2] The Clinical Research Sub-Committee was renamed the Clinical Methodology Sub-Committee (CMSCo). We were pleased to welcome Marina Altmann de Litvan (Montevideo, Uruguay) and Kay Long (New Haven, Connecticut, United States). Susana Vinocur-Fischbein left to join the revived Conceptual Research Committee. Mitchell Wilson departed and subsequently became the editor of *Journal of the American Pyschoanalytic Association.*

Marina Altmann brought a special commitment to clinical observation study groups and a research interest in metaphor. These fitted with the project of supporting practitioners in their local context to arrive at their understanding of clinical research rather than fruitlessly trying to impose a global prescription top-down. Thus, 'The Many Faces of Research in the Psychoanalytic Consulting Room' was held in São Paulo, Brazil, in October 2016.[3] The third conference, 'Facts, Metaphor and Interpretation in Clinical Practice', was held in Montevideo, Uruguay, in October 2017. Liana Pinto Chaves and Rudi Vermote worked with Marina so that learning might be carried forward from one conference to the next.

In late 2017, when I left the CMSCo, I was confident and pleased that its work would be carried forward and developed with Marina Altman as its chair. This substantial volume shows that expectation to have been right. This book contains the papers presented at these two conferences and much else besides. That it does owes everything to the work of its editor

Marina, as well as to the contributions of Liana Pinto Chaves. Its papers contain some of the best understanding pertaining to the perennial question of how we learn about the subject matter of psychoanalysis. It is a subject matter that exists independently of psychoanalysis itself. Maintaining the quality of how we learn about it is vital. Improving on that quality can only be achieved millimetre by millimetre, whereas diminishing it comes more easily.

I want to acknowledge my personal debt of gratitude to all my colleagues on the CRSCo/CMSCo. I learned a lot from all of them. Many became friends. There were few instances of irresolvable difference. Yet, in time, one sees that these, too, are grist to the mill of the work; they have a high-density value but a long latency.

References

Bronstein, A. (2015). Panel report, IPA Congress Boston 2015: Knowing and not knowing one's own mind. Is an unconscious at work? *The International Journal of Psychoanalysis*, 96(6), 1663–1665.

Chaves, L. P. (2012). Recent contributions from clinical research: On mental processing, on dreams and dreaming, and on the role of phantasies about parental couple relationships. *The International Journal of Psychoanalysis*, 93(3), 750–751.

Chaves, L. P., & Taylor, D. (2013). Examining today's theory of thinking in the light of the analysis of a patient unable to gain from his environment. *The International Journal of Psychoanalysis*, 94(6), 1180–1182.

Fonagy, P., Kächele, H., Leuzinger-Bohleber, M., & Taylor, D. (Eds.). (2012). *The significance of dreams: Bridging clinical and extraclinical research in psychoanalysis*. London, England: Karnac.

Part I

From clinical practice to clinical research

Chapter 1

The mysterious leap from clinical practice to clinical research

Liana Pinto Chaves

Part 1

What do average analysts think of clinical research? What do they think clinical research consists of?

We may intuitively grasp the idea that institutions (for example, the Tavistock Clinic in London, the Institute Alfred Binet in Paris, the Sigmund Freud Institute in Frankfurt, or the Karolinska Institute in Stockholm) promote research in its many expressions, supporting the analyst or psychotherapist with an institutional backup, facilities, and funding, while at the same time offering treatment to the community. But what about the individual psychoanalyst working in their consulting room?

The average analyst thinks almost exclusively like a psychoanalyst. The analyst who intends to do research needs to think simultaneously as a psychoanalyst and as a researcher.

And why is it so difficult to think in terms of research? We become analysts after many years of personal analysis and theoretical–clinical training, and it takes us many more years to become more at ease in our role as analysts, with a free transit between our subjectivity and that of the patient. We are aware of the dialogic character of the exchange that takes place in the transference–countertransference field created between the two protagonists of the analytical scene. To think in terms of research seems to amount to an extra effort, in addition to the fact that many analysts think of the term *research* with a degree of suspicion or prejudice. It is no longer acceptable to hold the naïve idea that every analyst is a researcher, as we frequently hear, but it is not easy to abandon common sense. Further theoretical knowledge and expertise are necessary to acquire the mind of a researcher.

The complexity of the epistemological and methodological considerations concerning the scientific status of psychoanalytical knowledge baffles the clinician. These considerations (natural science versus hermeneutics, induction, deduction, abduction, causal evidence, causes or meanings, data selection, verifiability, etc.) may seem like Greek to the clinician; they demand familiarity with certain concepts to be able to follow the discussion, not to mention to

DOI: 10.4324/9780000000002-2

participate in the discussion of a growing body of work, with an extensive bibliography. One could say that acquaintance with the discussion is a career in itself. It is precisely for that purpose that the Clinical Research Subcommittee of the International Psychoanalytical Association was created: Its aim was to promote discussion about the whole area of clinical research and make it more accessible for clinicians.

Our ancestors, the authors who became our references, wrote their excellent insightful texts that inspired generations of the subsequent analysts. Nowadays, with the growing discussion on the nature of clinical research, it looks as if there was a necessity for a special knowledge, a certain training, in order to build an attitude with regards to research.

André Green (as cited in Sandler, Sandler, & Davies, 2000, p. 24), with his usual rigour and dryness, said,

> Up till now, the great contributors to psychoanalytic theory (Freud, Abraham, Ferenczi, Rank, Melanie Klein, Bion, Winnicott, Lacan, Hartmann, etc.) have all enriched our knowledge with their work stemming from their single mind and from the working through of their own experience with their patients.

And then he moved on to say that 'there is no single major discovery for psychoanalysis which has emerged from research' (as cited in Sandler et al., 2000, p. 24). We do not have to agree with him and feel despondent, despite his stature.

All of us would agree that what is done in a session has to do with the discovery of the unconscious aspects present in the material, the suffering of the patient that keeps them entrapped in the repetition, and the central aim is the progress of the therapeutic process. But there is a great distance between this view and the understanding of the dynamics of the process becoming research. And then comes the question: How can it be systematic (as we expect research to be) if we are dealing with changeable states of mind?

Freud's (1923/1955, p. 235), opening paragraph, now almost centenary, in 'Two Encyclopaedia Articles' is usually the point of departure for the rich body of knowledge that has accumulated over the years, concerning the nature of the analytical endeavour and quoted by most authors:

> Psychoanalysis is the name (1) of a procedure for the investigation of mental processes which are almost inaccessible in any other way, (2) of a method (based upon that investigation) for the treatment of neurotic disorders and (3) of a collection of psychological information obtained along those lines, which is gradually being accumulated into a new scientific discipline.

This statement is valid to this day and it has remained the most succinct expression of what would later develop into an intense and fruitful debate in the last 30 years about the nature of psychoanalytical knowledge and its status among the sciences – to a great extent thanks to the enterprising spirit of Joseph Sandler, with his proposals of discussions around fundamental topics and the relationship of psychoanalysis to other fields of research. There is already a corpus of consolidated debate about clinical and conceptual research.

A brief statement by Anna Ursula Dreher (2016) helps in building the bridge:

> In a general understanding, clinical research in psychoanalysis subsumes all research activities directly linked to the core: the analytic situation. The aim of these different research activities and their different methods is to describe and to explain what happens in this analytic situation.

Part 2

I would now like to take as an example the work of Björn Salomonsson, from the Swedish Psychoanalytical Society, better known for his work on psychoanalytical psychotherapy with infants and parents done at the Mama Mia Child Health Centre in Stockholm. He is also a researcher at the Karolinska Institute. I will resort to a paper of his and will try to follow it in some detail to get closer to what I think would help us to 'see' what clinical research is and how it evolves, first in the consulting room and then in the work done after the sessions. To my mind his work is a good illustration of the title of Ricardo Bernardi's chapter: 'Moving From Clinical Inquiry to Clinical Research' (Chapter 6, this book). And he also spells out in each one of his papers 'a clear definition of the questions' (a point stressed by Bernardi, Chapter 6, this book) he proposes to tackle.

In other words, to my view, his work as clinical researcher can dialogue fruitfully with the work of Bernardi as conceptual researcher. Bernardi focuses on why and how the investigation of mental processes can be considered clinical research, and Salomonsson provides us with the opportunity to follow and grasp these two dimensions.

The paper we are going to use as an illustration, 'Infantile Defences in Parent–Infant Psychotherapy: The Example of Gaze Avoidance' (Salomonsson, 2016) is part of an ambitious project that investigates whether the psychoanalytical concepts we use for older individuals are applicable to babies as well. Earlier papers, which were part of this project and many of which published in the *International Journal of Psychoanalysis* with very engaging titles, dealt with infantile sexuality, 'Has Infantile Sexuality Anything to Do With

Infants?' (Salomonsson, 2012); transference, 'Transferences in Parent–Infant Psychoanalytic Treatments' (Salomonsson, 2013); and primal repression, in the book *Psychoanalytic Therapy With Infants and Parents: Practice, Theory and Results* (Salomonsson, 2014). They attempt to cover a range of classical concepts in psychoanalysis. In all of these papers he puts the huge question: 'Can we really speak of the infant as being a subject?' (Salomonsson, 2016, p. 66). He acknowledges: 'Undoubtedly, such a project is fraught with heuristic difficulties' (Salomonsson, 2016, p. 66), considering that he is dealing with a 'person' before it becomes a proper person.

Salomonsson is an analyst who lives the therapeutic process with his patient(s), formulates questions, goes after the answers to those questions, does clinical research simultaneously with the therapeutic process (the famous Freudian conjunction), and, through informed analytical discussion of those phenomena and hypotheses and in the light of analytical theory, he builds his clinical reasoning.

The clinical material in this paper on infantile defences is about a mother with a 3-month-old baby girl who has difficulties in their relationship. The baby had an initial satisfactory development in the first 3 weeks of life but started to have colic attacks, and the mother was unable to comfort her. The baby started to avoid mother's eyes, which led the mother to depression, after a very loving and tender beginning. The baby looks at everything and everybody, except the mother.

I will not attempt to summarise the very detailed and sensitive clinical narrative constructed by Salomonsson, how he gradually collects the history of the mother during the sessions with all of the many important experiences. You will have to take my word. I invite you to read the paper: 'Infantile Defences in Parent–Child Psychotherapy: The Example of Gaze Avoidance', (Salomonsson, 2016). For our purpose today it suffices to say that initially he received mother, father, and baby and then concentrated on mother and baby. The therapy was planned to last 5 months, initially in a frequency of four times, then two, and finally one time per week, as the initial complaint resolved.

Salomonsson (2016) reflected on the possible psychodynamics of gaze avoidance. His guess is that the emotional stress during the weeks of colic laid the ground for the baby forming a negative internal image of the mother. This was complicated by the fact that the mother herself had difficulties when looking people in the eyes, presumably linked with her low self-esteem. According to Salomonsson, this created a representation in the baby's mind of a bad mother figure summarised in the phrase: 'If I avoid looking at it, I feel better' (Salomonsson, 2016, p. 97).

This guess (his word), which we could call an informed speculation, can also be considered a hypothesis, an assumption, and the starting point of the therapeutic process and the clinical research. He warns: 'Evidently this formulation is but a clumsy and speculative verbalization of a representation that was pre-verbal yet impacting the girl's behavior' (Salomonsson, 2016, p. 97).

Throughout the sessions the analyst sometimes addresses the mother and sometimes addresses the baby, and after a particular intervention, the girl starts looking into the mother's eyes. As the atmosphere becomes serene, more and more material come out, dealing with the mother's relationship with her own mother.

Salomonsson's theory to account for his analytical observation and clinical experience was inspired mainly by Freudian, Kleinian, and Winnicottian perspectives. I will quote him more extensively here:

> The mechanism, I assumed, was as follows: Her perceptions of Mum had been influenced by the pain and distress inherent in the colic and Mum's ways of handling her. These perceptions were then subjected to splitting mechanisms and projective distortions. This caused a terrifying internal maternal part object to emerge. Any contact with the external Mum, above all looking into her eyes, entailed a risk for Kirsten to get in emotional contact with the feared internal object. Thus, *her aim was not primarily to evade contact with her mother's eyes but to avoid having a scary emotional experience.* This process was also fuelled by how the mother perceived the girl; she was desperate about the colic and the gaze avoidance and accused herself of having caused at least the latter. This made Mum tense when she was with Kirsten. (Salomonsson, 2016, pp. 71–72)

The hypotheses about the mother's internal situation could be investigated in the usual way in therapy, through associations and interpretations. But what about the baby's internal world? He then proceeds to discuss the question of the baby as a subject, to which he responds affirmatively, after revising the relevant literature and describing the steps in the treatment that led to the dissolution of the symptom and the reestablishment of a more harmonious contact between mother and baby.

He describes the baby's conflicts like this: 'I love my mother; she always comforts me. No, she doesn't. She is helpless when I'm helpless. She can't take my pain away at once. I close my eyes because I want her out of my life' (Salomonsson, 2016, p. 76)

His questions as a researcher were the following:

1 Can the baby defend herself against a representation? In his words: Can such a young psyche muster psychological defences?
2 From the perspective of the baby as a subject, 'Can we ask if psychoanalytic concepts can describe her internal world and its links with her behavior?'

He concluded that gaze avoidance was not a solipsistic symptom but was part of a relationship disorder. Because the baby was seen as a subject and a very active, participative partner, the analyst addressed her directly, following the classic analytic description of a defence. There were three subjects in the room (the baby with her distress and her symptom, the mother with her guilt and depression, and the analyst with his countertransference), and the acknowledgement of this led to the affective breakthrough and to a behavioural change in the baby.

Being a finely attuned analyst and concerned with issues regarding research, he gives us the opportunity of following the progression of his work in a twofold movement: from the clinical experience to the theory and back from the theory to the experience. Given his exceptional clarity, we can follow his naturalistic observational capacity and the discoveries made in the clinical situation in the classical tradition of the single case.

Again, but in other words: I took this particular paper as an example of how phenomena that are found in the consulting room give rise to questions that will be systematically considered under the light of the continuity of the psychoanalytical process submitted to theoretical reflection/ consideration.

I think Salomonsson achieved exactly what Bernardi preaches with regards to clinical research: The first task is to identify significant clinical facts and then to gather and attribute meaning to a set of data that, until then, seemed disconnected (Bernardi, Chapter 6, this book).

And Bernardi adds:

> Transparency is also essential in the clinical field. In this case, replicability does not imply the repetition of identical clinical situations, which are unique, but rather the possibility of conceptual reproduction. This means traceability of the inferential process that goes from observation to conclusions. In this way it becomes possible to compare one author's observations and conclusions with those of others. (Bernardi, Chapter 6, this book)

Analysts who work with severe pathologies, or difficult cases, curiously make it easier to follow them in their work and the maturing of their knowledge about these cases and to have an idea of how they do clinical research, probably to a great extent because of the enormous pressure on them. I have in mind Anne Alvarez, Björn Salomonsson, and Joshua Durban, among others, who work with autistic, psychotic, traumatized children and adolescents.

The same could be said of times when there is intense passionate discussion, exchange, and research going on in the consulting rooms, leading to the production of important psychoanalytical work – for instance, the importance of the work of the Kleinian group in London on psychosis in the 1950s (the work of Rosenfeld, Segal, and Bion) following Melanie Klein's recent developments on schizoid mechanisms.

I hope I have succeeded in conveying the gist of Salomonsson's work both as a psychoanalyst and as researcher. In addition to working with the single case in a more traditional way, he is engaged in extraclinical research with groups of mothers and babies, comparing their treatments, with follow-ups, interviews, questionnaires, and measurements. He is a full researcher. And I hope I was able to bring some of the aspects of clinical research to your attention. I think Salomonsson offers us a model of research that does not sacrifice the importance of subjectivity and singularity of the cases studied, a prejudiced view that many people hold to this day.

Part 3

To conclude, I would like to mention something about the São Paulo Regional Conference, the second of a series of three proposed by the Clinical Research Subcommittee, which was called 'The Many Faces of Clinical Research' and was held in 2016. The first one took place in San Francisco and was called 'Says Who? Evidence, Fact, and Belief in Clinical Psychoanalysis'. The São Paulo conference's logo was a keyhole – the keyhole of Freud's house in Maresfield Gardens. Its meaning was not immediately evident; it was a bit hermetic and condensed, I must say. The intention was to conjure up the idea of something that happens behind doors, something for which we were not invited and do not have access to or, to use Ron Britton's idea, a room in which we can only enter with our imagination – the mythical primary scene of the intimacy of patient and analyst. The idea of this conference was to do this imaginative exercise: how other colleagues think about the clinical phenomena.

References

Dreher, A. U. (2016). Film of advertisement for the São Paulo conference on clinical research held in 2016. Retrieved from https://www.youtube.com/watch?v=Xp07gayXM Co&feature=youtu.be

Freud, S. (1955). Two encyclopaedia articles. In J. Strachey (Ed.), *The standard edition of the complete psychological works of Sigmund Freud* (Vol. XVIII). London, England: The Hogarth Press. (Original work published 1923)

Salomonsson, B. (2012). Has infantile sexuality anything to do with infants? *The International Journal of Psychoanalysis*, 93(3), 631–647.

Salomonsson, B. (2013). Transferences in parent–infant psychoanalytic treatments. *The International Journal of Psychoanalysis*, 94(4), 767–792.

Salomonsson, B. (2014). *Psychoanalytic therapy with infants and parents: Practice, theory and results*. London, England: Routledge.

Salomonsson, B. (2016). Infantile defences in parent–child psychotherapy: The example of gaze avoidance. *The International Journal of Psychoanalysis*, 97(1), 65–88.

Sandler, J., Sandler, A. M., & Davies, R. (2000). *Clinical and observational psychoanalytic research: Roots of a controversy – Andre Green & Daniel Stern*. London, England: Karnac.

Chapter 2

What is clinical research in psychoanalysis?

Some comments on its scientific background

Anna Ursula Dreher

Introductory remarks

To the question 'What is clinical research in psychoanalysis?', there are so many substantial answers that no further variant should be added here. Instead, the discussion of some epistemological and methodological themes of this research field may help clarify possible answers. On the one hand, these themes are about questions generally preceding each research, such as scientific worldviews or respective pre-assumptions of the state of the world. On the other hand, these themes are about concrete decisions in each research project, about the chosen view of the research subject, about the research aims, and about the choice of methods, in order to be able to achieve the aims. Worldview, subject, aims, and methods influence each other; decisions on one topic have effects on the other topics. It is more than useful not only to be aware of one's own position on these pre-assumptions but also to formulate them explicitly. Such transparency may clarify that and why there can be well-founded decisions other than one's own and may – this is the hope – facilitate a critical and productive discourse between researchers of different scientific beliefs and between researchers and clinicians.

Nowadays, scientists often tend to justify their research activities by the canon of scientifically recognised *methods* only. The selection of the 'right' methods should justify the scientific nature of their research. I do not want to proceed from there. Research is defined not only by the choice of methods but also by its *scientific worldviews with its ontological pre-assumptions*, its *research subjects*, and its *aims*. Accordingly, I will regard the field of clinical research taking all of these issues into account. The methods actually used in the context of clinical research come from different sources: from psychoanalysis itself, from the neighbouring disciplines of medicine and psychology, from the natural sciences, from qualitative social research, etc. Methods are, on the one hand, tools for the collection and the analysis of data, but they themselves can also be the subject of scientific assessment, reflections, and discussions. Methodological considerations quickly make it clear how method, subject, and aims are interrelated: insofar as they deal with the

DOI: 10.4324/9780000000002-3

question of whether a method fits the subject, the hypotheses and the data to be researched at all, and to what extent the intended research aims can be achieved with this method.

Such considerations are particularly useful when there are competing proposals or even controversial beliefs as to which methods should best be used in the specific field of research. Two small examples: Those who have the aim of finding causal natural laws must use experimental methods, because causal hypotheses can only be tested by means of experimental designs. Those who aim to extract patterns or types from single cases – for example in the sense of 'deep and thick descriptions' (Geertz, 1973) – tend to use descriptive, reconstructive, and interpretative methods.

Epistemological and methodological themes and reflections may be far from clinical practice, sometimes even far from research practice, but they build the philosophical and scientific background of all research. The explicit as well as implicit or so-called hidden assumptions concerning these themes may have immense consequences: *which paradigm of* clinical research is implemented and practiced and *how* useful the results for the improvement of our theories, models, and concepts are – and, last but not least, also for the improvement of our clinical work and for the benefit of our patients.

Usages of the term *clinical research*

The term *clinical research* is widely used in sciences and has various meanings inside and outside psychoanalysis. Inside, the understanding of clinical research ranges from our traditional 'conjunction of cure and research' and systematised procedures of clinical reasoning up to brain scanning of patients under treatment conditions, from qualitative studies up to quantitative–experimental designs of treatment processes and outcomes, etc. Furthermore, extraclinical research methods from infant and developmental research, from conceptual or historical research, from neuroscience or ethnopsychoanalysis, can also play a role in the context of clinical research. In a traditional understanding, for some analytic authors the term clinical research *only* refers to the analyst's activities in and around the analytic situation on the basis of analytic methods. Of course, our central theoretical ideas about nature, structure, and functioning of the psyche have been inferred from traditional analytic–therapeutic work. But what do we call the searching and groping attitude of the analyst? I think any *practicing analyst* may be called an explorer or an investigator of the patient's psyche, especially the patient's unconscious dynamics in the setting of the analytic situation. Of course, this exploring and investigating part of the analyst and their clinical reasoning play an important role in each research process. However, the contributions of the treating analyst are unfortunately only necessary, but not sufficient, elements of a research process. If you call the analyst a *researcher,* there is the risk of a misunderstanding: Nowadays, the term *research* in the contemporary understanding of scientific communities must satisfy methodological criteria. Scientific research therefore is no longer possible as a 'one-person endeavour', practiced by the treating analyst alone, but is a social project, embedded in a scientific community, driven by ideas and hypotheses, data, methods, and results but also driven by communication, discourse, and, last but not least, criticism from those who have other ideas or different analytic or scientific opinions. Other researchers than the treating analyst can act with gain, and methods other than the analytic ones could be used for research purposes.

This means that I use the term clinical research in a broad understanding, not in the traditional and narrow sense – including all research activities by analysts and researchers related to relevant clinical phenomena in the analytic work with patients. I see the analytic situation as a privileged – not the only– place of *discovery* of clinical phenomena or of generating ideas, as well as a privileged place – not the only– of *justification* of all sorts of new psychoanalytic concepts and thoughts related to the analytic practice. What a scientific research project looks like in concrete terms, which other researchers are involved, and which methods are used are decisions that are based on epistemological and methodological considerations.

Science, research, and 'psychoanalysis between nature and culture'

It is commonly understood that the secured assets of scientific knowledge are sedimented in concepts, theories, and models, and research is seen as the most important motor for scientific progress in general. But what does *scientific* mean? Some fundamental controversies on clinical research are based on the differing beliefs about science and how it should be practiced (see Dreher, 2010). When discussing such sensitive issues, one has to bear in mind that all epistemological and methodological themes – whether regarding world-views, hidden assumptions, theories, procedures for testing hypotheses, aims, choice of methods and concepts etc. – are *not* genuine psychoanalytic themes but fundamentally general scientific topics and they belong to intellectual history. To this end, one must leave the domain of psychoanalysis and reflect on what others have to say, especially the philosophy of science. The ideas of how clinical research could be conducted scientifically are constantly changing. Some more or less prominent trends of the last decades may serve as illustrations; for example, empiristic, behaviouristic, cognitivist, and recent neuroscientific research paradigms have been suggested as methodological prototypes – unfortunately often claiming to have the sole representation. If one is to acknowledge that there is no 'one and only' mode of science and scientific research but several competing, partly complementary views about what science is and how scientific research works, then one would easily find ways and means to accept different psychoanalytic research approaches to explore the analytic situation as subject of research. However, this only works as long as these views are made explicit and thus become subject of critical scientific discourse.

Not everyone can accept a broad and open-minded understanding of the maxims preceding each research, because it affects fundamental questions of science and its status. The Anglo-Saxon world, for example, with its evaluative distinction between 'science, humanities, and arts', introduces an historically and culturally grown, narrow understanding of scientific that many others would not share in this rigorous way. Researchers who regard only natural sciences as 'true' science will rate methods and aims from psychoanalysis or from cultural, social, and historical sciences as 'unscientific' and, therefore, as less acceptable. This historically and culturally based differing boundary between science and non-science in research issues has, over the past decades, unfortunately been a dominant background factor in many discussions of clinical research. And it can, at the same time, be seen as an example of how massively different worldviews and specific methodological beliefs can complicate discourse and prevent acceptance of divergent opinions. Someone with a *nomothetic* worldview tends to look for causal explanations and the general in all cases and wants to find decontextualised universal laws, which – like the laws of physics – apply independent of culture and history. Someone with an *ideographic* worldview, however, tends to look for the particular in every unique case and sees each case embedded in historical, cultural, and social contexts. The differences between the two worldviews, which correspond to the nature–culture dichotomy, give rise to a methodological question: Do we seek *causes* for behaviour or *reasons* for actions, or do we seek both? Two everyday examples may illustrate this. A cause for crying might be a grain of sand in the eye, a reason for crying might be that someone is mourning. A cause for laughing might be that someone is being tickled, a reason for laughing might be that someone just understood a joke. Psychoanalysis, this is easy to discern, deals with both, with causes and reasons as well as with facts and meanings.

I therefore agree with an allocation of psychoanalysis that played an important role in the Green-Wallerstein debate; there, psychoanalysis is seen as a science *between nature and culture* (Green, 2005; Wallerstein 2005a, 2005b). Since its beginnings, psychoanalysis has always gained by moving in this field of tension; that is to say, paying attention to the nature of human beings in the form of physicality, genetic predispositions, innate drives, ecological givens, and programmes designed by evolution and, on the other side, paying attention to the *culture of human beings*; to the results of family, social, and cultural socialisation; to language and to historical and economical givens. It has always been of particular interest *how* nature and culture *interact* in individuals and form biographically grown human psyches – and that, of course, remains the great challenge of researching these psyches *in a scientifically satisfying way*.

Clinical research: Preceding epistemological and methodological questions

With methodological questions it is not useful *not* to give an answer, because 'no explicit answer' usually means that one takes an implicit or hidden position on them. That one cannot scientifically consider the world without any unprovable assumptions Popper has already shown (1934/1959): there are *no theory-free* data in empirical sciences. Data are always collected in the light of theories and ontological assumptions about what reality is and how it works. Theories direct our view to reality. For example: There is no behaviour of a patient that is 'transference' by itself; there is only behaviour that can be 'seen as' and 'understood as' transference in the light of psychoanalytic theory and in the context of a concrete analytic treatment. Anyone who does not share the theoretical background of psychoanalysis and who does not know the concrete clinical context cannot recognise transference phenomena in a patient's behavioural flow. In the same way, there is also no *epistemologically free and methodologically free* research regarding worldview, subject, aims, and methods. Only explicit answers clarify positions and enable discourse and the search for better solutions. I will formulate ten pertinent topics as questions. And I think more than one answer is possible in each case.

1 How to deal with the mind–body problem in clinical research?

The oldest and most relevant epistemological problem regarding the relation between psyche and soma leads to these questions: What actually exists in reality and what can be a subject of scientific research at all? Do only physical entities – matter, energy, and information (here: in the physical sense) – exist? Or do entities like mind, psyche, and soul also exist there? And if both exist and are accepted as subjects for science, what is their relationship? Can mind or psyche be completely reduced to physical processes, as a strictly reductionist position would see it? Or are mind and psyche merely epiphenomena like smoke on a fire, as others see it?

Psychoanalytic ideas actually suggest that the relationship between immaterial psychic phenomena and the physical brain, between psyche and soma, follows an interactionist model. Both are partly independent subjects of scientific research, but the brain and the body can influence the psyche, and the psyche can influence the brain as well as the body. Psychoanalysis sees the psyche not only as an immaterial interface between biological hardware and external physical and cultural world but as an inner virtual psychological space with its own structures and processes – and methods for research have to do justice to this fact. Scans, for example, can only capture material phenomena such as electrical or biochemical processes but not psychic representations or subjective meanings. And even if, for example, one knows where and how the representation of the mother is sedimented in the brain, one cannot see on the pictures *how* this representation is psychically configured, whether it is a loving or a neglecting or a 'dead' mother in Green's sense (see Green, 1999). This sort of information (here: in the psychological sense) can only be made accessible through inference and interpretation. A small example concerning the difference of the sorts of information: the results of a pregnancy test (yes or no) may transmit only one bit of information, but they can have life-changing psychological meaning for the people concerned. However, one's own belief about the problem of how immaterial phenomena can arise from matter explicitly or implicitly influences the scientific position, as well as the answers to methodological questions.

2 What is our most important subject of research?

The focus of 'psycho-analysis' is, as the term implies and even if it may sound trivial, the analysis of the human psyche, which we believe can be clinically and scientifically investigated. Already the labelling of the *psychic* aspect of human beings in sciences causes problems: Would it be better to talk about *psyche* or *mind* or *soul* or just *brain*? Would it be wise to equate psyche=-mind=brain? The terms psyche, mind, and brain have different references and meanings. Therefore, already the choice of a label for the subject of research is an epistemological decision with methodological consequences. The only material and physical object is the brain in the skull, the hardware for the immaterial upper software categories like mind and psyche – and, by the way, also for personality, character, intelligence, etc. Whoever speaks of mind usually refers to cognitive and emotional information processing. It is assumed that these processes are formed by evolution and determined by the environment and that they operate structurally in the same way in all brains, which is why it can make sense to build a computer model of 'the' human brain or 'the' human mind. Whoever speaks of soul usually refers to spiritual and religious aspects of being human. But those who speak of *psyche* primarily refer to the subjective and private inner worlds of individuals and to interpsychic interchange between humans. Our psychic realities, our individual inner virtual realities, so to speak, are formed in biography by nature and culture. And we assume that the psyche is as individual as a fingerprint or DNA. Notwithstanding this, the systematic access to the psyche has some unruly and nasty properties, but this should be seen as a challenge rather than an obstacle for research (see also Dreher, 2015).

3 What does empirical *mean in clinical research?*

In the sciences there are different extensions of what can be understood by *empirical*. Natural sciences have a narrow understanding. Only observable or measurable behaviour or electric or chemical brain activities are empirical. Psychoanalysis has a broad understanding of empirical. All intra- and inter-psychic phenomena, all psychic mechanisms and processes are empirical; they are not metaphysical ideas, even if these phenomena are not directly observable, neither from the third-person perspective of the analyst or scientist nor from the first-person perspective of the patient. Unconscious processes can only be accessible indirectly through inference and interpretation. By the way, this is similar to dark matter and dark energy in physics.

No realist would question that physical facts exist. Searle (2010) gives reasons why 'social facts', the products of subjective attitudes of human beings, are also just as real and objective as physical facts. In an analogous way, it is useful for psychoanalysis to speak of *psychic facts*; for example, the 'facts of life'. An empiricist occasionally contradicts the independent existence of psychic facts, which paradoxically contradicts the subjective experience of most people. Practically anyone of us has evidence for what it is like to be in a psychic state, like being angry, happy, jealous, injured, etc., or what it is like to have feelings of attachment to a friend, or what it is like to love or hate someone. Instead of assuming different ontological domains, different unrelated worlds, so to speak, I would like to speak of 'one world' for physical, social, and psychic facts, so that the psychic facts psychoanalysis deals with could also fit in the 'one world'.

4 Which realities are to be taken into account?

However, the possible methodological access differs, depending on whether one explores physical reality, social reality, or – like us analysts – psychic reality as research subject. The clinical situation brings together these three aspects of reality that differ in their epistemological characteristics and methodical approaches. First, there is the one shared external physical reality that is the same for all people. Second, there are different and specific social and cultural realities, shared by social and cultural groups. And third, every human being also has their own psychic reality, which is not simply an inner representation or image of external realities, be they physical or social. Of course, physical and social realities influence psychic reality, but psychic reality also influences the subjective perception of the external world. Elements of psychic reality can be projected into both social and physical reality and can individually distort it. External reality follows natural laws; social and cultural realities follow social and cultural rules, norms, and legal laws. Psychic realities are essentially determined by biographical history and dynamic unconscious processes. And, as Freud has already shown, neither the rules of logic nor the rules of space and time apply in some parts of this inner world, which is why the sources of fantasy and creativity lie here.

Since time began people have been fascinated not only by the external world, accessible through perception, but also by their internal world, accessible through introspection and dreams. A look at intellectual history up to modern times illustrates the countless attempts of myths, religions, art, and, in the end, human sciences to approach the mysteries of human inner life, to understand all kinds of intrapsychic phenomena better. The focus of analytic clinical research is primarily on all of these internal psychic phenomena and their intersubjective dynamics and only secondarily on the manifest behaviour. In contrast, the focus of clinical research in cognitive therapy is on observable behaviour and on the representation of the external world in the mind.

5 Who are we talking about?

The emphasis on the research subject 'psyche' has consequences for how we see our patients. In first line we do not see 'mental disorders' with ICD (*International Classification of Diseases*) or DSM (*Diagnostic and Statistical Manual of Mental Disorders*) codes, nor do we see 'abnormal behaviours' or 'abnormally functioning brains'. But what we do see are children, adolescents, men, and women with their distress and their problems, their sufferings and psychic pain, with their biographically grown personality; and they have their individual family, social, cultural, ethnic, religious, and economic provenances and backgrounds – just like us analysts. Of course, patients can be classified on the basis of theoretical models as disturbed or mentally ill or as showing abnormal behaviour. And, of course, they have brains that may function in a deviant mode – but the border between 'normal' and 'abnormal' or 'deviant' is based not only on naturally given categories but essentially on cultural conventions, always including normative, historically contingent, and culturally dependent aspects. But, first of all, our patients are human beings who meet with us analysts; that is, there is, in the specific analytic situation, an interaction of two individual actors with their respective subjective modes of functioning. Of course, patient and analyst have different roles, specified by a fundamental asymmetry. Analysts are to follow the professional rules of analytic neutrality and abstinence and should – this is the reasoned expectation – distinguish themselves by clinical experience and competence. Only when these conditions are met is the kind of space created in which phenomena can show and unfold, onto which we then direct our clinical as well as our clinical research attention.

6 Which perspectives are to be taken into account?

The subject of clinical research is to investigate what happens 'in' the patient, 'in' the analyst, and 'between' them. From a technical point of view, it can therefore be useful to distinguish a number of perspectives: first, the two first-person perspectives of patient and of analyst: What do both see and experience? What do they say? And what do they do? Then, the two second-person perspectives: How does the analyst think the patient sees them? How does the patient think the analyst sees them? Psychoanalysis understands these two perspectives as interwoven in a network of defence and resistance, transference, countertransference, role-responsiveness, etc.

The treating analyst is simultaneously in multiple roles. Analysts are inside the analytic situation, simultaneously 'actor', 'diagnostic instrument', and 'method'. Outside the analytic situation, they are 'reporter' – also about themselves – *and* possibly objectifying researcher. The treating analyst may therefore be required to adopt *further* perspectives. When thinking about, reasoning, or reporting on the treatment, analysts take a decentred third-person perspective; they must be able to adopt a distanced, reflected, and occasionally critical attitude towards themselves and their treatment. This stance is similar but *different* from another third-person perspective, the objectifying third-person perspective of a researcher. One of the criticisms of the so-called conjunction research, with its view of the analyst at the same time as therapist *and* researcher, concerns a possible confusion of both third-person perspectives.

Each researcher must make his or her own choice as to which of these perspectives is to be considered. It can be necessary and useful that other researchers support the analyst in a kind of maieutic function and help to save, to structure, and to process the clinical material (see, e.g., Thomä & Kächele, 2006) – thereby meeting not only clinical but also scientific requirements.

7 What belongs to clinical data?

For the analyst during analysis and also for the clinical researcher who researches, clinically relevant phenomena – as basis for research – may show in manifold modes. They show in overt behaviours; in gestures and facial expressions; in emotions; in feelings and affects; in libidinous, aggressive, or other motives; in dreams, free associations, or narratives; in fears or intuitions, by following courtesy and cultural rules or by violating such rules, intentionally or unconsciously. And last but not least – and this is not very astonishing in a talking cure – they show in language, in all of its aspects: in syntax, semantics, and pragmatics of what was said and in phonology and prosody, in when and how it was said and in what was not said.

The expressing of the psychic pain and suffering of the patient and the analyst's responsiveness to it and containing and interpreting it play an essential role: These are phenomena that are characterised by the perception of behaviour and of conscious phenomena but also by sensations of *preconscious and unconscious processes* going on in and between the two protagonists. Analysts try to verbalise these processes that only in part show in behaviour. They infer them on the basis of nonsensory perceptions by their special sort of introspection but remain the sole authority for these clinical data. Analysts follow up their inklings and densify them to assumptions, abductions, and hypotheses. They try to grasp how this tentative search again and again leads to impasses or obstacles and they often carefully elicit the interweaving of their concepts with their clinical data describing this process in micro-moments. This dependency of important data from the analytic process on that which analysts report 'from their psyche' is certainly a great challenge for clinical research.

The question concerning the data is even more intricate: The analytic situation is not only complexly composed of a multitude of – technically speaking – *channels or variables*, it also has a *holistic* aspect, which can not only be captured by variables. It also has to do with the identification of 'well-formed *Gestalten*' and with the elaboration of figure and background, of signal and noise. However, analysts have a professional means of dealing with such a totality and with such – again technically speaking – an abundance of information and with reducing this complexity for themselves. By means of their analytic attitude – expressed in terms such as equally suspended attention, reverie, attention to countertransference reactions, or listening without memory and desire – they have a relevance filter, especially for unconscious aspects. Thus, for example, one of the important aims of clinical research is to make these clinical data – the analyst's intuitions, speculations, and inferences – transparent and explicit. It is worth the trouble, because this is the place from which clinical research traditionally starts. And this is where, from its beginnings, the gold of psychoanalysis has been mined.

8 Which language games are used?

Which language is used in the context of clinical research? English, many would say, is the lingua franca of research. The question, however, does not refer to communication between researchers but to the adequate language used to talk about our research subject. Which language game is best to describe clinical phenomena? Our traditional analytic concepts have largely been introduced by Freud to especially grasp these phenomena. That was a long time ago, and now, in the course of theoretical development, there is a multitude of analytic dialects worldwide, hard to overlook. Many analysts are reminded of the Babylonian confusion of language (Dreher, 2019). The question, however, is aimed at another plurality, because in the field of clinical research there are three language games to choose from:

- The traditional analytic dialects from various schools with which analysts usually talk about their patients and which are regularly used in case studies, such as Freudian, Bionian, Kleinian, etc.
- The language games according to the ICD and DSM, the classification systems for psychic disorders, which must be used for example, in the

context of health systems and which are often also used in research reports.

- Below these two language games, in research there is another level, that of operationalisations and measurement scales, with the help of which clinical phenomena should be identified, classified, and measured.

If, for example, Kleinians or intersubjectivists report on their cases or if a therapy researcher wants to record transference phenomena, for example, using the CCRT method (the core conflictual relationship theme method; Luborsky & Crits-Christoph, 1990), then everyone talks about transference – but whether they always mean the same phenomena and whether they refer to the same clinical evidence remains to be questioned. But if a concept has different definitions and meanings for different groups, this not only makes communication difficult – inside and outside psychoanalysis – but also hinders the transfer of results from research into clinical practice. Our classic formulations of analytic treatment aim at making the unconscious conscious, mitigating the superego's austerity, etc., and tend to be preferably used to this day within the analytic community – they should appear in useful outcome studies, too. Practically all of our traditional treatment aims (see Sandler & Dreher, 1996) are little suitable to meet those criteria of the medical systems that today must be used in many countries in order to prove the efficacy of psychotherapy. This may also be because the classical aims are formulated by means of metapsychological metaphors, which are no longer highly appreciated today.

The diversity of meanings of almost all psychoanalytic concepts used in our language games is a great irritation and a barrier, which unfortunately is not always seen by everyone. It is not uncommon to get the impression that some authors argue like Humpty Dumpty in *Alice in Wonderland*: The concept I use has exactly the meaning I myself give to it here and now. But at least in the research context it would be useful if the meaning of concepts in question was made explicit. It would also be helpful if there were translation aids for clinicians who usually do not learn more about the scales quoted in reports than that they are reliable – there is often no information about clinical validity.

9 Single cases or random samples?

Who are the 'test persons' in clinical research? From a nomothetic world view, every patient in a study – and every analyst, by the way – is only one element of a random sample that should be as large and representative as possible for a specific population. Such a population could, for example, be patients with bipolar affective disorder belonging to the F31 category according to ICD-10 or analysts belonging to Freudian, Kleinian, Kohutian, etc., traditions. When samples are examined, usually only statistical characteristic values such as correlations, means, variances, etc., are of interest; most individual characteristics from the cases disappear to error variance.

From an ideographic point of view, individual cases are examined in which both the specific of the individual case as well as the general are of interest. This general can appear as a structure or pattern over many cases. However, in this proceeding the aggregation works quite differently, not top-down by defining populations, drawing random samples, and randomised assignment to treatment conditions but bottom-up by overlaying and aggregating many individual cases to identify common structures, patterns, and types under which single cases can be subsumed.

Classic single-case studies in psychoanalysis are 'solitaires' in the field of clinical research; they are a holistic, 'all-inclusive' kind of report that presents simultaneously all sorts of clinical data, theoretical ideas, and conceptual reflections. Of course, from a methodological point of view, such dense descriptions of single cases have some weaknesses:

- Individual cases permit only limited statements; generalisations beyond the individual case are not possible at first.
- Individual cases are normally communicated as narratives; they usually contain verbal data, rarely quantitative indications.
- The description can be imprecise; the psychoanalytic concepts are elastic and usually have school-specific meanings.
- The amount of clinical information reported is naturally very limited. The report represents only a small subset of the complex clinical events. For example, usually only short dialogue passages are given, which are also often smoothed out in language. Nonverbal clues rarely appear in narratives, and mostly only then if the analyst considers them clinically relevant.
- The selection of the reported information is the sole responsibility of the treating analyst; there is a risk of 'contamination' through subjective biases; for example, biases because the analyst wants to present their work in a favourable light or because they can see things not at all or only distorted.

The limited generalisation can be overcome by overlaying and aggregating a larger number of single cases, through a way similar to the nomothetic approach. It may apply to natural sciences that measured values and numbers are always exact and words opaque or ambiguous but, in the current state of measuring technique, for analytic research it is often a prejudice that numbers are better than words. In analytic research so far, we have only been able to *measure* a few phenomena well, and that means, above all, reliably *and* clinically valid. The dangers of subjective biases and distortions can be reduced by involving other researchers in the selection of data or by comprehensively documenting some channels with technical tools. That the analyst is only a part of the material does not have to be a mistake; nevertheless, the dual role of analyst and researcher must be discussed and reflected upon.

10 What type of truth is appropriate?

The claims of scientific research are not only well justified descriptions and explanations but also that the assertions are as 'true' as possible. Researchers appreciate the truth; no one wants their ideas or research results to prove false. But 'truth' in the sciences is understood in different ways. That a scientific statement is true does not depend on the belief of a researcher but on the condition that the criteria for truth are fulfilled. However, there are four different criteria for truth discussed in sciences, and truth in everyday life is not even covered by these criteria:

- The correspondence theory of truth is *preferred* in the natural sciences; theories and models should be an as good image as possible of that part of the world to which it refers. As a result, theories and models should allow the best possible prognoses to be made.
- The consistency theory of truth is *preferred* in formal sciences; theories or models should be logically free of contradictions.
- The coherence theory of truth is *preferred* in sciences working with narratives and interpretations. All indices should be integrated coherently and plausibly into an overall framework.
- The consensus theory of truth is *preferred* in sciences that give special weight to a 'dominant opinion'. When majorities change, the beliefs considered true and right also change.

Correspondence theory is not suitable for researching the psyche because the psyche does not represent either physical or social realities as accurate realistic images. Different from ear and eye, the psyche is not a camera or tape recorder. What is sedimented in the psyche as mechanisms and psychic representations is the result of lived subjective experience and manifold subsequent reworkings and new creations. Idealisation, for example, consistently ignores negative aspects; denial does not even let some things in; projective identification splits into good and bad parts; and the psychic reality of narcissists is only loosely connected with the external reality, etc. In the context of an analytic treatment, the scientific concepts of truth play only a subordinate role for the analyst 'as analyst'. What is regarded as 'true' between patient and analyst is oriented towards the everyday understanding of truth and results from a consensus between both and shows itself in the narrative they have jointly developed. This is mainly influenced by the analyst's clinically coherent picture of the patient and their biography. If, on the other hand, the analyst acts 'as a researcher', they can decide, according to their worldview, which scientific truth criteria they want to satisfy. This will essentially depend on the scientific community in which the research project is located – and from the dominant opinion in the respective scientific society.

To conclude ... Many roads lead to Rome

I have attempted to sound out the epistemological and methodological terrain of clinical research and to discuss it from an explicitly psychoanalytic point of view. Our research subject psyche is not only difficult to grasp clinically and by research; it is also a difficult field to work on *methodologically*. There are analysts who regard psychoanalysis as a handicraft or an art and who, therefore, want to keep a distance from science. However, most analysts think that psychoanalysis should participate in scientific discourses, and that precisely means that our clinical research also orientates itself towards scientific standards. At the least, when it comes to the proof of efficacy in health systems, one is confronted with scientific criteria such as those formulated in evidence-based medicine. 'Conjunction research' was historically a successful idea but does not fully satisfy the requirements of modern research in some scientific aspects, particularly concerning systematisation, objectivity, completeness, and control. The paradigms of evidence-based medicine meet these requirements but are subcomplex – in particular, they do not capture unconscious phenomena and do not take into account any sort of context. I am aware of the great pressure from the medical system in many parts of the world to adopt a point of view that is orientated at rules of natural sciences and of empiristic methods. I have discussed some methodological problems and cliffs that, unfortunately, cannot be ignored if one takes seriously that not only behavioural or mental but also psychic phenomena are to be investigated. Certainly, one can repress or deny these cliffs, but, as we know, they do not disappear. If one is to do *psychoanalytic* clinical research successfully, one has to negotiate them critically; that is, one has to sharpen again and again one's own methodological position in order to do justice to our subject matter *between nature and culture*.

Epistemological and methodological reflections and decisions belong to clinical research but are not research yet. In order to select a research paradigm, a design, or a set of methods regarding a concrete research question, it is helpful to take an explicit stand concerning the ten questions listed above. I do not give any practical indications, but a number of consequences can be derived for clinical research in psychoanalysis in general:

- We take notice not only of behaviour but also of the *meaning of behaviour*. Behaviour can be recorded by observation; meaning can only be recorded by inference and interpretation.

- We take notice not only of behaviour but also of *action*. If one looks at actions, one should also consider conscious and unconscious intentions as well as the individual, social, and cultural contexts.
- We not only examine 'monads' like patient or therapist but we also take notice of the relevance of *dyadic interaction* in this special analytic situation.
- We try to be as objective as possible; 'objectivity' is understood as intersubjectively consensual. But we also take notice of the relevance of *subjectivity* of patients, analysts, and even researchers.
- We accept all sorts of *relevant clinical data*, quantitative as well as qualitative and verbal data, even if this means applying different strategies for data collection and data analysis.

Psychoanalytic research might even benefit from the use of different scientific belief systems and methodologies, because this would enable it to critically weigh and select the best of several scientific worlds. To put it concisely: The devalued hermeneutic methods like interpretation and rational reconstruction should keep their place besides experiment and measurement in the analytic research landscape. Clinical research is actually not an end in itself but should serve the improvement of clinical practice and, thus, the better treatment of patients and should contribute to further understanding of the human psyche.

At the very end is a barely noticed *epistemologically* problem, perhaps even the most difficult one in human sciences. In addition to the questions of best scientific access there is the problem of self-reference of all sorts of research: Whoever explores the psyche of others is always exploring themselves, be that as an analyst or as a researcher. There is no extra-human point of view on humans. All research findings about the psyche or mind or brain of patients also hold for the analyst's or researcher's psyche, mind, or brain. So, what is left in answer to the question posed in the title: In the same way as the core competency of psychoanalysis is the analysis of the psyche, there can be no psychoanalytic clinical research without reflecting the intricacies when exploring this psyche scientifically, if psychoanalysis wants to keep its identity.

References

Dreher, A. U. (2010). Pluralism in theory *and* in research – And what now? A plea for connectionism. In M. Leuzinger-Bohleber, J. Canestri, & M. Target (Eds.), *Early development and its disturbances: Clinical, conceptual and empirical research on ADHD and other psychopathologies and its epistemological reflections*. London, England: Karnac.

Dreher, A. U. (2015). Psychoanalytic research with or without the psyche? Some remarks on the intricacies of clinical research. In S. Boag, L. Brakel, & V. Talvitie (Eds.), *Philosophy, science, and psychoanalysis*. London, England: Karnac.

Dreher, A. U. (2019). Inside Babel. In A. M. Schloesser (Ed.), *A psychoanalytic exploration on sameness and otherness: Beyond Babel?*London, England: Routledge.
Geertz, C. (1973). Thick description: Toward an interpretive theory of culture. In *The interpretation of cultures: Selected essays*. New York, NY: Basic Books.
Green, A. (1999). *The dead mother: The work of André Green*. London, England: Routledge.
Green, A. (2005). The illusion of *common ground* and mythical pluralism. *The International Journal of Psychoanalysis*, 86, 627–632.
Luborsky, L., & Crits-Christoph, P. (1990). *Understanding transference: The core conflictual relationship theme method*. New York, NY: Basic Books.
Popper, K. R. (1959). *The logic of scientific discovery*. London, England: Hutchinson & Co. (Original work published 1934)
Sandler, J., & Dreher, A. U. (1996). *What do psychoanalysts want? The problem of aims in psychoanalytic therapy*. London, England: Routledge.
Searle, J. (2010). *Making the social world: The structure of human civilization*. Oxford, England: Oxford University Press.
Thomä, H., & Kächele, H. (2006). *Psychoanalytische Therapie: Forschung*. Heidelberg, Germany: Springer.
Wallerstein, R. S. (2005a). Dialogue or illusion? How do we go from here? Response to André Green. *The International Journal of Psychoanalysis*, 86, 633–638.
Wallerstein, R. S. (2005b). Will psychoanalytic pluralism be an enduring state of our discipline? *The International Journal of Psychoanalysis*, 86, 623–626.

Chapter 3

Commentary by Judy Kantrowitz

Anna Ursula Dreher's chapter, 'What Is Clinical Research in Psychoanalysis?' (Chapter 2, this book), fills an important gap in our understanding of this topic. By keeping a clear focus on the subject and aim of a study, she makes explicit that considerations of the method of exploration must be in the service of the goal of the project. When the field of study is clinical psychoanalysis, then the questions we want to address are the ones to improve our theories, models, and concepts and the ways in which we practice for the benefit of our patients. She then specifies the methods that are and are not appropriate for our field and details why some methods are applicable and others are not. She provides a sophisticated overview of ideas about how clinical research can be conducted scientifically and underscores how such ideas change with changes in current interests in the field; for example, the current focus on neuropsychological research.

One can only applaud her 'broad and open-minded' appreciation of science as encompassing psychoanalysis; cultural, social, and historical fields; as well as natural science. She explicates how one's worldview leads to different kinds of interests; for example, seeking universal laws or an interest in 'the particular in every unique case' in its particular context. She asks: Do we 'seek *causes* for behaviour or *reasons* for actions, or do we seek both?' (p. 000). How stimulating those questions are! They direct our attention to the particular and how theory building could emerge from pursuit of this way of developing our inquiries – the both/and, not either/or, way of thinking. Her ideas are also bidirectional: Seeking causes and reasons can lead to the development of theory, and theory can lead us to seek specific kinds of data. 'There is also no *epistemologically free and methodologically free* research regarding worldview, subject, aims, and methods' (p. 000). And for each of these big ideas she provides vivid illustrations.

Dreher's ability to weave together overarching ideas about the nature of clinical research and the specifics of clinical problems to study stimulates the reader. Her presentation makes one believe that we do not need to be stuck in the quagmire of controversy that often paralyses creative endeavours. Her disinclination to close down thinking to single answers means

DOI: 10.4324/9780000000002-4

that ideas can expand our understanding of the world and ourselves. Over and over in her text, we can see how her creative mind expands the reader's thinking: the mind-body problem:

> Psychoanalysis sees the psyche not only as an immaterial interface between biological hardware and external physical and cultural world but as an inner virtual psychological space with its own structures and processes – and methods for research have to do justice to this fact. (p. 000)

A brain scan cannot reveal the quality of mothering. A pregnancy test reveals the fact of pregnancy or not, but the experience of the impact of this information is a different matter.

Dreher's questions get bigger and bigger. She wants us psychoanalysts to explore our psychic realities formed by our nature and our culture and how it is always unique – we share a common outline of what makes a person, but who we each become is someone specific, different from all others. No wonder our work is so challenging – and stimulating, impossible, thrilling – and we know something happens, but how? And why?

Through this insightful, clearly reasoned essay, Dreher again and again makes the cogent point: One's method of studying a phenomenon depends on the particular nature of what is being studied. There are similarities and differences in our field of study from other sciences: 'Unconscious processes can only be accessible indirectly through inference and interpretation. By the way, this is similar to dark matter and dark energy in physics' (p. 000). She reminds us that physical and psychological realities require different methods of study. Psychoanalytic research is primarily focused on 'internal psychic phenomena and their intersubjective dynamics and only secondarily on the manifest behaviour' (p. 000) in contrast to the fact that 'clinical research in cognitive therapy is on observable behaviour and on the representation of the external world in the mind' (p. 000).

Dreher underscores how research in psychoanalysis becomes further complicated because we as psychoanalysts are not, and cannot be, purely objective observers. Despite our training in which we learn to be neutral and abstinent in our work with our patients, our psyches inevitably become part of the intersubjective process. Here I would add that we learn more and more about the human psyche and our own over the years. What is neutral for one patient is not for another. For example, to remain silent with a self-critical patient will not be experienced as neutrality but rather as joining the patient in their self-directed criticism (Kris, 1990). Abstinence means not using the patient for any personal benefit for the analyst, but it does not mean being cold and distant.

Though the treating psychoanalyst has information that no other person can provide in terms of what transpires, Dreher makes it clear that the treating analyst's perspective cannot have the objectivity of a third-person observer. Therefore, it is 'necessary and useful' to introduce other researchers who are not personally involved in the process to corroborate, contradict, or expand the perceptions of the treating analyst, 'thereby meeting not only clinical but also scientific requirements' (p. 000). But in line with the complexity and sophistication of her thought, she adds that the researcher who is not part of the dyad also has a psyche that will contribute to what is and is not perceived.

Dreher's description of the clinical data we study makes vivid and alive what it is that we as psychoanalysts listen and respond to. Part of our data is behavioural, conscious, and easily observable, but we are trained to look and listen for *preconscious and unconscious processes in our patients and ourselves*. We recognise these phenomena by what is present in affect as well as words and by what is absent in silence, in impasses, and in enactments when they occur. We explore our reactions as well as our patient's. Our process is free association, and the aim is for the patient to become freer in accessing thoughts and feelings, freer to know and to tell us. As Dreher states, we try to grasp the whole situation, using our clinical tools of listening with an analytic attitude, 'equally suspended attention, reverie, attention to countertransference reactions' (p. 000). Clinical research needs to make all of these seemingly effable phenomena 'explicit and transparent'.

And Dreher does not skirt the extra problem in research in psychoanalysis that different psychoanalytic theories each have their own language and the same words may have different meanings within a different theory. When scales are used to categorise a concept, reliability of ratings is important, but without information about clinical validity the data are meaningless. Over and over again she makes it clear that clinical research in psychoanalysis cannot be meaningfully undertaken in the way studies in natural science can, because our data include more than what is observable; for example: 'Behaviour can be recorded by observation; meaning can only be recorded by inference and interpretation' (p. 000). 'If one looks at actions, one should also consider conscious and unconscious intentions as well as the individual, social, and cultural context' (p. 000). We examine not only the psyche of the patient and the analyst but also 'take notice of the relevance of *dyadic interaction* in this special analytic situation' (p. 000). 'We try to be as objective as possible; "objectivity" is understood as intersubjectively consensual. But we also take notice of the relevance of *subjectivity* of patients, analysts, and even researchers' (p. 000). And all sorts of data may be studied as long as they are clinically relevant. Dreher ends this chapter by reminding us that the observer always affects the observed.

I cannot add to what Anna Ursula Dreher has presented. I can only state my admiration for her comprehensive summary of what is and what is not relevant when undertaking research in psychoanalysis. Her definitions leave room for many approaches but also require of us that we understand why certain methods fit our concepts and others do not and that we be rigorous in our self-scrutiny about our research endeavours, carefully formulating what we are trying to study and what data are relevant, asking ourselves whether we have employed a method suited to our questions, and trying to stay as aware as we can of the influence of our subjectivity. This is a tall order, but it is the way for our work as well as the field of psychoanalysis to be respected.

Reference

Kris, A. O. (1990). Helping patients by analyzing self-criticism. *Journal of the American Psychoanalytic Association*, 38, 605–636.

Part II

Different perspectives on clinical research

Chapter 4

Researching subjectivity

Single-case studies and psychoanalytic knowledge

Robert Douglas Hinshelwood

The research that produces psychoanalytic knowledge faces a number of problems not encountered in natural science, medicine, or the more objective experimental psychology. The psychoanalyst uses subjective data and a subjective instrument for making observations. That determined reliance on the subjective raises suspicion, but as the hallmark of psychoanalysis, it needs defending. Almost all psychoanalytic knowledge has come from the clinical setting and cannot be abandoned without losing a large part of our framework for thinking about our work. It is therefore worth considering the serious criticisms we face in a project to tighten the rigour of our research and the confidence in our knowledge. This chapter will list the problems arising from subjectivity and then attempt to show how we may deal with them. The claim is that the problems can in fact be resolved with careful thought, observation, and a logic designed specifically for research into the psychoanalysis of subjective data.

As the philosopher Richard Rorty advised:

> [P]sychoanalysts [must] stop asking (obsessive?) questions like 'Is psychoanalysis a science?', 'Was Freud a scientist or a littérateur?', 'Are psychoanalytic claims objectively verifiable?' … The founders of great and influential intellectual traditions quite often did not know quite what they were doing. The enduring impact of their work may have little to do with their original intentions. (Rorty, 2000, p. 822)

Despite Rorty's advice, there still remains a question: What is specific about psychoanalytic knowledge? And, in particular, how can we make a sceptic stop and think about our forms of evidence? Do we in fact need evidence and a logic comparable to natural science?

Freud thought that psychoanalysis was a natural science: 'that the psychical is unconscious in itself enabled psychology to take its place as a natural science like any other' (S. Freud, 1938/1964b, p. 158). However, because our studies use the data of subjectivity, and are based on experiences in, and of, relationships with others, we do not have objective

DOI: 10.4324/9780000000002-6

measurements. In addition, and significantly, both our research and our everyday practice are carried on in the same clinical setting. And this, rightly, raises doubt about conflict of interest when research coincides with the pressures to effect cures.

So, how should we argue for our knowledge?

Outcome and R&D

Currently, mental health institutions and insurance schemes want evidence that the treatments work. Pharmaceutical companies are therefore involved in two phases of research – first, the development of new drugs and treatments and, second, testing their use (outcome studies).

We are inevitably linked with this medical approach and pressed to show the effectiveness of our treatments. And, indeed, we ourselves would like to have confirmation; we would not want to subject people to long treatments that are barely justified. Strident demands for outcome data on psychoanalytic treatments conform to those addressed to the pharmaceutical industry. However, it is not always possible to achieve this for psychoanalytic treatments in the way it is for medical ones. Assessment of personality change has to be quite different from assessment of symptom change (Hinshelwood, 2002). Because the measures for the two criteria – personality change or symptom change – are different, we cannot necessarily compare like with like. Despite this, there have in fact been important clinical trials of psychoanalysis and psychoanalytic psychotherapy over many years; for instance, there is the extensive bibliography compiled by Milton (1992) and the recent definitive assessment of psychoanalytic psychotherapy for depression (Taylor, 2015).

However, there is also the first phase of research. Pharmaceutical companies conduct a lot of research prior to the outcome trial of a drug. That earlier phase is a long and expensive process called R&D (research and development). Such basic research is quite distinct from the assessment of effectiveness

In the same way, in psychoanalysis, a great deal of basic research has had to go on, too. It is 120 years since Freud's key analysis of his Irma dream in 1895, which produced the first significant understanding of the Unconscious and the way it works. So, we too have had that long phase of research. It is, however, very different from pharmaceutical R&D. In psychoanalysis we call it *conceptual research* (Dreher, 2000). The accumulation of our basic concepts and knowledge is very important. It produces the knowledge that is and must be the basis for use in our clinical work. For psychoanalysis, research and development is the creation of the concepts of psychoanalytic knowledge, rather different from the production of a new drug. Moreover, as mentioned, our knowledge development relies on testing our concepts in the very same setting – our clinical practices – quite different from the distance between research and practice with medical treatments.

I shall here consider the basic research in psychoanalysis that is equivalent to the R&D that goes into producing a drug.

Critical appraisals of psychoanalytic knowledge

Today the concepts we use in our practice and theory are most powerfully under scrutiny. Cogent and responsible criticisms of psychoanalysis, as well as irresponsible ones, have been quite liberated ever since the earliest days of Freud's work. One simplistic argument used against psychoanalytic knowledge is that because our methods of research are so different from those of natural science, they cannot be valid. Freud was therefore a charlatan (Cioffi, 1970; Crews, 1993; see also Forrester, 1997). More serious critiques have developed since the 1950s (Hook, 1959; Popper, 1959). A lot is at stake.

There appears to be a crisis over our clinical work as the source of our knowledge, and we are now tempted to turn to other disciplines: experimental psychology – for instance, the mother–infant interaction (Mahler, Pine, & Bergman, 1975; Stern, 1985) – or to the cognitive sciences (Solms & Turnbull, 2002). The intention is to gain *objective* confirmation of what we already believe and use. There is nothing wrong with reaching out to other disciplines for corroboration, but nearly all psychoanalytic knowledge has come originally from clinical work. Unless we defend that form of knowledge production, we might otherwise have to accept that it is not up to standard, and therefore we would have little left! Indeed, it is necessary for our practice that we retain a confidence, so that we can continue to use our knowledge. I want to make the case that the clinical method of gaining psychoanalytic knowledge is still valid and therefore usable clinically, without having to back away into objectifying our data, however useful that may be in a supplementary way.

The solid foundation of natural science is the causal link between events and the capacity to create conditions for definitive testing of the link. This is true for psychoanalysis, too, though not the whole truth. Many analysts, in reporting their work, do point to causal evidence by following the response to their interpretations that can guide their mistakes and successes. An accurate interpretation *causes* an immediate response, which contrasts with the response to an inaccurate one. In this line of argument, there is some kind of outcome data, though not in the terms usually required. It is the outcome of making an interpretation. The timescale is very different; it is a micro-timescale. For instance, Breuer and Freud (1895) demonstrated his hypnotic treatment to Freud by describing how Anna O's symptoms changed after an abreaction. Later S. Freud (1900) accepted that an interpretation was correct if a coherent meaning for a dream (and later a symptom) could be found. Anna Freud (1936) relied on an interpretation enabling the emergence of material from the preconscious; Klein (1926) watched for a release of inhibition in play after interpreting the child's anxiety. Later we will consider Henry Ezriel's (1956) criterion of a movement from the required relationship in the transference to an avoided relationship. And even the hermeneutic tradition, which emphasises meanings rather than causality, does think that meaning-making and narrative-telling cause *some*thing.

However, evidence-based arguments like these do not always convince others, not even other psychoanalysts looking from the perspectives of other schools of psychoanalysis. The subjectivity with which we observe and assess this kind of change gives rise to the suspicion that the analyst's own professional interests distort what he observes. When different psychoanalysts with different background theories have different perspectives from which to assess the response to an interpretation, they frequently assess the response to an interpretation by using the theories that are to be tested by the response. It seems potentially a 'Heads I win, tails you lose' situation, and 'most welcome to our opponents', as Freud ironically noted (S. Freud, 1937/1964a, p. 377). The variation in the way the responses to interpretation are looked at is a difficulty in the way we debate with each other – let alone those outside our field.

The logical status of a subjective 'science'

There is no point in dismissing the better-informed criticisms. Those criticisms need to be acknowledged and then provoke us to consider how psychoanalytic knowledge must gain validity and how we might strengthen our arguments.

The common demand on us is to convert the subjectivity of individuals into data that can be regarded as if it were objective. The hope is to convert subjective experience into measurable data that can be handled like the quantitative methods of natural science. Defending the *subjective* nature of psychoanalytic work and research is less usual. However, Glen Gabbard (2000) said, rousingly:

> In an era of quick-fix managed care approaches and rampant biological reductionism, we can derive a great deal of gratification from the fact that we still see value in the unique subjectivity of the person who comes to us for help. (pp. 713–714)

So, we could at least see what we could achieve if we retained our fundamental reliance on our unique subjective 'data'.

One thing we achieve is a whole raft of philosophical and practical problems! But though they are significant and many, it does not necessarily mean they are not solvable. My assessment as I argued at length in *Research on the Couch* (Hinshelwood, 2013) is that the problems *can* be resolved. We can respect our own specific kind of subjective data and still achieve serious research and knowledge production. It may be called the science of subjectivity (Heimann, 1991; Meissner, 1999) because our methods diverge from the pattern of natural science, but it does not mean we cannot be logical and convincing. Logic and conviction do not have to be the exclusive partners of objectivity.

So, first of all, I will list the problems that would need to be solved in order to claim that our knowledge production is rigorous. Then I will consider in brief the approach we could follow for each of those problems. Some can be resolved more easily than others. But I do not offer as complete an answer as may be necessary here. Further details and examples can be found in *Research on the Couch* (Hinshelwood, 2013).

The problems

What, then, are the problems? Here is a list of the fundamental conceptual and practical issues:

1 *Subjectivity*: The suspicion of subjectivity is the most common problem from which the others tend to flow. The doubt arises from the conflict that exists between careful observation on the one hand and the wish to see what confirms one's own opinions on the other. Subjectivity is experienced rather than measured, though it may have a variable intensity. In addition, the means of gathering the data of subjective experience is via an instrument that is equally subjective; it is the mind of the psychoanalyst.
2 *Research as testing*: Science itself has changed over the years, and notably since Freud died. And this has had a knock-on effect on what is required of psychoanalytic (or any) research. Freud depended heavily on inductive thinking to justify his theories scientifically. That view of science has changed since those claims. More rigour and a different kind of logical justification tend to be required now. Popper (1959) developed a logical model of science, ruling out inductive thinking and emphasising the deductive testing of theories, to which he claimed psychoanalysis was unable to conform (Popper, 1963, 1976). In natural science, that logical method is a hypothetico-deductive one, which was laid out in Popper's (1959) classic treatise. Psychoanalysts on the whole trained in an intuitive clinical method are not always comfortable to follow along that logical road.
3 *Single-case studies*: The conventional research design in other related disciplines, notably medicine and experimental psychology, is to use large samples of subjects, with an equal sample of control subjects. The experimental sample contrasts the actions of one variable that is present with the control sample where the variable is absent. With large enough samples the expectation is that other, and unknown, variables will cancel

each other out. That method is not open to the psychoanalyst – his samples are too small. And the method of large sampling research aims to eradicate the individual characteristics of each subject, whereas individuality is what psychoanalysis uniquely focuses on.

4 *Causes or meanings*: One strategy often adopted for coping with the criticisms is to make the alternative claim that psychoanalysis is not so much about knowledge but about meanings and narratives, instead. Then we enter an unfortunate contest *within* psychoanalysis – a contest between science and hermeneutics. That is to say, we have conflicts about whether we look for causes or for meanings in our patients.

5 *Distortion of data selection*: Then there are further problems about how we select data when we observe from the conceptual positions of different schools and thus select different kinds of data. We should worry that our own minds observe what we wish to find; that is, data to confirm our pet theories. As psychoanalysts we are more aware than most of the subtle and unconscious forms of wish fulfilment. Thus, we have the circular problem that the pet theories we have in mind are used to select the material we use to confirm those pet theories. So, when different kinds of clinical material are selected by different psychoanalysts, we cannot compare their different kinds of evidence. We end up with a debate in which the protagonists cannot engage sufficiently with each other's point of view. This is true on a greater scale when trying to compare psychoanalytic data with that from other psychological or other therapeutic disciplines.

These very significant criticisms are indeed valid questions to raise. We might wonder whether we can in fact justify our methods. Nevertheless, I wish to show that it is worth going on to challenge these criticisms. In fact, I think we can meet them all, even though the arguments that are needed are sometimes quite extensive and demanding of our clinical skills. I propose to deal briefly with each of these obstacles. In so doing, we probably need to be clear that psychoanalysis has to place itself outside the objective natural sciences, though not beyond respect for our rigour and convincing logic. In acknowledgement of this, I prefer to regard – and term – our work 'knowledge production' rather than to call it science. I hope the answers I give, and discussions, will indicate that we do not have to give up confidence in our knowledge, and those inside the psychoanalytic world as well as outside should remain confident of continuing to use and test what we know.

1 Subjectivity

Our field of observation is a subjective one; it is *personal experience*, conscious, and, especially, unconscious. So, our facts are *not* comparable to those of natural science, dealing as it does with the objective world of matter. As Robert Caper (1988) said, ours are 'immaterial facts'.

Experiences cannot be measured by the usual parameters of length, breadth, intensity, substance, etc.

The instrument with which we make our observations of immaterial facts is itself immaterial; it is the subjectivity of the psychoanalyst's mind. It is about *our* experience. Of course, how else *could* we observe some other person's subjectivity? We have therefore to contend with the immateriality, the un-measurability, the emotional conflicts of interest, the volatility of the relations with our kinds of research subjects, and the propensity of the human mind to distort perceptions and memories.

What follows are the necessary conditions for a confidence in the subjective knowledge we need for our work.

2 The research logic of testing knowledge

This is the most fundamental of the issues with which psychoanalytic research must deal. Is there a specific logic that leads to a conviction that some piece of knowledge is valid? In the subsequent sections we will examine the various elements of the procedure, but here the question is more epistemological – what counts as knowledge itself? Freud thought that was easy enough to answer, as we saw earlier; he thought that psychoanalysis was 'a natural science like any other' (S. Freud, 1938/1964b, p. 158). That view has fallen out of favour.

It can be similar to, though it is not in fact one of, the natural sciences. We should claim that there can be many forms of knowledge production. To get a general view of what knowledge is, we can look back to the ancient view derived from Plato and before. In *Thaetatus*, Plato (1987) stated that knowledge is opinion plus an argument to justify the opinion. So, our issue is the kind of argument(s) researchers use and, in particular, what arguments psychoanalysts have. Popper's (1959) reformulation of scientific logic describes a move beyond induction to a deductive approach, which seems to be a process that the more developed and mature sciences come to. There is no reason why it should not be time for a corresponding move for our more developed psychoanalysis, however distant psychoanalysis is from natural science.

Induction

Freud's arguments were the kind traditionally accepted in medicine in his time. They were inductive ones. Typically, several occurrences with something in common lead to a generalisation – a theory. If the sun rises every day in the east, then it can be (inductively) generalised that every day will begin with the sun rising in the east. Darwin (1859/2009) found specimens in nature that showed a common pattern that allowed him to generalise the theory of natural selection. Further occurrences of a generalisation add incremental support to the theory. This process of generalisation from a collection of instances is called *induction*. Freud depended heavily on this logic. One more case showing that the analysand had an Oedipus complex added to the confidence that Oedipal theory is correct (S. Freud, 1916). Much clinical research continues on that basis; another instance of the metapsychological theory strengthens that theory. However, this kind of claim has been superseded by a more rigorous logic.

Deduction

The change has been the increasing emphasis on a *deductive* method. In that design, we deduce certain predictions from a theory and then make observations to test whether the prediction can be confirmed. This deductive method provides stronger support than the inductive one. It is now called the hypothetico-deductive method and has become the most prominent – the brand leader, perhaps – following Karl Popper's *The Logic of Scientific Discovery* in 1959:

> I developed further my ideas about the demarcation between scientific theories (like Einstein's) and pseudoscientific theories (like Marx's, Freud's, and Adler's). It became clear to me that what made a theory, or a statement, scientific was its power to rule out, or exclude, the occurrences of some possible events – to prohibit, or forbid, the occurrence of these events. Thus the more a theory forbids, the more it tells us. (Popper, 1976, p. 41)

Popper's (1959) logical model for science emphasised the theories that could be ruled out. The deductive testing of theories requires that a scientific theory should be risky; so that it can be ruled out. A theory must generate predictions that could be shown to be wrong and thus disconfirm the theory. A good theory survives this test. Therefore, unlike induction, which aims to support a theory, the deductive method aims to dispose of it. If it is not at risk of being disposed of, then it is not a scientific theory.

As Thomas Kuhn (1962) noted, scientists wish to conserve their theories rather than give them up (just like psychoanalysts), so in practice we can observe sudden jumps in the progress of knowledge in all disciplines, when the evidence has overwhelmed the conservationists. In psychoanalysis perhaps the significant example is how ego-psychology hung on for a couple of decades after cracks began to appear in its theoretical structure in the 1970s (for instance, Fromm, 1971).

Popper's (1959) view was that psychoanalysis could not conform to the demand for risk, because he thought that all responses to interpretation could be turned into support for the theory. In particular, if the patient agrees, that is fine; if he disagrees, that is resistance. However, we know that the patient's agreeable response is no reason to assume he is not resisting, and we will take that into account later. The more important consideration is whether our subjective data can be used for the hypothetico-deductive research design. Unhappily, if our theories can conform to this logical challenge, then they risk being ruled out! And that, of course, is unsettling for most of us. Our very commitment to a school of theory tends to make us reluctant to risk a deductive, predictive method, although, as indicated, this is not unlike natural scientists.

The deductive method has a specific protocol, which starts by taking a theory and deducing what sort of phenomena it would lead to. These are the research predictions. So, under the conditions in which the theory applies, one can predict what observations will conform to a prediction. Then observation tests whether the prediction is in fact confirmed or not. That evidence is then regarded as robustly empirical, and insofar as the predictions are confirmed, the hypothesis is robust, too. If the prediction is not confirmed, then the theory has failed and is ruled out. So, if we can make predictions and find reliable observations, then our theories are risky.

Testing, science/psychoanalysis

Let us consider examples. In the scientific arena we can consider Arthur Eddington's test of Einstein's theory of relativity (Dyson, Eddington, & Davidson, 1920). This theory predicted that the course of a ray of light will be bent when it passes through a gravitational field. Eddington tested that prediction by looking at the direction of light from a distant star as it passed near the mass of the sun. In order to observe a star close to the sun, he set his experiment during an eclipse of the sun – in 1919 in India, actually. He then measured the apparent displacement of a distant star during the eclipse when the sun was obscured. The displacement of the star (at the moment it could be observed) was measured. The position was indeed displaced, indicating that the path of the light had been bent by the gravitational field of the sun. The theory of relativity predicted the apparent displacement of the star. The observations could have confirmed or disconfirmed that the star appeared displaced. In fact, in this instance the observations confirmed the displacement and Einstein's theory was not dismissed.

Now, a comparable debate within psychoanalysis: In 1921 Sandor Ferenczi (1921) argued on theoretical grounds that nervous tics were autoerotic phenomena occurring with no object towards which the impulse was aimed. This was countered in the same year by Karl Abraham (1921), who made the opposite generalisation. Abraham (1921) predicted that cases of nervous tics would exhibit an underlying object relation. In fact, Abraham (1921) presented no case, and so at that stage no observations existed to test the prediction. But in fact, shortly after, a case was presented. That case was an observation showing a tic, underlying which was an unconscious object relation (Klein, 1925/1948). Thus, a clinical observation could resolve with a deductive method that Ferenczi's prediction could be ruled out just as Eddington's test of relativity supported his prediction.

3 Single cases

In principle, just because medicine and psychology use large-sample research design, we are not necessarily committed to that. In fact, it might be quite justifiable to keep to our single-case design. Interestingly, we noted Eddington's deductive test of Einstein's theory. Preexisting Newtonian theory was thus disconfirmed – and it was disconfirmed by a single experiment. And in fact there are many examples of a single case design in scientific experimentation. Just one experiment can effectively test a theory.

Marshall Edelson (1985) is one example of a psychoanalyst who has defended the possibility of psychoanalysis using single-case studies. In arguing for a more deductive approach he wrote:

> The [psychoanalytic] case study does not necessarily imply deviation from the canons of scientific method and reasoning. It should not be relegated to the context of discovery. The case study can be an argument about the relation between hypothesis and evidence. (Edelson, 1985, p. 611)

If we made efforts to write up our cases in specific ways, specifying that deductive relation between hypothesis, prediction, and evidence, we might find that psychoanalysis can conform to the same logical shape as Eddington's test of relativity. In fact, we might find psychoanalysis is actually more like natural science than medicine is!

We have seen how Ferenczi (1921) made a risky claim of the kind that Popper demanded for science. Ferenczi argued theoretically for a generalised hypothesis. That was risky. The theory that nervous tics are autoerotic implies that all cases of tic must be of this type. None will have an underlying object relationship. Ferenczi's risk is that someone finding even one case of a tic, indicating a relationship, destroys the generalisation. When eventually a single case was presented, showing a case of nervous tic that did not conform to his generalisation, Ferenczi's prediction was not confirmed. That single case invalidated Ferenczi's generalisation – it simply could *not* be generally true about tics.

Thus, a single-case research design can yield definitive evidence in the test of a psychoanalytic theory. The important feature of this example is that for a single case to be effective, there must be a clear issue with a yes or no answer. It might be called a binary question. Generalisations are potent sources for offering such definitive yes or no answers. It needs no more than a single deviant case to show a generalisation does not cover all of the cases. An effective way of testing a theory is to make a prediction that is a generalisation of the theory. This is then risky because a single case could rule out the generalisation and the theory.

Here we are interested in the *structure* of the logic that allows such a definitive result. This use of a single-case study design to test generalisations is an opportunity for psychoanalysts as much as natural scientists. Psychoanalysts frequently promote theoretical generalisations, their metapsychology. They are exactly the kind of risky knowledge that is vulnerable to a nonconforming single case. I suggest that this is a good sign, and we should explore how much that can be exploited.

4 *Causes versus meanings*

Now to consider the debate about causes or meanings: Is psychoanalysis concerned with scientific causation or with hermeneutic meanings? There is no doubt that Freud thought that psychoanalysis dealt in meanings – ever since he asserted in 1900 that he had discovered the meaning of dreams (S. Freud, 1900/1953). Today, every time we make an interpretation, we are attempting to create conscious meanings out of unconscious ones. But we are *also* interested in causing effects. Though we deal in meanings, which we call interpretations, we expect those meaning-filled interpretations to have an effect. We are interested in *both* causes and meanings. Meanings have effects. As Edelson (1986) said, 'It is a common mistake to suppose that because psychoanalysis is concerned with meanings or purposes it is not concerned with causal explanation' (p. 102).

In a psychoanalysis, we observe both meanings and causality!

Because the meanings of our interpretations rely on our psychoanalytic knowledge, the response to interpretation is a verdict on the knowledge we use to make our interpretation. So, on occasions when the interpretation offers a meaning that does not cause a significant response, we must consider whether the knowledge we used was valid. To see how such a disconfirmation of an interpretation can be achieved, see section A Clinical Example of Checking Observations.

There is an important point to understand. On the one hand, the psychoanalytic process in a clinical session resembles an experiment (Ezriel, 1956) in that it consists of a process: (a) first, initial conditions are established, (b) then an intervention is made, and, (d) finally, the consequences are observed. On the other hand, we make meanings. That is a very different activity to scientific experiments, as just outlined. The meaning is what we use to make the intervention; that is, (b) in the above sequence.

To summarise this research process, the intervention we make in a session is a *meaning* – it is the interpretation based on some metapsychological idea. The meaning is that which is preoccupying the patient before we give the interpretation.

Then, we observe a *causal process* – that is, the change in the specific meaning from before the intervention to after it. Now a very brief example from the literature. The patient was a man who was particularly submissive in the analytic relationship. He had lost his father during adolescence when the patient had been in a particularly rebellious phase. The patient's meaningful narrative is that he will be rebellious in the transference and the analyst will die. The point is that in the present the patient feared his own rebelliousness and ensured that he was submissive in case that rebelliousness should cause his analyst's death too. For reasons of safety, therefore, the patient made his unconscious complaints distantly, about the government.

Then, interestingly, after the analyst interpreted this, the patient's associations were complaints about the Tavistock Clinic, where the psychoanalyst was working. Thus, the effect of the interpretation was a change. It was not a change in the exact meaning but a change that moved the narrative a little nearer to the point of anxiety – the complaints about the clinic *after* interpretation were much closer to the analyst than the complaints about the government *before* the interpretation. It implies that in the transference, the anxiety resulting from his rebelliousness had become a little less frightening. The change was a topological one, a degree of movement from unconscious anxiety towards a conscious one.

This example comes from Henry Ezriel (1956), a psychoanalyst-researcher of an earlier generation. The causality is that the response to the interpretation was a move to addressing more closely the anxiety that this patient feared in the transference. He could more nearly address his rebellious complaining about the analyst. The change in this patient's meaningful narrative was that the balance of his rebelliousness versus his regret began to change in favour of the regret, and his fear of his own rebelliousness diminished, so it could allow the rebellious complaints to come closer to the present. Such a change after the interpretation confirmed the interpretation and the metapsychology from which the interpretation was derived.

Ezriel emphasised this here-and-now process of change within the session. As he said, 'Only such forces as exist at a certain time can have effects at that time' (Ezriel, 1956, p. 35). The logical structure is comparable with a scientific experiment. But the nature of the intervention was radically different, being a meaning. The latter is immaterial and subjective.

Some changes do *not* confirm an interpretation. Because the prediction can be made in this very precise way – to bring the anxiety closer to the here and now – it allows us to predict precisely which change confirms the interpretation. Any other change is a response to something non-psychoanalytic – a change that might be called a false positive.

Meanings are involved in the vital process of creating an interpretation. Causality then tests that interpretation and the metapsychological meaning behind the interpretation. We do not have to choose between meanings and causes. Both are aspects of our clinical and experimental work.

Interestingly, we use different sets of theories for the two different kinds of observations. Metapsychological theory informs our observations of meanings to infer and interpret. And, quite separately, we observe the process with what is known as clinical theory – transference and the anxiety defence structure. That separation of theories draws on Wallerstein's (1990) distinction:

> [O]ur clinical interventions (apart from differences of style and of theory-drenched languages) reflect a shared clinical analytic method, rest on a shared clinical theory of defence and anxiety, of conflict and compromise, of transference and countertransference, and evoke comparable data of observation, despite our avowed wide theoretical differences. … [But] these comparable observational data get 'explained' by us ultimately through widely differing theoretical explanatory frameworks. (p. 11)

Thus, the theory to which we mostly give our agreement (clinical theory) can be deployed to test the theories (metapsychology) about which mostly we disagree. There is therefore a potential opportunity for an agreement over the causal process, which then tests our major metapsychological differences.

5 Data selection

The final problem is the selection of the pieces of clinical data suitable to test our theories. This last one is unfortunately the most complex issue. The serious problem is that we observe with an instrument that is identical to the field of observation. Our instrument is our own experience through which we observe our patient's experience. That instrument is composed, in part, by the very theories under dispute and that we seek to defend. We tend to look for different bits of meanings according to the conceptual school we are loyal to. And our loyalties are often very strong and driven by powerful emotional attachments.

Following what I have said above, it is clear that we make two sets of observations. The first observation before the interpretation is directed towards constructing a meaning, which becomes the interpretation. That first observation will be an understanding of some anxiety that the patient is unconsciously presenting but keeping in a latent state. After interpretation of the anxiety, the second observation follows the fate of the interpreted meaning in terms of some predicted shift towards a closer manifestation of the anxious narrative in the transference, in the session.

Ezriel (1956) thought of this as a set of 'operational criteria' – some initial 'required relationship' before interpretation is overtly invited in the session in order to hide some 'avoided relationship' that the patient fears, unconsciously, to threaten some catastrophe (like the death of the analyst in the example given earlier).

Checking for distortions

The problem that remains to be solved is the most difficult. It is the distortions due to our instrument (our own minds) simply picking bits and pieces from the sequence of the associations that suit what we would prefer to find. Perhaps there is no completely foolproof way of avoiding the distortions of this kind of observer bias. And to be frank, the experiments of natural science are not always free of such distortion either; we can cite the work of Cyril Burt's falsified work on the average IQ measures of different human races (Joynson, 1989). Nevertheless, we can go a long way towards validating such subjective observations. The method I have discussed elsewhere (Hinshelwood, 2013) needs further examination, but it is one that could be useful not only for research data but for ordinary clinical purposes, too. Indeed, it tends to be used in an intuitive way by careful clinicians anyway. The suggested protocol has three parts to it; in effect, there are three checking devices:

- Before the interpretation, we need to make parallel observations: (a) First we listen to the patient's association to discern a narrative meaning and (b) we observe through our own experience the countertransference we have in the session in terms of the meaning of the relation between us. These two observations need to have a similar meaning; moreover, only when they do coincide with a single meaning do we have an interpretation worth making to the patient. In other words, the meaning we extract from the associations needs to be checked against the countertransference and vice versa.
- Then, on the basis of this observation of a meaningful narrative, we make a prediction of the kind of change expected. It will predict a similar narrative but a change in the narrative towards the avoided relationship that more strongly expresses the unconscious anxiety.
- Finally, we give the interpretation of the unconscious anxiety and then make observations in the same way: (a) We listen again to the associations for their narrative meaning and (b) we observe as before the countertransference for what it says of the relation between us. We require the same confluence as before so that we only assess the interpretation when:

    a the meanings from both associations and countertransference coincide; and b the narrative revealed is an evolution of the narrative identified initially and used for the interpretation.

The postinterpretive narrative meaning must be observed in terms of the preinterpretive narrative. In other words, the metapsychological theory must be the same in each case, so that the narrative meaning is much the same but with a degree of modification. It must not be a completely new narrative. This change in the predominant narrative is illustrated well in the example above from Ezriel's (1956) case – the change from a distant Oedipal murderousness to a somewhat less distant one. That change in the narrative is what Freud called 'working through'.

But the metapsychology may change after the interpretation. For instance, if the narrative before the interpretation appears to be about an Oedipal exclusion and then afterwards it is a completely different narrative about, shall we say, a helping doctor who fails to touch their patient in the right place, then something has gone wrong. The intervention has been based on a theory that is not applicable to the initial material. That intervention is inaccurate, has misunderstood the material, and has interrupted (not touched) the patient's preoccupation at that time. The example to follow will give actual examples of an interpretation not relevant to the patient's anxiety, and one that is relevant. Thus, the metapsychology on which the interpretation is based is under test at that moment when used to understand the patient. This can then be used for finding the relevance of theories from any school of metapsychology.

A clinical example of checking observations

The model of clinical observation is complex and needs a clarifying illustration. The vignette below shows an interpretation that does not produce a change in line with the conditions set out. So, the interpretation was wrong, because the narrative meaning that was identified before the interpretation must have been incorrect. In the session, after a reconsideration, a different meaning was identified, and so a new interpretation was made. That second interpretation *did* show a change that matched the criteria. The change therefore matched the prediction of a move closer to the meaning in the transference, and so the interpretation could be regarded as correct.

> This a 45-year-old professional man, Mr. X, who came for a second analysis because of feelings of depression and an awareness that he did not always follow good sense, including, for instance, resorting to cocaine. He was quite omnipotent in many respects, which led him to be unreliable, sometimes alarmingly. He was diabetic, but his lifestyle led to taking his insulin irregularly, and from time to time he had hypoglycaemic spells. He told me this often happened unexpectedly, and he was

> somewhat casual about it, leaving me far from casual and wondering what I would do if it happened in a session. In addition, he frequently went to sleep in his session, with loud snoring and, more alarmingly, sleep apnoea. This also worried me. I was often beset by the sense that I did not have the capacity to make a helpful analytic impact on his problems with the resources that I had.
>
> In one mid-week session, Mr. X told me of a meeting he had had with a friend with whom he was working on a project. The friend did very little towards the project, rarely contributed what he had agreed to do, and was in fact a very unreliable man. My patient was extraordinarily fond of and loyal to this friend. I found myself thinking what an unreliable patient I had, who sometimes even went to sleep on the project I was conducting with him. I felt a mixture of irritation that I was struggling to make headway with his analysis; at the same time, I thought a patient has a right to use his analysis to express his problems in his own way – and he was certainly doing that, I thought.
>
> His material is a story about an unreliable friend, causing frustration in a loyal relationship; and I said something about unreliable friends, comparing how we both struggled to keep a project going, him with his friend, and I with him. I said the frustration of his work with his friend demanded a loyalty and tolerance, and he may be anxious about my tolerance of how he made use of the analysis.

I had thought that the association told a story about his unreliability, that connected with my irritation in the countertransference. This suggested my interpretation which articulated a supposed (and repressed) anxiety that my tolerance may be limited. This implied he avoided overstepping that limit, and we could deduce a *prediction* – that his concern at my intolerance will become clearer and less repressed. Did it?

Continuing,

> Characteristically he was silent, and then he started snoring until he woke with his apnoea and a nasty gasping intake of breath. He remembered what he had been talking about, and the interpretation, and he courteously acknowledged the link I had made. I felt he was reassuring me, even patronising me a little. He continued to tell me how he had worked with his friend all evening and well into the night. He explained how the friend needed a lot of encouragement and reassurance, and his own role was to be very tolerant whilst doing most of the work.
>
> This does not confirm the prediction, since he did *not* express more directly a concern about *my* tolerating *his* unreliability. In fact, rather the opposite – he had gone to sleep! Afterwards, I felt him soothing me, and he did not express more of the concern about my tolerance, as predicted.

> Actually, there was some change. He went to sleep and then expressed a courtesy and reassurance. This, however, was not the predicted change – towards a stronger expression of concern that I may be intolerant. So, the interpretation I made was wrong. To be sure, sleep could be a response to the anxiety, maybe greater anxiety, and it might have been a greater repression. But it was not the *predicted* change, which would have been a more manifest anxiety with *less* repression.

So, I continued to listen to the material – he had continued by telling me how his friend needed so much reassurance and encouragement. Then I could see another story, told twice; first in the countertransference and then in the material:

- In the countertransference, I felt encouraged; and
- then in the material I heard that story repeated as his encouragement of his friend. So, continuing with my notes:

> I interpreted that he was trying to tell me that he felt he had to be very tolerant of my limited abilities to contribute to the analysis in the way he had expected and needed. Yet I said he felt very loyal to me, and so he had to keep things going himself.

Then we can predict that if he was concerned about the way I worked with him, a more explicit expression of that concern would emerge. And, indeed, the response did seem to be along those lines:

> This time he did not go to sleep. He changed the subject and said he had been very interested in two insects flying in the room where he had been working, and he had been trying to estimate the difference in the buzz of each, which gave him some thoughts about the project he was working on – it was a musical project. I was heartened by his change of topic because it made me think that something was moving on.

What I saw here was a change that seemed significant. This change was in line with the expectation (a prediction) that a lack of cooperation would move towards a more cooperative narrative. There was indeed material about cooperation – the two insects buzzing around together. And moreover, from the other perspective, the countertransference, I did feel more heartened and encouraged. I felt a more cooperative and hopeful feeling, as I listened to the story of the buzz between the two of us 'busy bees'.

Discussion

This vignette provides an illustration of the discrimination between an accurate observation of data and an inaccurate one. The nature of this double observation is a kind of triangulation. From two angles the point can be fixed. In this case the meaning is fixed by the observations of both the associations and the transference–countertransference. The fixed point is what is meaningful to the patient at this moment. I have shown how that meaning is important for research purposes as well as the clinical/therapeutic purpose. For research data, this protocol is for observations of meanings at two points in relation to the interpretation. Each observation is a double one, a triangulation. It should appear in a case presentation at two points when claiming the validity of metapsychological meaning and narratives.

There are complications that may create confusions. The cause–effect sequence is a process that can be read as a narrative itself – If I do this, then that happens. But that kind of narrative in psychoanalysis is a narrative *about* a meaning or, more specifically, a narrative about *the change or development of a meaning*. So, even though the meaning may be a narrative, like the Oedipal story, the fate of that meaningful narrative in a session is also a story. We can consider that the causal narrative is the analyst's narrative, whilst the meaning that an interpretation is about belongs to the patient.

Another complication is the negative therapeutic reaction. This always has to be taken into account. It has for long been an important pitfall and the opportunity for dispute amongst psychoanalysts. Whether a negative therapeutic reaction is merely a failed interpretation or an acting out of a negative transference towards the analyst is a dispute I will not go into here (but see Hinshelwood, 2013).

Conclusions

The intention of the research design described in this chapter has been to stick closely to the clinical method, to clarify the steps by which the data is collected and understood and then used. These steps are based on the analyst using his personal sensitivity, just as he does in the clinical work. The advantages of the analyst's subjectivity and intuition are vastly greater than objective observation of behaviour, language, and conscious reports from the patient. It is, however, difficult to maintain such a rigorous clinical process, and maybe we have to rely on short vignettes from within sessions. But a short vignette can be very revealing of the accuracy of meanings, as in the illustration given, and, as it is also argued, single cases can provide clear answers with confidence.

Examples have been given of the precise selection of data in the analytic process, of the kind of changes that can test the metapsychology of an interpretation. It is necessary to refer elsewhere for an example of a comparison between the conceptions of two different schools of metapsychology. The paper on comparing repression and splitting as related concepts used by different groups of analysts shows how, with careful operationalising of the two concepts, they *both* can be shown to have a valid relevance (Hinshelwood, 2008). For those interested in greater detail on the scope of this design, it may be necessary to turn to this paper (Hinshelwood, 2008) as well as the book *Research on the Couch* (Hinshelwood, 2013).

This research design is one possible way of justifying psychoanalytic knowledge by using the traditional setting from which almost all knowledge has originally come. It is one attempt to defend psychoanalysis from the criticisms that its knowledge cannot be tested and so cannot be valid. The knowledge can be validated. And that validity comes from our having a standard setting in which a process occurs. So, we already closely follow a pattern that can reveal causal relations and can therefore use a deductive method of testing. This may not be the only method for testing our form of knowledge production and for comparing different conceptual frameworks with each other. We may even need different methods to do different kinds of testing jobs. But this chapter has tried to show that, in principle, it is possible to design a convincing logic to justify knowledge of subjective experiences. It has emphasised that the radically different nature of our data – subjective experience as opposed to material measurements – implies a need for caution and for extensive debate amongst the schools of psychoanalysis, to which this book is dedicated. So, if nothing else, it may encourage better and easier research designs to evolve in the investigation of subjectivities.

Although, as Richard Rorty said, 'Psychoanalysts [must] stop asking (obsessive?) questions like "Is psychoanalysis a science?"' (Rorty, 2000, p. 822). We do have to face critics with some sort of answers to their questions. It could be best to accept the argument that our reliance on subjective processes and data puts us outside the boundary of natural science. But that does not mean that psychoanalytic research has to be less logical or convincing, provided that we are clear about the conditions for the logical steps we take. Thus, one could say that psychoanalytic research is not science but it is very similar. Its methods of research must differ in significant respects; but then the methods of various natural sciences differ amongst themselves anyway, according to their field of enquiry and the nature of their data.

We should therefore not give up our method too easily and turn to those of other sciences. Of course, results from other disciplines may be of value, but we need to examine first more meticulously what *our* method is and why it is in fact just what we need.

References

Abraham, K. (1921). Contribution to a discussion on tic. In K. Abraham (Ed.), *Selected papers on psychoanalysis*. London, England: Hogarth.

Breuer, J., & Freud, S. (1895). *Studies on hysteria. Standard edition of the complete psychological works of Sigmund Freud* (Vol. 2). London, England: Hogarth.

Caper, R. (1988). *Immaterial facts*. New York, NY: Jason Aronson.

Cioffi, F. (1970). Freud and the idea of a pseudo-science. In R. Berger & F. Cioffi (Eds.), *Explanation in the behavioural sciences*. Cambridge, England: Cambridge University Press.

Crews, F. (1993). The unknown Freud. *New York Review of Books*, 40(19), 55–65.

Darwin, C. (2009). *On the origin of species*. London, England: Penguin. (Original work published 1859)

Dreher, A. U. (2000). *Foundations for conceptual research in psychoanalysis*. London, England: Karnac.

Dyson, F. W., Eddington, A. S., & Davidson, C. (1920). A determination of the deflection of light by the sun's gravitational field, from observations made at the total eclipse of May 29, 1919. *Philosophical Transactions of the Royal Society A*, 220(571–581), 291–333.

Edelson, M. (1985). The hermeneutic turn and the single case study in psychoanalysis. *Psychoanalysis and Contemporary Thought*, 8, 567–614.

Edelson, M. (1986). Causal explanation in science and in psychoanalysis – Implications for writing a case study. *Psychoanalytic Study of the Child*, 41, 89–127.

Ezriel, H. (1956). Experimentation within the psychoanalytic session. *British Journal for the Philosophy of Science*, 7, 29–48.

Ferenczi, S. (1921). Psycho-analytical observations on tic. *The International Journal of Psychoanalysis*, 2, 1–30.

Forrester, J. (1997). *Dispatches from the Freud wars*. Cambridge, MA: Harvard University Press.

Freud, A. (1936). *The ego and the mechanisms of defence*. London, England: Hogarth Press.

Freud, S. (1900). *The interpretation of dreams. Part I. The standard edition of the complete psychological works of Sigmund Freud* (Vol. IV). London, England: Hogarth.

Freud, S. (1916). Lecture XXI The development of the libido and the sexual organizations. In *Introductory lectures. The standard edition of the complete psychological works of Sigmund Freud* (Vol. XVI). London, England: The Hogarth Press.

Freud, S. (1953). The interpretation of dreams. In J. Strachey (Ed.), *The standard edition of the complete psychological works of Sigmund Freud* (Vols. IV and V). London, England: The Hogarth Press. (Original work published 1900)

Freud, S. (1964a). Constructions in analysis. In J. Strachey (Ed.), *The standard edition of the complete psychological works of Sigmund Freud* (Vol. XXIII). London, England: The Hogarth Press. (Original work published 1937)

Freud, S. (1964b). An outline of psycho-analysis. In J. Strachey (Ed.), *The standard edition of the complete psychological works of Sigmund Freud* (Vol. XXIII). London, England: The Hogarth Press. (Original work published 1938)

Fromm, E. (1971). *The crisis of psychoanalysis*. London, England: Penguin.

Gabbard, G. O. (2000). On gratitude and gratification. *Journal of the American Psychoanalytical Association*, 48, 697–716.

Heimann, P. (1991). Some aspects of the role of introjection and projection in early development. In P. King & R. Steiner (Eds.), *The Freud-Klein controversies 1941–1945*. London, England: Routledge.

Hinshelwood, R. D. (2002). Symptoms or relationships (Comment on Jeremy Holmes', 'All You Need Is CBT'). *British Medical Journal*, 324, 288–294.

Hinshelwood, R. D. (2008). Repression and splitting: Towards a method of conceptual comparison. *The International Journal of Psychoanalysis*, 89, 503–521.
Hinshelwood, R. D. (2013). *Research on the couch: Single-case studies, subjectivity and psychoanalytic knowledge*. London, England: Routledge.
Hook, S. (Ed.). (1959). *Psychoanalysis, scientific method, and philosophy*. New York, NY: New York University Press.
Joynson, R. (1989). *The Burt affair*. London, England: Routledge.
Klein, M. (1926). The psychological principles of child analysis. In *The writings of Melanie Klein: Volume 1. Love, guilt and reparation*. London, England: Hogarth.
Klein, M. (1948). A contribution to the psychogenesis of tics. In *Contributions to psycho-analysis*. London, England: Hogarth. (Original work published 1925)
Kuhn, T. (1962). *The structure of scientific revolutions*. Chicago, IL: University of Chicago Press.
Mahler, M., Pine, F., & Bergman, A. (1975). *The psychological birth of the human infant*. London, England: Hutchison.
Meissner, W. W. (1999). The self-as-subject in psychoanalysis. *Psychoanalysis and Contemporary Thought*, 22, 155–201.
Milton, J. (1992). Presenting the case for NHS psychotherapy services – A working bibliography. *Psychoanalytic Psychotherapy*, 6, 151–167.
Plato. (1987). *Theaetetus* (R. H. Waterfield, Trans.). London, England: Penguin.
Popper, K. (1959). *The logic of scientific discovery*. London, England: Hutchinson.
Popper, K. (1963). *Conjectures and refutations*. London, England: Routledge and Kegan Paul.
Popper, K. (1976). *Unended quest: An intellectual autobiography*. London, England: Fontana.
Rorty, R. (2000). Pragmatism. *The International Journal of Psychoanalysis*, 81, 819–823.
Solms, M., & Turnbull, O. (2002). *The brain and the inner world*. London, England: Karnac.
Stern, D. (1985). *The interpersonal world of the infant: A view from psychoanalysis and developmental psychology*. New York, NY: Basic Books.
Taylor, D. (2015). Treatment manuals and the advancement of psychoanalytic knowledge: The treatment manual of the Tavistock Adult Depression Study. *The International Journal of Psychoanalysis*, 96, 845–875.
Wallerstein, R. (1990). Psychoanalysis: The common ground. *The International Journal of Psychoanalysis*, 71, 3–20.

Chapter 5

Discussion by Charles Hanly

I find myself in strong agreement with not a few of Hinshelwood's arguments. The exception is his reliance on Popper in excluding the importance of inductive inferences in generating psychoanalytic knowledge and his abandonment of Freud's understanding of the nature of psychoanalytic knowledge. I am in basic agreement with Hinshelwood (Chapter 4, this book) who, like Popper (1934/1959), holds that from any adequate descriptive or explanatory (causal) idea in psychoanalysis there can be inferred what observations would falsify it no less than what facts would support it. Analysts, while analysing no less than when theorising, should be on the lookout for negative instances. In psychoanalysis negative instances are associations or transferences (clinical facts) that run counter to the expectations of the hypotheses guiding their interpretations. Verification (establishing levels of probability) depends on the possibility of falsification. In order to observe affirmative or negative facts, we need guiding ideas but, in order to know what is, we must be able to allow our observations to falsify our ideas and learn what is not. Popper (1934/1959) claimed that psychoanalysis is doomed to be a pseudo-science because the psychoanalytic idea of resistance is always available to be used to explain away each and every negative instance. And, of course, the cause of a negative instance in psychoanalysis – a verbal denial or no change when a theoretically and experientially plausible interpretation of a symptom is given – may be the effect of the patient's resistance or it may mean that the interpretation does not currently tally with what is now most urgently going on in the patient or that it is not ever going to tally because it is mistaken. In doing analysis, analysts have to be able to nonjudgementally accept whatever transferences come into play, and they must also be able to use the experience-based ideas they have of the patient, while tolerating the possibility that they may turn out to be false. Tolerance for the uncertainty involved in having one's ideas tested in this way needs to be and can be integral to the analytic attitude. The recognition of resistance at work in conflicted psychic processes does not cause analysts to invariably use it to avoid contrary observation of facts.

Nor is Popper immune, by his own standards, to a philosophical version of pseudo-science in his failure to study and digest the negative instances to

DOI: 10.4324/9780000000002-7

be found in Freud's development of psychoanalytic theory. For example, if psychoanalysis is a pseudoscience, then Freud considers only confirming evidence for his theories. But Freud (1915/1957) willingly accepted negative instances. Therefore, psychoanalysis is not a pseudoscience and Popper is in error. By the way, the argument I have just formulated is a valid hypothetical argument that denies the consequent and the antecedent. One of several examples is Freud's discovery that his seduction theory was not a universal cause of neurosis (Hanly, 2014). It would appear that Popper kept himself quite ignorant of Freud's work; otherwise, he would have come upon Freud's (1915/1957) paper titled 'A Case of Paranoia Running Counter to the Psycho-Analytic Theory of the Disease'. Grünbaum (1984) criticised Popper for this specific error and, more generally, Grünbaum refuted Popper's rejection of inductive reasoning. It is little wonder that Popper rejects inductive reasoning and satisfies himself with a deductive proof that psychoanalysis is a pseudoscience that turns out to have a demonstrably false premise given the facts. Neither was Popper able to comprehend the epistemological and methodological significance of Freud's (1916–1917) differentiation of the manifest dream in which the meaning of the dream is not to be found and which may very well be influenced by the patient's ideas about what they believe the analyst wants to hear and the latent dream in which the meaning of the dream is to be found in the unconscious wishes, memories, and phantasies that cause it and which belong only to the patient, even when the patient does not want to own them. Nor does Popper do justice to Freud's (1938/1964b) pointing out, actually cited and appreciated by Hinshelwood (Chapter 4, this book), that it is not the patient's agreement or disagreement that decides matters of fact in psychoanalysis; it is change of what kind and how much and for how long or not in the analytic process after interpretations are made. This failure in Popper's philosophical thinking to attend carefully to negative instances of his hypothesis about psychoanalysis raises a basic question for me about the utility of Popper's (1934/1959) epistemological ideas for a psychoanalytic epistemology despite my agreement about a downscaled (when compared with Popper's limitation of knowledge to what is known to be false) notion of the importance of falsifiability as a criterion for an adequate scientific hypothesis. Freud (1950) treated his seduction theory as falsifiable, despite his initial pride in it, and employed inductive reasoning using evidence of absence of change and recurrence of symptoms to show that as a universal theory it was false. I shall argue below that the most serious flaw in reliance on Popper is the abandonment of induction.

Unfortunately, in my view, Hinshelwood follows Popper on this basic question:

> Freud depended heavily on inductive thinking to justify his theories scientifically. That view of science has changed since those claims.

> More rigour and a different kind of logical justification tend to be required now. Popper (1959) developed a logical model of science, ruling out inductive thinking and emphasising the deductive testing of theories, to which he claimed psychoanalysis was unable to conform (Popper, 1963, 1976). In natural science, that logical method is a hypothetico-deductive one, which was laid out in Popper's (1959) classic treatise. Psychoanalysts on the whole trained in an intuitive clinical method are not always comfortable to follow along that logical road. (Chapter 4, this book)

I would rather say that analysts should not rely on intuition but should test intuitive ideas against facts of clinical observation and that inductive verification justifies not following Popper's proposed 'logical road'.

But, before turning to the basic disagreement, let me cite two further important points of agreement. Hinshelwood rejects the phenomenological, hermeneutic, and relational idea that meaning and causality are dichotomous (Hanly, 1979). Psychoanalysis is simultaneously a search for meanings and a search for causes. The meaning of a dream, symptom, or inhibition is to be found in the unconscious wishes that cause them. Also, in agreement with Hinshelwood (Chapter 4), I think that interpretations are grounded in hypotheses that imply predictions of what will happen, if the hypothesis is true. These predictions can be tested against the effects of the interpretations on the psychic functioning of the patient inside and outside the analysis, as illustrated by Hinshelwood's examples of a shift in a patient's displacement of anger and in the correction of an interpretation he had made in a clinical episode. Among these predictions, some of the most important are predictions of what the patient's childhood pathogenic memories will turn out to have been. They have often been called 'retrodictions' when interpretations are considered from a genetic point of view or 'constructions' by Freud (1937/1964a). In analysing, the analyst makes predictions about what the patient will be able to recall in the next days, weeks, and months of what happened that was pathogenic in the past and what defensive processes are likely to be running interference with their recollection.

Perhaps it is worth noting for the phenomenological sceptics among us that these hypothetical and deductive thought activities may not be even explicit in the analyst's attentive listening and observing. We need to be receptive observers of shifts from session to session of our patient's affects, desires, aversions, and moods. The cultivation of this attentive receptivity is akin to focusing a microscope. It focuses the analyst's mind on the patient and opens it to the relevant observations that can be made. For example, 'The patient's cheerfulness seems forced. I wonder if he is protecting himself and me from something painful. What could it be?' These thoughts are more likely to be experienced in the analyst's thinking not as hypotheses and predictions as such but as questions, doubts, uncertainties, and hunches. However, inherent in them are implicit hypotheses such as 'when patients force themselves to be cheerful, probably they are not'. It is this implicit hypothesis that guides the analyst's thought to observe more of the patient's associations, to sieve through accumulated relevant preconscious memories of the patient's way of dealing with painful affects thus far and to reflect on the transference implication of protecting the analyst from pain. The first task is to form an adequate impression of whether and, if so, how forced and defensive the patient's cheerfulness is. The second task is to speculate about why. This process may be largely preconscious (but not unconscious because that would activate the analyst's primary process thought activity) and may result in one or more interpretive possibilities that could arrive in the analyst's conscious mind 'somewhat out of the blue'. In the situation we are considering, the interpretation could be as simple as, 'I wonder if you are trying to be more cheerful than you actually feel?' Again, implicit in this interpretation there is a hypothetical prediction 'the interpretation of the defensive intensification of an affect may allow the warded off affect to become conscious or, already being conscious, communicable to the analyst in the patient's associations'. If this interpretation does not have its predicted result (actually experienced by the analyst as something hoped for) and the patient's forced cheerfulness persists in the session, the analyst will probably be led by this to continue his search for and make trial of other interpretations, each of which will have the implicit logical hypothetical and deductive–predictive structure. I agree that the logical structure is at work preconsciously even when it is not conscious and even when the analyst is not familiar enough with logic to explicitly state to themselves why this process of thought is logically valid; that is, given that the implicit prediction has turned out to be false, then the hypothesis on which the interpretation is based is also probably false. But I do not agree that this description of the role of deductive thinking in clinical psychoanalysis enables us to dispense with inductive reasoning or that an exclusive reliance on Popper's hypothetico-deductive logic is feasible as a methodology for psychoanalysis clinically or theoretically. Before turning to this basic issue, let me consider a crucial related epistemological question.

Freud considered his clinical use of patient's free associations to be capable of the same objectivity as the microscopic smearing technique he had used in his study of neurons in eels when a student of biology. To say to a male patient suffering from a delusional accident phobia, 'You loved, admired and needed the protection of your father, but you also wanted to get rid of him so that you could have your mother for yourself' is to describe an important psychic experience of the patient's childhood that is no less objective than Freud's description of the eel neurons that established that they were structurally and functionally identical with human neurons contrary to the then 'creationist' belief. Hinshelwood (Chapter 4) thinks of the analytic observer as using his subjective psychic processes to observe the subjective psychic processes of patients. This description is unexceptionable as a description of the fact that each person has only their own psychic functions with which to experience self and the world, but 'subjectivity' in this context refers to the ontological subjectivity of the individual psyche. Each person's experience, thoughts, feelings, and wishes are their own. Psychic life is sustained by the brain inside each person's head. True enough, but the structure, functioning, and contents of the psyche are, of biological necessity, at least sufficiently adapted to reality (objectivity) despite the animistic thinking that replaces what is with what is wished for. From birth, biological hunger makes the neonate able to differentiate the breast that nourishes from the quasi-hallucinated image of the breast that does not. Therefore, epistemological objectivity and subjectivity are differentiated from the ontological subjectivity of our psychic life (Hanly & Hanly, 2001). If the fact of ontological subjectivity makes psychoanalytic observation somehow unscientific, it will have had the same effect on Galileo's telescopic observation of the materiality of the moon!

Popper (1934/1959) claimed that all experience (observation) is 'theory laden'. If theory laden means 'our ideas (theories) constitute what we experience', then the observations that appear to falsify hypotheses may well be themselves epistemologically subjective; that is, contaminated by an adherence to a contrary theory. This hypothesis would explain Popper's inability to grasp that Freud had observed negative instances of the clinical predictions of his seduction theory and had abandoned his original claim of universality for his seduction theory. The fact that Freud looked for negative instances (clinical observations that would falsify his first aetiological theory of the neurosis) falsifies Popper's (1934/1959) claim that psychoanalysis is a pseudo-science as mentioned previously. However, if theory laden means 'a guide to observations that would verify or falsify the theory in question', then Popper's use of the descriptor 'theory laden' is misleading. Is it possible that Popper's descriptor has contributed to misleading those analysts who, spurred on by the popularity of postmodern relativism by legitimate anxiety about clinical objectivity and therapeutic effectiveness, have seriously exaggerated the epistemological fallibility of psychoanalytic clinical observation in a contradictory attempt to improve it? The subjectivist argument claims that, in order to be objective, it is first necessary to accept that all clinical observations are epistemologically subjective (Hanly, 2019). Therefore, it is important to differentiate between using ideas to guide the search for observational evidence for or against the truth of psychoanalytic hypotheses despite psychological difficulties that can stand in the way of doing so (critical realism) and the epistemological claim that ideas inevitably constitute the observations made, rendering them epistemologically subjective – the observational reflection back to us of nothing but our own ideas. Ironically, subjectivist epistemologies in psychoanalysis provide grounds for Popper's (1934/1959) claim that psychoanalysis is a pseudo-science because psychoanalysts can only 'find' in their patients what they already believe are the causes of their difficulties in life even before they lie down on the couch and begin the tasks of free-associating and forming transferences. I do not wish to minimise the problem for psychoanalysis posed by the need for gurus and ideologists in psychoanalysts. These needs bring about the theory-laden observing and thinking that fractures what should be mainstream psychoanalysis into often contradictory 'schools'. Let me turn now to the basic problem with Popper's (1934/1959) hypothetico-deductive method.

Deduction does not guarantee truth. A deduction may be valid, but the conclusion thus derived may well be false. Whether or not it is true will depend on the truth of the premises. How can we know whether or not the premises are true? Could the premises be true because they can themselves be deduced from yet other premises? They could only be true if the premises of these other argument are true. Valid deducibility does not guarantee truth. Sooner or later the premises on which conclusions deductively depend have to be shown to be true by inductive reasoning. Deductive validity does not establish truth. Therefore, the truth of any body of empirical knowledge, any knowledge based on facts of observation or experiment, depends on inductive reasoning. The same turns out to be true of deductive systems of geometry, as we now know. The history of ideas is littered with the wreckage of deductive proofs (e.g., Descartes' [1986] innate ideas and Kant's [1781/1929] a priori conditions for external perception) that space is as postulated by Euclid (rectilinear and independent of mass), but as Hinshelwood's (Chapter 4, this book) citation from astronomy shows, it is highly probable that space is Riemannian (curved relative to mass) except for applications in the construction of buildings and the surveying of small areas where, for example, Euclid's Pythagorean theorem works well enough but does not work well in predicting locations even of planets in the solar system.

Predictions derived from a hypothesis can deductively and validly prove that a hypothesis is false, but the truth of the prediction cannot validly prove that the hypothesis from which it is derived is true. Thus, in the case of Hinshelwood's astronomy example, the prediction falsified the Newtonian prediction of the light's path through the sun's gravitational field and it confirmed Einstein's special relativity prediction. But it is deductively invalid to derive the truth of Einstein's hypothesis, on which the prediction was based, that space curves in the vicinity of mass from the truth of the prediction derived from it. Such an inference is a logical fallacy called 'affirming the consequent'. Popper's (1934/1959) deductive method deductively demonstrates what is false but fails to establish deductively what is true. (It is for this reason that Popper is so well satisfied with knowing what cannot be or happen.) Then how do we find out whether or not space curves relative to mass? Physicists find out the highly probable truth of the hypothesis by means of inductive inferences from many confirming observations of the behaviour of diverse objects in gravitational fields. Einstein's relativity theory has a high probability but it is not deductively proven to be true, even when its probability has been recently increased by the discovery of the gravitational waves predicted by it. For relativity theory could always be subsumed in a somewhat different theory that would explain what relativity theory now explains, just as relativity physics better explains what Newtonian mechanics explained but do more by unifying relativity theory and quantum mechanics, which relativity theory cannot itself accomplish (Rovelli, 2014). Claiming that relativity theory has been proven (i.e., demonstrated with certainty) goes far beyond the probability that the inductive inferences on which it is based allows. Such a unified theory would be yet more probable, but it could also be replaced by a yet more inclusive unified physics theory.

It does not follow that deductive reasoning is not useful in the construction of psychoanalysis. For example, Freud (1905/1949) was able to use homosexuality in adult men and women to show that the biological aim of libido is not uniquely defined in terms of reproductive sexuality but in terms of pleasure which may take a variety of forms during childhood and in adult sublimations. Elsewhere (Hanly, 2014) I have articulated the deductive elements in Freud's major modifications of psychoanalytic theory in conjunction with his use of inductive reasoning. In all theorising, deductive and inductive reasoning are interdependent, although inductive reasoning is the more fundamental because it is based on reality testing.

But let us return to clinical psychoanalysis. A university-educated, professionally employed, married but childless woman in her late 20s suffering from severe frigidity fell silent four times in a weekly analysis after an early phase of some months of telling her analyst about problematic aspects of her current life and its history. Her silence on the couch reminded her analyst of two silences in her childhood about which she had earlier informed me. Her parents had divorced during her early latency. Her mother refused to allow her to visit her father if his new wife was present. Her father refused the condition and never saw or spoke to her again except for a single visit when, at her request in her early teens, she saw him once in his office for a brief awkward, unsatisfying visit. She was an only child living alone with her mother, who punished her for misdemeanours by withdrawing from her and not speaking to her for long periods until she would tearfully beg her mother to relent and promise obedience. My surmise was that this cruel punishment arose from the mother's awareness of the disloyalty of her daughter's longing for her father. Now she was coming to deprive her analyst of her speech. Over a number of weeks, I interpreted to her that in being silent she was wanting me to know how painfully unloved her parent's silences had caused her to feel, how frightened she was that her analyst might treat her refusal to speak with a like parental silence or even terminate her analysis, and how angry she was for her being subject to this threat. Given her silence from the beginning to the end of her sessions there was nothing in the here and now of the analysis to guide me but her silence and her initial snippets of the history of traumatic silences in her life that I must, at all costs, not repeat. I assumed that she wanted me to know by suffering a resistive but communicative sample of the painful parental silences she had suffered because of the abandonment of her by her father for his girlfriend and the punishment of her mother, all the while hoping that I would forgive her for her projection of it into her experience of me in the transference; that, nevertheless, she feared her disobedience would result in repetitions at my hands; and that she was profoundly and vengefully angry with me (her silent parents) in the transference. From this clinical hypothesis interpretations can be derived; for example, 'You badly wanted your father's attention and approval; his withdrawal and refusal to see you was painfully depriving'; 'Your mother's anger at him deprived you of your father and she punished you with withdrawal into silence when you only had her to turn to'; 'I sometimes wonder if you are very anxious about what you may have to say, if you let yourself speak'; 'I wonder if the anger you had toward your parents, you now have toward me, and its intensity frightens you'. The basic prediction was that these and the like interpretations would enable the patient to begin to free-associate. This prediction was born out by what followed. What followed was not only a slow shift into communicating verbally as she gained confidence that my analytic silence involved attentive nonjudgemental sympathetic listening to her and an effort to identify sympathetically with her experience as she began to free-associate again. Also, psychologically substantive confirming phantasies began to find expression in her associations. She had been encouraged by her husband to seek analysis because of her unrelenting sexual frigidity since their marriage. These phantasies emerged: I was cheating on her or on my students and most likely both; she wanted her husband to force her to stop coming to analysis; I would deserve it because no one can be a university professor and also a psychoanalyst; she wanted her husband to beat me within an inch of my life. She remembered that after drinking too much at a party, on the way home in the car she had raged and wept, imploring her husband to seek out her father and kill him. She had been unable to remember anything of this the next morning. The expression, interpretation, and analytic working through these and other like phantasies and phobias were sufficient to enable her to proceed to a successful analysis that 3 years later had cured her sexual frigidity.

But what does this clinical result prove? That the interpretations and the analyst's attitude toward the patient implicitly expressed in them (Hanly, 1994) appear to have brought about a crucial change in her engagement in the analytic process. But these facts do not, by themselves, prove that they caused the desirable change that occurred. Accepting, what is reasonable in my view, that 'hoping' during the session can be legitimately construed as implicitly 'predicting', the occurrence of what was predicted does not prove causality despite providing reasonable grounds for clinical encouragement. The reason that this is so is not psychological; it is logical. The hypothesis is 'if the analyst interprets x, y, and z, the patient will begin to free-associate again' (the major premise). The observation is that the patient gradually resumed free-associating when these interpretations were employed (the minor premise). This hypothetical deductive conclusion is invalid because the minor premise affirms the consequent. What we have is not a proof of truth justified by hypothetical–deductive prediction but a probability based on these facts of observation derived from one analysis. What we now need is further evidence that the same result occurs in patients who suffer the same impasses in order to increase the probability that it was the interpretations that were effective in bringing about the change.

Because we cannot deductively prove that the hypotheses that guided my interpretations that released the patient from anxious and angry resistance to free-associating are necessary and sufficient causes of what happened, what can we infer from this observation of change and according to what rules of inference? Mill's (1843/2002) method of agreement allows us to affirm a minimal probability that the interpretations caused the change in the patient's engagement in the analysis. One way in which this probability can be enhanced is by enumerating and eliminating other potentially relevant causes. The probability that we are observing a causal relation will be increased if other possible causes can be eliminated. Two such possibilities are Grunbaum's (1984) favourites: suggestion and placebo. In this case, suggestion can be ruled out insofar as I did not greet her silence with encouraging statements and promises about the benefits of free-associating, moralistic statements about the patient's obligation to herself to tell me what thoughts and feelings she was having, threats of an early termination, and the like. To be sure, there was an implicit encouragement in the nonjudgmental interpretations of traumatically painful experiences past and present. They were sympathetic and reasonable reconstructions based on her initial several weeks of relating her history and complaints. One of the inescapable necessary but not sufficient conditions of making psychoanalytic clinical observations is the requirement of a decent and respectful human clinical relationship dedicated to honesty and truth. Grunbaum's (1984) criticism of what he calls Freud's 'tally argument' mistakenly claims that suggestion or a placebo cannot be ruled out in principle and that, therefore, inductive enumeration cannot be used to augment or diminish the probability of the truth of the therapeutic causality of psychoanalytic interpretations.

But questions of placebo and suggestion are not questions of principle. They are empirical questions about how the analyst has conducted the analysis, whether or not there is evidence of a disruptive countertransference, what interpretations were made or considered but not made, and the like. Whether or not there is a placebo at work is similarly a factual issue. In this case it can be ruled out simply because, if the change – the patient's return to free-associating – was the result of a placebo, which typically has a relatively short life, she would have reverted to this form of resistance soon enough, but she did not. She worked hard with remarkable honesty and success in her free-associating and transferences. This inference that contradicts Grunbaum's (1984) criticism of the tally argument is a valid deductive inference known in logic as *modus tollens*. Far from being a placebo, the interpretations had the effect of enabling the patient to continue free-associating even when the memories and wishes that were emerging were deeply painful to her. Contrary to Grunbaum (1984), suggestion and placebo can be ruled out depending on the facts of the analytic process. Their possibility should always be considered. The reader will also notice that I acknowledge theoretically and practically that opportunities for deductive reasoning arise in our clinical thinking. My view is only that deductive reasoning is not sufficient to prove the hypotheses that guide our clinical work and that we must rely on inductive reasoning as well in order to establish their reliability, or their degree of probability.

Another group of possibilities for relevant hypotheses are to be found in alternative psychoanalytic theories that have differing clinical theory and interpretive implications. For example, self psychology and contemporary relational psychology have an alternative theory of the Oedipus complex with a narcissistic aetiology in a failure of adequate parenting. It is essential to enumerate these alternatives because their consideration provides a method for evaluating their efficacy by means of the consequences of their use in making interpretations in changes occurring or not in the analytic process and ultimately in determining what interpretations and what theories are most probable. Other possibilities include alternative treatment modalities from medication to behavioural modification. Inductive enumeration is not such a Sisyphean enterprise as it may appear to be because each of the enumerated possible causes must be relevant; that is, there are good reasons to think that they might cause the changes in the analytic process and the patient's life we clinically observe, and there is evidence that they have been active in bringing about the observed improvements in the patient's psychic functioning.

Thus, in my view, despite major agreements with Hinshelwood (Chapter 4), my fundamental disagreement is with his Popperian assumption that inductive reasoning is not needed for the construction and testing of psychoanalytic knowledge. I persist in this view, even though it is also true that the humanity of the analytic relation to patients makes it difficult to form the control groups that might best establish causal relations between interpretations and symptom remission or cure based on Mill's (1843/2002) joint methods of similarity and difference. Contrary to Scriven (1959/1990), the ethical humanistic standards of psychoanalysis prohibit any experiment that would assign suicidally depressed patients to a control group deprived of treatment or with a phony treatment. Granted, this constraint limits the use of control groups that would be logically and scientifically helpful for psychoanalysis as a science. Nevertheless, what inductive reasoning from observations cannot provide to psychoanalysis cannot be provided by abandoning inductive reasoning and replacing it with the hypothetico-deductive reasoning proposed by Popper (1934/1959).

References

Descartes, R. (1986). *Meditations on first philosophy with selections from the objections and replies* (J. Cottingham, Trans.). Cambridge, England: Cambridge University Press.

Freud, S. (1949). Three essays on the theory of sexuality. In J. Strachey (Ed.), *The standard edition of the complete psychological works of Sigmund Freud* (Vol. VI). London, England: The Hogarth Press. (Original work published 1905)

Freud, S. (1957). A case of paranoia running counter to the psycho-analytic theory of the disease. In J. Strachey (Ed.), *The standard edition of the complete psychological works of Sigmund Freud* (Vol. XIV). London, England: The Hogarth Press. (Original work published 1915)

Freud, S. (1964a). Constructions in analysis. In J. Strachey (Ed.), *The standard edition of the complete psychological works of Sigmund Freud* (Vol. XX). London, England: The Hogarth Press. (Original work published 1937)

Freud, S. (1964b). An outline of psycho-analysis. In J. Strachey (Ed.), *The standard edition of the complete psychological works of Sigmund Freud* (Vol. XXIII). London, England: The Hogarth Press. (Original work published 1938)

Freud, S. *(1950).* Extracts from the Fleiss Papers. *In*J. Strachey (Ed.), *The standard edition of the complete psychological works of Sigmund Freud* (Vol. XXIII). London, England: The Hogarth Press.

Freud, S. (1916–1917). In J. Strachey (Ed.), *The standard edition of the complete psychological works of Sigmund Freud* (Vol. XXIII). London, England: The Hogarth Press. (Original work published 1915-1917)

Grunbaum, A. (1984). *The foundations of psychoanalysis.* Berkeley: University of California Press.

Hanly, C. (1979). *Existentialism and psychoanalysis*. New York, NY: International Universities Press.

Hanly, C. (1994). Reflections on the place of the therapeutic alliance in psychoanalysis. *The International Journal of Psychoanalysis*, 75, 457–467.

Hanly, C. (2014). The interplay of deductive and inductive reasoning in psychoanalytic theorizing. *The Psychoanalytic Quarterly*, 83, 897–916.

Hanly, C. (2019). The problem of pluralism in psychoanalysis. In P. M. Sandler & G. P. Costa (Eds.), *On Freud's 'The Question of Lay Analysis'*. London, England: Routledge.

Hanly, C., & Hanly, M. A. F. (2001). Critical realism: Distinguishing the psychological subjectivity of the analyst from epistemological subjectivism. *Journal of the American Psychoanalytic Association*, 49, 515–532.

Kant, I. (1929). *Kant's critique of pure reason* (N. Kemp Smith, Trans.). London, England: Palgrave Macmillan. (Original work published 1781)

Mill, J. S. (2002). *A system of logic*. Honolulu, HI: University Press of the Pacific. (Original work published 1843)

Popper, K. (1959). *The logic of scientific discovery*. London, England: Hutchinson. (Original work published 1934)

Rovelli, C. (2014). *Seven brief lessons on physics*. New York, NY: Riverhead Books.

Scriven, M. (1990). The experimental investigation of psychoanalysis. In S. Hook (Ed.), *Psychoanalysis scientific method and philosophy*. New York, NY: New York University Press. (Original work published 1959)

Chapter 6

Moving from clinical inquiry to clinical research

Ricardo Bernardi

Research: *Untersuchung* and/or *forschung*

When Freud had to define psychoanalysis in an article for an encyclopaedia (Freud, 1923/1955), he described it as 'a procedure for the investigation of mental processes which are almost inaccessible in any other way' (p. 235), as a method for the treatment of neurotic disorders, and as a growing scientific discipline. This definition continues to be universally accepted in psychoanalysis, but there is less agreement when the nature of these three dimensions and the relationship among them tries to be accurately established. In what follows, I will focus on why and how the investigation of mental processes can be considered clinical research, on the one hand showing the differences between clinical research and extraclinical empirical research and, on the other hand, underlining the profound unity between them and the possibility of their mutual complementation. The scientific nature of research resides in the search for data that possess increasing validity, reliability, and significance and in methods of gathering and processing these data in a way that enables conclusions that are progressively more critically supported. My intention is to revise these requirements in the clinical field and to examine which paths for advancement are being explored at the moment and are more promising for the future.

Many languages have two different words to designate the activity aimed at achieving new knowledge. Freud used the German term '*Untersuchung*': '*Psychanalyse ist der Name 1) eines Verfahrenszur Untersuchung seelischer Vorgänge …*' (1923/1955, p. 235). That being said, in German there is also the term *Forschung* to refer to discovering new information or reaching new understanding. In a similar way, in English there is a distinction between *investigation* and *research*, or in French, between *investigation* and *recherche*. Let us examine the distinction between both terms. *Untersuchung*, or investigation (the latter has the same spelling in French and a very similar one in Spanish, *investigación*), refers to an activity of enquiry or exploration in a broad sense, because it can also be carried out by a police or administrative investigator. *Forschung*, research, or *recherche* refers to a systematic search that conforms to the methodological requirements of the scientific disciplines.[2]

DOI: 10.4324/9780000000002-8

I have pointed out that Freud used for his definition the broader term *Untersuchung* rather than the more specific *Forschung*. However, if we look at the whole of his work on the Psychoanalytic Electronic Publishing database (P-E-P Web, 2017), we will find that he used both terms with a similar frequency. The expression '*Psychoan* Untersuchung*' was used 38 times by Freud and '*Psychoan* Forschung*' was used 46 times (the asterisk indicates that the search includes all of the words that include that root). If we now turn to all of the English-language literature the Psychoanalytic Electronic Publishing database contains, we will find that between 1920 and 2017, the expression '*psychoan* investigation*' was used 1,091 times, and '*psychoan* research*' was used 2,410 times; that is, the latter was preferred more than twice as many times. If we look at the last 20 years, the proportion in favour of research jumps to 3/1 (370 to 1,186, from 1997 to 2017). Therefore, in psychoanalytic literature, at least in English, when the authors want to refer to the activity of searching for new knowledge, they seem to be inclined to the term that suggests a methodologically rigorous search, based on verification or empirical evidence of a systematic and replicable nature.

It is convenient, in my opinion, not to separate both meanings excessively. Spanish uses the same term for both forms of search, which has certain advantages in the case of psychoanalysis. We can say that all analysts investigate in the session, in the broad sense of the term (enquiry, exploration, *Untersuchung*), because we make use of a method that leads us into the discovery of the unconscious aspects of the material. In this way, the cocreation of 'dyadic truths', characteristic of any analysis and any analyst–patient couple, is produced (Jiménez, 2009). The central aim is the progress of the therapeutic process, and the advance of knowledge is the means to achieve this progress. This activity, as Liberman (1971) pointed out, takes place with the patient during the session, and it is therefore also called 'online' research (Leuzinger-Bohleber, Kallenbach, & Schoett, 2016) or 'research on the couch' (Hinshelwood, 2013).

The term *research, Forschung, recherche,* or, in Spanish, *investigación en sentido estricta* becomes more justified the greater the effort to improve the quality of the data collected and the way in which the conclusions are drawn. Clinical research can be complemented by the use of other methods outside the session (extraclinical or 'offline research').

Psychoanalysis is essentially a clinical discipline that is supported by its own method, but it can and should resort to a variety of other methodologies when the questions it seeks to answer so demand it.

Clinical and extraclinical research

Some authors, like M. Leuzinger-Bohleber (Leuzinger-Bohleber & Fischmann, 2006), distinguish clearly clinical research (carried out with the psychoanalytic method in the session) from extraclinical research, which studies the analytic materials or other related issues by using the methodologies characteristic of rigorous scientific research. This distinction is valid if we are interested in discriminating the methods employed. If, on the other hand, we are interested in underscoring the result or purpose sought, I would suggest 'research at the service of clinical work' for the full set of procedures that provide us with evidence that is useful for the comprehension of a problem or a situation that is relevant to psychoanalysis. The use of the term *clinical* in medicine can serve as an example. Strictly speaking, clinical enquiry is what the doctor does next to the patient's bed (*kline* in Greek) to gather together the symptoms and signs of the illness. We use the term *paraclinical* when we refer to the laboratory exams and the different kinds of procedures that complement the clinical enquiry and that contribute to the diagnosis, treatment, and study of the evolution of the patient. Both the clinical activity and paraclinical studies are meant to support each other in the rigorous research done by the basic sciences. From a broader perspective, all of these sources of knowledge are useful for the comprehension of the clinical situation of the patient. Their methods differ, but they are not in opposition. Evidence-based medicine is precisely the attempt to join individual clinical expertise and the best external evidence available (Sackett, Straus, Richardson, & Rosenberg, 1997).

In this chapter, I will try to show the deep unity and continuity there is between clinical research and systematic empirical research, without any attempt to deny the differences between them or the specificity of each method. This continuity is clearly perceived when we place the clinical field in the foreground. The clinical work is one, just like the patient is one. The comprehensive study of a patient with an illness, either somatic or psychic, includes all aspects that are relevant, whether they come from the auscultation, the psychoanalytic method, or the procedures originated in the basic sciences, the neurosciences included. From this point of view, the psychoanalytic perspective is part of a broader clinical approach, which includes the biological, psychological, and social levels. It is necessary to maintain this integrative interdisciplinary vision to avoid the present tendency towards fragmentation, which is sometimes manifest in an exclusively biomedical vision. We must avoid opposing an also unilateral psychoanalytic vision. Psychoanalysis should defend its specificity, not its isolation.

Different forms of clinical and extraclinical research

Depending on the kind of question and methodology employed, it is possible to distinguish between different types of research. A panoramic view shows an extensive field that is open for psychoanalysis and a fluidity and complementarity among the diverse possible approximations.

A study at the service of clinical work can be based on exclusively clinical data or it can resort to extraclinical data and methods. The tools used can be of a qualitative, quantitative, or mixed type. The research can be done in a naturalistic context, studying the phenomenon such as it takes place in real contexts, or in an experimental context, seeking higher control of the variables. There are prospective clinical studies, which follow the evolution of the phenomena as time goes by, or retrospective ones, which try to reconstruct stages prior to the present. The focus of interest can be the study of the therapeutic process or of its outcome or, as it is more and more frequently, the process–outcome relationship, in an attempt to understand the mechanisms of change. Studies of a statistical or epidemiological nature are indicated when information that can be generalised to the whole population studied is sought. On other occasions, however, the interest lies in single-case studies, combining different methodologies for the in-depth study of a given case. There are also special fields, such as the study of child development or the neurosciences, among others, which have their own requirements.

It is important to make it clear that there is no intrinsic superiority of one method over the other, valid for all cases or in all cases. What is really important is to find which method better suits the questions we are attempting to answer.

Central questions in clinical work

Clinical activity has always led the professionals in charge of a patient to raise certain basic questions:

1 *What happens to the patient?* In psychoanalysis, just as in any clinical discipline, we attend somebody because they ask for our help because of a problem that makes them suffer and constrains them and that has to be diagnosed; in other words, conceptualised. At a certain level, it is useful to resort to descriptions of a metaphoric or almost artistic nature, but when we need to move on to a more general and systematised perspective, it is necessary to turn to operationalised descriptions. Later in the text, I will refer to the excellent psychoanalytic diagnostic systems available today.
2 *Why does this happen to the patient?* Freud's complemental series serve as a guide for us in the study of the factors that predispose, trigger, and maintain mental disorders or protect us from them.
3 *How should we treat the patient?* Whether they explicitly formulate it or not, every analyst or therapist has an idea of the focal points that have to be dealt with in the treatment, and this vision is gradually modified and deepened as the treatment develops.
4 *What is the evolution of the patient?* The evolution is a crucial source of evidence in favour or against our therapeutic hypotheses. It focuses on the result obtained, which are obviously of interest not only to the professional but also to the patient.

The psychodynamic case formulation (Bernardi, 2016) offers a method for giving expression to the therapist's hypotheses on these four fundamental questions. In the psychodynamic field, case formulation was developed in a pioneer paper by Perry, Cooper, and Michels (1987), published many decades ago. It had an important development in other psychotherapeutic schools, such as cognitive behavioural. Only recently has it deserved reconsideration from a dynamic perspective (Bernardi, 2014a, 2016). Case formulation is in itself both a tool for clinical research and a field to be investigated (Eells, 2007). Psychodynamic formulation can be complemented with the study of the patient's transformations according to the Three-Level Model (3-LM) for observing patient transformations. This model is a guide or heuristics for clinical discussion groups (or for individual reflection) submitted by the author of this chapter to the International Pyschoanalytical Association Committee for Clinical Observation, which implemented its use in different regions (Altmann de Litvan, 2014). The 3-LM promotes group discussions of the different steps that lead to the clinical observation of the changes in the patient and to theoretical hypotheses that make their explanation possible, with a constant focus on restricting the group discussion to what can be supported by the clinical material. From the point of view of clinical research, both case formulation and the 3-LM can be considered advances in the direction of a higher subtlety and systematisation of the observations and towards processes of peer validation.

Questions awaiting an answer

Psychoanalysis has formulated convincing hypotheses on many of the problems that clinical practice poses. In certain cases, a consensual hypothesis has not been achieved and diverging responses appear, often strongly biased by theoretical assumptions. I will give only a few examples. Many theoretical and technical approaches consider it inconvenient or even detrimental to work in the way other approaches propose. But to what extent can we demonstrate the superiority, in the clinical practice, of the outcomes of one theoretical approach over a different one? What is the weight of each theory's own therapeutic factors as compared to nonspecific or common factors found in different approaches? These are some open questions that are usually responded to on the basis of authority or rhetorical–persuasive types of arguments, when, as a matter of fact, it is necessary to transform them into the object of research based on a rigorous conceptual scrutiny followed by a search for empirical verification. It is only in this way that debates based on critical–reflexive arguments (van Eemeren & Grooterndorst, 2004) are possible. It is not unusual that the more passionate a theoretical or technical discussion is, the lower the level of available evidence.

The conclusion is that much more rigorous research is needed in psychoanalysis and all types of research, including clinical, extraclinical, conceptual, historic, etc., and it is also necessary to allow these diverse forms of research to complement and reinforce each other.

Clinical facts

Some postmodern or poststructuralist schools have questioned the existence of 'facts' as such, stating that there are only narratives, conditioned by the historic, social, and cultural contexts in which they emerged. Without a shadow of a doubt, our knowledge is strongly influenced by contextual factors. The term *semantic holism* refers to the assumption that it is not possible to assert something that is not conditioned by the broader linguistic context to which it belongs. Our observations of facts are influenced by our theoretical lenses, by the historic time, and by numerous biases from various origins. But none of this abolishes the existence of facts. Being aware of the conditioning factors that influence our knowledge, far from making us dispense with the notion of clinical fact, forces us to multiply the paths that enable us to deepen, refine, operationalise, and systematise the observations we make and to critically revise our inferences based on those observations. I think this is the basis for clinical research.

The first task is to identify significant clinical facts; that is, to distinguish the 'selected facts' from the 'overvalued ideas' of the analyst (Britton & Steiner, 1994). The expression *selected fact*, borrowed from Bion (1967), who took it, in turn, from Poincaré, refers to elements that make it possible to gather and attribute meaning to a set of data that, until then, seemed disconnected. It is important, then, for us to become sensitive to this kind of fact.

Different procedures from qualitative research offer, in turn, numerous methodological contributions to improve the perception and conceptualisation of clinical facts. We can also indicate the proximity between clinical research and what has been called action research, because clinical observation takes place in the context of a therapeutic practice. It should also be pointed out how much empirical research has contributed to psychoanalytic practice and theory. This occurs not only in studies of process and outcome but also in multiple fields, such as, for example, the study of early relationships and infant observation (Altmann de Litvan, 2007).

I will now refer to the challenges we face in order to improve the quality of our clinical observations, conceptualisations, and inferences. I will then examine how clinical and extraclinical evidence complement one another.

Refining clinical observation: The analytic listening and the second look

The classical psychoanalytic method is a suitable tool to respond to the questions for which it was created; in other words, to explore, together with the patient, the unconscious meaning that unfolds at a certain moment of the session. Using this comprehension of what happens in the session as a starting point, we can propose different metapsychological models. As Freud (1914/1964) put it, the more general and abstract constructions of a theory are the top of a building, not its foundation. The foundation, Freud insists (1914/1964), is observation, and it is observation that can corroborate or falsify our speculations. Metapsychology must be considered from this point of view (Bernardi, 2014b).

Psychoanalytic observation includes a certain paradox. It aims at objective descriptions about the subjective or, to put it more accurately, about that which has not yet become subjective, because it is unconscious. The way in which we can gather together the objective and the subjective has always been problematic. Systematic empirical research seeks support in audio- or video-recorded clinical material to bring higher levels of objectivity into the observations. But interpersonal comprehension and its transmission through a direct account complement audio and video recordings, and it is not reasonable to disregard them. Objective recordings will, undoubtedly, continue to be perfected, and it is likely that, in the near future, 'online' recordings of the somatic variables of both patient and analyst will be included. But it is difficult, or rather impossible, for the comprehension that emerges between two people and that is conveyed through a direct narration to lose its value at any time in the foreseeable future. Psychoanalysis is not 'between' science and hermeneutics: it belongs to both fields and should make use of the resources in both.

In the analytic session, the psychoanalyst has at her disposal the means indicated by Freud: the patient's free association and the analyst's evenly suspended attention. As human beings, we have a natural sensitivity for apprehending unconscious emotional phenomena. This sensitivity, which human beings share with other mammals, is reformulated, but not suppressed, by language and finds expression in the representations of our internal world. This capacity – related to what Fonagy, Gergely, and Target (2002) have called 'mentalization' – shows us that we have the best possible scanner conceivable for the apprehension of the unconscious, but it also shows us that this scanner is an instrument that is very difficult to calibrate.

Adjusting the scanner

Different psychoanalytic theories prioritise different aspects of listening. For instance, whereas Kohut and the relational currents underline the achievement of a better empathic reception, the Lacanian perspective is attentive to the manifestations of the interplay of the signifiers. It is undoubtedly useful for every school to seek to perfect the elements that its own theoretical perspective contributes. But it does not turn out to be less useful, though it is less frequently put into practice, for analysts to experience perceiving a clinical material from the point of view of other theoretical approaches. Supervision or, better still, clinical discussion groups with colleagues who have different theoretical perspectives offers clinical research a valuable occasion for the comparison and examination of the contribution from each perspective, thus complementing the intra-theoretical vision with the intertheoretical one.

The analysis of the countertransference offers an inescapable path towards refining the listening (De León de Bernardi, 2000, 2010; Ogden, 1997). Traditionally, it has been assumed that countertransference should be used in a critical form, bearing in mind its quality both as an instrument and as a possible resistance on the part of the analyst. In the words of Hanna Segal (cited by Hunter, 1994), countertransference is a good *servant* but a bad *master*. This implies that the analyst should make use of their countertransference, taking care not to confuse their unconscious aspects with those of their patient. But not everybody agrees with this position, which we could call critical or moderate. Whereas some schools, like the Lacanian, emphasise the resisting nature of the countertransference, denying its usefulness in the analysis, other schools prioritise the value of everything that occurs in the mind of the analyst as a response to the unconscious of the patient.

Ferro (2012, p. 260), inspired by Bion and the notion of 'dynamic field' from the Barangers, has proposed to develop, to the extent possible, the capacity for containment, for *reverie*, and for tolerance for the uncertainty in the analyst, inviting the analyst to produce a 'transformation into dream' of what the patient says. This implies a narrative deconstruction of the material from the session, de-concreting it, followed by a 're-dreaming' of the communications of the patient, making use of resources that go beyond conscious thinking.

Different clinical observation groups have tried to promote an openness to the unconscious in the analytic listening. The groups interested in the specificity of psychoanalysis stress the free association of the analyst. Likewise, in its first level of analysis, the 3-LM stresses the internal resonance of the clinical material in the participants, which has certain points of contact with the transformation into dreaming that Ferro (2012) proposes. However, in this model, this first stage is followed by a second look in search of a more critical reflection in the other levels.

As can be seen, these proposals sensitise the listening, but they also increase the likelihood of biases originated by the subjectivity of the observer, whose unconscious is certainly more interested in the fulfilment of their own wishes than in the faithful observation of reality. It is necessary, therefore, for the analyst to be attentive to two poles. On the one hand, they have to be a participant in the process they are part of (the analytic field) and that later, in the second look, they can observe with a more objective attitude, which allows them to become aware of their own participation in it (Baranger, Baranger, & Mom, 1983). Without the right balance between these two poles, the analyst either remains very distant from their patient or the door is open for a folie à deux between them. Clinical discussion groups help correct both situations, but it should not be forgotten that collective delusions can be produced. One of the challenges of clinical research is to combine the richness of the subjective participation with both the objectivity and the confirmation by third parties required.

Calibrating the scanner

Research work moves one step forward when we manage to go deeper with the listening of the unconscious emotional aspects in a first step and then, in a second step, we revise in a critical and systematic form what has been observed, seeking higher validity and reliability.

The 'second look' on the analytic field proposed by Baranger et al. (1983), which I have previously mentioned, makes it possible for us to move forward in that direction. Baranger et al. (1983) indicated that the analytic process inevitably leads to the configuration of 'bastions'; that is, situations where the analyst does not manage to adequately discriminate from their patient or to maintain their role, which gives rise to chronic enactments (Cassorla, 2005) and hinders the progress of the analytic process. In those moments, the analyst must shift their look, leaving behind the predominating attitude during the first look, focused on the communications from the patient, in order to adopt a broader perspective aimed not only at the patient but also at their own participation in the analytic process. In this 'second listening', their role as an observer comes to the foreground, in an attempt to objectively evaluate the way in which both participants are involved in the analytic process. I consider it extremely useful, from the methodological point of view, to hold this dialectic shift in the analyst between their role as a participant and their role as an observer of the process.

The second look can be broadened so that it also includes other aspects. Two of them are key elements of clinical research: the significance of the analytic moment as regards the overall psychopathology of the patient and its significance in the flow of time of the analysis, considered both prospectively and from the perspective of the a posteriori (*Nachträglichkeit*) reconstruction (Bernardi, 2014b). This expansion of the field of research opens the doors to diverse clinical studies on the changes that are produced in the analysis and the possible underlying mechanisms. It also makes it possible to put the different predictive hypotheses of the analyst to the proof. As indicated by Jiménez (2009), when working with their patient, the analyst is not primarily concerned with finding theoretical explanations to the situations emerging in the analysis; rather, first of all, they are concerned with making predictions on the effects that their interventions will have. We can take one step forward if we make these predictions explicit and compare them with the patient's evolution. In short periods of time of the analysis, it is possible to test the interpretation with the help of a series of indicators, as Etchegoyen (1986, 2001) proposed. The 'listening to listening', suggested by Faimberg (1996), examines the way in which the patient receives our interpretations from a perspective that takes into consideration the 'retroactive attribution of meaning' (*après-coup* in French; p. 668). It is less frequent in the literature to find the examination of long periods of analysis, which requires the development of special perspectives, such as those proposed by the 3-LM. It is useful to let the facts come to us with all of their metaphoric force and then, in successive levels, to reformulate them in a language that enables us to examine their validity and reliability more rigorously and, in a third level, to examine the clinical support for the theoretical hypotheses that seek their explanation.

Metaphoric, operational, and systematic approaches to clinical concepts

Certain human experiences need metaphors and figures of speech in order to be expressed. They evoke the memories of scenes from literature and from art that help us understand the meanings of those experiences. They are part of the interaction that arises in the analytic field between the analyst and the patient (de León de Bernardi, 2013a, 2013b). During the discussion at the first level of the 3-LM, certain expressions frequently stand out in the collective listening. For example, 'The patient felt like a little porcelain doll', or 'The patient lived in his Batcave', or 'He felt as if living like a robot' summarise an essential aspect of a clinical case better than any other description. They are part of the 'selected fact' that gathers together and gives sense to a multitude of other data and behaviours and makes them more meaningful.

When we want to conceptualise these phenomena making use of more general categories, new demands have to be met. In the first place, it is necessary to identify the essential dimensions of the phenomenon and then to define them operationally; that is, to specify the operations or procedures that allow us to define the heart of the concept in shareable terms. There is a tension or conflict between these procedures and the metaphoric richness that we have previously discussed. Sometimes the operationalisation is rejected because it implies impoverishing the phenomenon because only its essential characteristics are considered, and other valuable or evocative aspects are left aside. This is clearly the case sometimes, but it is the reason why operationalisation is useful, just as a radiograph is useful because it only takes into account certain contrasts.

Fortunately, there are excellent psychodynamic diagnostic manuals today that allow us to make use of operationalised concepts that encompass the main characteristics of personality. I am referring to the *Operationalized Psychodynamic Diagnosis OPD-2* (OPD Task Force, 2008) and to the

Psychodynamic Diagnostic Manual: PDM-2 (Lingiardi & McWilliams, 2017). Despite having different conceptual structuring, both manuals essentially agree on the main characteristics used to evaluate the functioning of personality. The same is the case with the Level of Personality Functioning Scale, which, as I have discussed elsewhere, was incorporated into the *Diagnostic and Statistical Manual of Mental Disorders*, fifth edition, Section III (American Psychiatric Association, 2013), devoted to alternative models (Bernardi, 2010). From this point of view, the dimensional aspect of the personality disturbances – in other words, the degree of severity of the disturbances – is a central aspect for the diagnosis and its psychopathological formulation. This dimensional aspect of the personality disturbances is centrally considered in the proposal made by the World Health Organization (2018) in a new version of the *International Classification of Diseases, 11th Revision (ICD-11)*.

Inferential processes in clinical work and in empirical research

Once we have collected the significant clinical data and we have conceptualised and systematised them, the following step is to find the interpretation that best suits them and makes it possible to provide a sense of what happens in the analytic process. This implies an inferential process where many different operations are at play. Whereas in systematic empirical research one seeks a clear definition of the questions, a simplification of the variables, and a parsimonious progress, clinical judgements must find the best possible explanation for complex phenomena, with multiple variables that cannot always be clearly identified and defined.

In an inference or in a clinical judgement, it is always easy to discover the deductive processes first. The initial comprehension of a problem sets into motion hypotheses that arise from theoretical assumptions, though an inferential process that can be described as 'top-down' or descending, as it attempts to understand certain problems emerging from the clinical practice with the help of certain general principles previously formulated. The constant temptation for the clinician is to let themselves carried away by their theoretical assumptions and suppose that they always offer the best explanation to all of the problems they can be presented with. The more narcissistically invested these theoretical assumptions are and the stronger the sense of affiliation or belonging to a given group or school of thought the analyst experiences, the stronger their conviction that these assumptions offer the only valid form of comprehension possible. For this purpose, it is not infrequently necessary to force the facts so that they can fit the explanation proposed.

For clinical research to actually take place, it is necessary to counterbalance this tendency with a reverse movement, 'bottom-up', that can start from the clinical facts and can go in pursuit of the hypotheses that best fit them. For this to happen, it is necessary to create room for doubt when the first hints of comprehension arise in us and to be attentive to those aspects of the material for which we have no fully convincing explanations. In this way, it is possible to formulate alternative hypotheses. For instance, we can wonder, 'The patient behaved in this way because of an aggressive impulse or are they showing needs for affect that they do not manage to express otherwise?' In these cases, inferential processes that C. S. Peirce (1931–1958) called 'abductive' are at stake. This happens in the field of medicine (Ridderikhoff, 1993) and in psychoanalysis (Leibovich de Duarte, 2000; Pichon-Rivière, 1967). For Peirce, there are three basic forms of inference, which are deduction, induction, and abduction. In the latter, the inferential process moves in search of a leap in the direction of what the previous experience allows us to consider the best possible explanation. A clinician will frequently say, 'I find this case similar to that other one, in which it turned out that. …' Together with the abductive processes, there are deductive processes in play (Hinshelwood, 2013). Special interest deserves the eliminative induction (Edelson, 1983), not essentially different from abduction, where the less likely hypotheses are gradually discarded. Something similar happens in medical clinics in the field of differential diagnosis.

Abductive processes are related to what was discussed previously in connection with the selected facts. Abduction is based on the identification of the essential aspects of clinical situations, which enable the beginning of the inferential bottom-up or ascending process and then the search for the more convincing explanation. The inferential process promoted by the 3-LM essentially follows this path: In the first level, the analyst is asked to expand and refine their perception of the most significant aspects of the clinical facts, which provides the 'anchor points' to evaluate the transformations in the patient. In the second level, there is an attempt to find the conceptual formulation that can best provide an abstract expression for the clinical findings. Finally, in the third level, there is a comparison between the possible explanatory hypotheses for the changes that have occurred in the patient, seeking those that best account for the clinical material.

This procedure reveals the existence of a common ground between analysts with different theoretical orientations (Bernardi, 2017). In the first level of the analysis of the 3-LM, certain parts of the material promote a shared resonance among the participants of the group, regardless of their theoretical preferences. It is also possible to find elements in common in the forms of conceptualisation, though this is less frequent. The shared aspects are easily visible in the third level, when the theoretical explanations are based not so much on official or public theories (Bleger, 2012; Sandler, 1983) but rather on each analyst's implicit theories and the personal mini-models that the analyst operates on in their clinical practice; that is, the conceptual, referential, and operative schemas described by Pichon-Rivière (1998). It is interesting to confirm that whereas the discussions in which the top-down inferences predominate, favouring the weight of the theoretical principles, tend to lead to collapses in communication, when the clinical groups face the clinical problems that the material presents and the participants resort to their personal operative models, it is easy to find shared aspects among them, despite their theoretical discrepancies. The clinical common ground among analysts with different perspectives is therefore verified both at the level of the shared resonance of the clinical material and at the level of the operative schemas, demonstrating that a productive dialogue is possible under these circumstances (Bernardi, 2017).

In sum, clinical reasoning implies a twofold movement: from the theory to the experience and from the experience to the theory. At the heart of this twofold movement, we can find the abductive processes that support the operative hypotheses that inform everyday clinical practice. The capacity to consider, to a greater or lesser extent, alternative hypotheses and the clinical and theoretical aspects to which value is attributed in order to choose from those hypotheses give rise to different inferential styles that can vary from analyst to analyst (de León de Bernardi, 2018). This field of research is relevant both for a better comprehension of clinical practice and for psychoanalytic education.

In epistemology, it is frequent to distinguish between the context of the discovery and the context of the justification. The former admits all kinds of hypotheses, of very varied origins, as can be seen in the proliferation of theories that define present pluralism. The latter, on the other hand, demands putting these hypotheses to the test in a rigorous way and discarding those that are not supported by experience. But in the clinical field, it is very difficult, if not impossible, to find evidence or arguments that allow the conclusive demonstration that any given hypothesis is false. Clinical material can admit more than one theoretical explanation, though clearly not any explanation whatsoever. But it would not be fair to assume that this is exclusively a problem of the clinical field. The problem is more general, because no scientific discipline can aspire to flawless unquestionable knowledge. It has been pointed out that an underdetermination of theory by evidence is to be found in every field of knowledge, because theories always exceed what their empirical grounds authorise. It is partly a holistic underdetermination, because it is not possible to corroborate any hypothesis in isolation without compromising the rest of the theory and its related auxiliary hypotheses. Besides, alternative theoretical explanations are always possible (contrasting underdetermination), and the future can bring new and better hypotheses that show the limitations of the present ones (transitory underdetermination).

Triangulation

Accepting this type of underdetermination does not mean to say that an absolute indetermination has to be admitted, which would justify a sceptical position. On the contrary, the existence of a margin of underdetermination forces us to do our utmost to achieve the best possible rationale for our hypotheses, no matter how partial or transitory the result can be. I have previously referred to different forms of improving clinical observations, their conceptualisation, and the inferences that sustain their interpretations. I would now like to discuss the value of the triangulation of observers, data, methods, and theories as a strategy for reinforcing the validity of our hypotheses. As is the case in navigation or topography, to triangulate means to look at the same phenomenon from different angles, which amplifies the breadth, diversity, and impartiality of the observation. By comparing results obtained from different sources in the face of a specific problem, certain conclusions turn out to be confirmed, whereas others are weakened or suggest the need for new approaches. Triangulation, in this sense, serves in some cases as a filter paper and in other cases as a magnifying glass. Some opinions argue that psychoanalytic hypotheses should be supported only by the psychoanalytic method, but there is no reason for excluding evidence in favour or against that can come from other sources.

Single-case studies are a privileged form of showing how the confluence of diverse approaches is possible in the study of a given clinical material. The case of a patient called Amalia X is the best-known single-case study, and the clinical material was analysed with different procedures (Kächele, Schachter, & Thomä, 2008). In the research on Amalia X, whose treatment was fully recorded by Thomä and Kächele, the traditional narrative of the case was accompanied with studies based on specific methodologies applicable to every area investigated. For example, to explore the transference, they made use of Luborsky's method for the study of the core conflictual relationship theme. The way in which Amalia reacted to separations was the object of a special study, as was the case with the emotional insight, the series of dreams, etc. From the point of view of language, linguistic studies on verbal and emotional vocabulary were applied, together with the Mergenthaler therapeutic cycles model, among other procedures.

We can find another example in the use of systematic clinical observation or empirical tools for the analysis of a patient's first interviews (Rodríguez Quiroga de Pereira, Borensztein, Corbella, & Marengo, 2018). In their study, initial interviews were studied at four levels of analysis. To the traditional clinical report they added a systematic clinical study for which they used the 3-LM, a diagnostic evaluation with the Shedler-Westen Assessment Procedure (Shedler & Westen, 2006), and a computer-assisted analysis of texts as indicators of the response to the treatment in order to study the referential activity (Bucci, 1997).

The triangulation of observations turns out to be particularly useful when certain clinical conclusions need corroboration. For instance, the treating analyst's or therapist's capacity to accurately evaluate the changes in the patient has been challenged by different authors (Bystedt, Rozental,

Andersson, Boettcher, & Carlbring, 2014; Hannan et al., 2005; Hatfield, McCullough, Frantz, & Krieger, 2010). To advance in the discussion of this problem, it seems useful, first of all, to provide analysts or therapists with procedures and training in patient observation and, secondly, to triangulate clinical observation with other assessment tools. Vinocur de Fischbein (2018) combined the study of the evolution of the patient with the 3-LM and with the Symptom Checklist 90 by Derogatis. It has been indicated that single-case studies have not yet received enough attention within the field of research (Roussos, 2007).

Replicability

Research has to be replicable, because this is the only way in which its results can be corroborated by the scientific community. However, at present we are witnessing what has been called a 'crisis of replicability'. Many observations and experiments on which hypotheses that have been accepted are based do not succeed in being replicated. This situation becomes more serious as we move from the exact sciences to the biological sciences and the social sciences, and psychology in particular, where the absence of replicability is higher (Fanelli, 2012). In medical sciences, many studies of therapeutic efficacy are now under scrutiny, and it has been claimed that many research results are no more than the presentation, under the form of exact measurements, of the investigators' biases (Ioannidis, 2005). Some of these biases may be intentional, whereas others are the result of methodological errors. The vulnerability to biases in many fields of research has been pointed out by Kahneman (2011). The problem also arises in the field of empirical studies of the process and outcome of psychotherapy. Leichsenring et al. (2017) related the absence of replicability in this field to the existence of biases in research that originates in the selection and processing of the data or that reflect the affiliation or theoretical preferences of the investigators. The best guarantee against voluntary or involuntary errors is to be as transparent as possible, granting the greatest possible access to the data and the methodologies employed in the studies, both those that corroborate their hypotheses and those that obtain negative results.

Transparency is also essential in the clinical field. In this case, replicability does not imply the repetition of identical clinical situations, which are unique, but rather the possibility of conceptual reproduction. This means traceability of the inferential process that goes from observation to conclusions. In this way, it becomes possible to compare one author's observations and conclusions with those of others. In clinical discussion groups, it is essential for participants to indicate on which parts of the clinical material they support their hypotheses. By doing so, theoretical or technical discrepancies become alternative hypotheses about the clinical material, each one of which has to show the clinical or extraclinical evidence on which it is supported. This results in an expansion and enrichment of the field of study. It is thus brought to light how collective the task of scientific research is. It is inevitable, as I mentioned earlier, for our theoretical assumptions to be part of the lenses through which we look at the clinical material, but it is also true that when we glimpse how the material is seen through our colleagues' lenses we become more aware of that ultimate reality, which, though always elusive and unreachable, always invites us to find new forms of approaching it. When we reach this point, we can say that we have come close to the very heart of clinical research.

Notes

1 A first version of this chapter was presented at the international conference Trabajando desde la Clínica. Metáfora e Interpretación (Working from Clinical Practice. Metaphor and Interpretation), organised by Uruguayan Psychoanalytical Association and the International Psychoanalytical Association Research and Clinical Observation Committees, in Montevideo, Uruguay, in October 2017, and it was published in 2018 as *¿Qué es la investigación clínica?* ('What Is Clinical Research?'), in F. M. Gómez (Ed.), *Psicoanálisis latinoamericano contemporáneo*. Buenos Aires, Argentina: APA Editorial.

2 It is interesting to note that in English a clinical investigator is different from a researcher. For example, in a randomised controlled trial, the investigator is not in charge of the methodology of the research; rather, they are the person who must verify compliance with the stipulated plan, respect for the rights and safety of the patients, etc.

References

Altmann de Litvan, M. (2007). Infant observation: A range of questions and challenges for contemporary psychoanalysis. *The International Journal of Psychoanalysis*, 88, 713–733.

Altmann de Litvan, M. (Ed.). (2014). *Time for change: Tracking transformations in psychoanalysis – The Three-Level Model*. London, England: Karnac.

American Psychiatric Association. (2013). *Diagnostic and statistical manual of mental disorders* (5th ed.). Arlington, VA: American Psychiatric Association.

Baranger, M., Baranger, W., & Mom, J. M. (1983). Process and non-process in analytic work. *The International Journal of Psychoanalysis*, 64, 1–15.

Bernardi, R. (2010). DSM-5, OPD-2 y PDM: Convergencias y divergencias entre los nuevos sistemas diagnósticos psiquiátricos y psicoanalíticos. *Revista de Psiquiatría del Uruguay*, 74(2), 179–205.

Bernardi, R. (2014a). La formulación clínica del caso. Su valor para la práctica clínica. *Revista de Psiquiatría del Uruguay*, 78(2), 157–172.

Bernardi, R. (2014b). The Three-Level Model (3-LM) for observing patient transformations. In M. Altmann (Ed.), *Time for change: Tracking transformations in psychoanalysis – The Three-Level Model*. London, England: Karnac.

Bernardi, R. (2016). La formulación clínica del caso: Su valor para la práctica clínica. In *La formulación psicodinámica de caso. Su valor para la práctica clínica*. Montevideo, Uruguay: Grupo Magro Editores – Universidad Católica del Uruguay.

Bernardi, R. (2017). A common ground in clinical discussion groups: Intersubjective resonance and implicit operational theories. *International Journal of Psychoanalysis*, 98(5), 1291–1309. Bion, W. R. (1967). *Second thoughts*. New York, NY: Jason Aronson.

Bleger, J. (2012). Theory and practice in psychoanalysis: Psychoanalytic praxis. *The International Journal of Psychoanalysis*, 93, 993–1003.

Britton, R., & Steiner, J. (1994). Interpretation: Selected fact or overvalued idea? *The International Journal of Psychoanalysis*, 75, 1069–1078.

Bucci, W. (1997). *Psychoanalysis and cognitive science: A multiple code theory*. New York, NY: Guilford.

Bystedt, S., Rozental, A., Andersson, G., Boettcher, J., & Carlbring, P. (2014). Clinicians' perspectives on negative effects of psychological treatments. *Cognitive Behaviour Therapy*, 43(4), 319–331.

Cassorla, R. M. (2005). From bastion to enactment. *The International Journal of Psychoanalysis*, 86(3), 699–719.

de León de Bernardi, B. (2000). Contratransferencia: una perspectiva desde Latinoamérica. *Revista Uruguaya de Psicoanálisis*, 92, 71–104.

de León de Bernardi, B. (2010). Transferencia, contratransferencia y vínculo: Enfoque clínico. *Revista Uruguaya de Psicoanálisis*, 111, 168–181.

de León de Bernardi, B. (2013a). Field theory as a metaphor and metaphors in the analytic field and process. *Psychoanalytic Inquiry*, 33, 247–266.

de León de Bernardi, B. (2013b). Metaphor, analytic field, and spiral process. In S. M. Katz (Ed). *Metaphor and fields: Common ground, common language, and the future of psychoanalysis*. New York, NY, and London, England: Routledge.

de León de Bernardi, B. (2018). Teoría del campo, segunda mirada y procesos inferenciales del analista. In F. M. Gómez (Ed.), *Psicoanálisis latinoamericano contemporáneo*. Buenos Aires, Argentina: APA Editorial & Lugar Editorial.

Edelson, J. T. (1983). Is testing psychoanalytic hypotheses in the psychoanalytic situation really impossible? *The Psychoanalytic Study of the Child*, 38, 61–109.

Eells, T. D. (2007). History and current status of psychotherapy case formulation. In T. D. Eells (Ed.), *Handbook of psychotherapy case formulation*. New York, NY: Guilford.

Etchegoyen, R. H. (1986). *Los fundamentos de la técnica psicoanalítica* [*The fundamentals of psychoanalytic technique*]. Buenos Aires, Argentina: Amorrortu.

Etchegoyen, R. H. (2001). Algo más sobre el testeo del proceso clínico. *Subjetividad y procesos cognitivos*, 1, 34–59.

Faimberg, H. (1996). Listening to listening. *The International Journal of Psychoanalysis*, 77, 667–677.

Fanelli, D. (2012). Negative results are disappearing from most disciplines and countries. *Scientometrics*, 90(3), 891–904.

Ferro, A. (2012). Creativity in the consulting room: Factors of fertility and infertility. *Psychoanalytic Inquiry*, 32(3), 257–274.

Fonagy, P., Gergely, G., & Target, M. (2002). *Affect regulation, mentalization, and the development of the self*. New York, NY: Other Press.

Freud, S. (1955). Two encyclopaedia articles. In J. Strachey (Ed.), *The standard edition of the complete psychological works of Sigmund Freud* (Vol. XVIII). London, England: The Hogarth Press. (Original work published 1923)

Freud, S. (1964). On narcissism: An introduction. In *The standard edition of the complete psychological works of Sigmund Freud* (Vol. XIV). London, England, The Hogarth Press. (Original work published 1914)

Hannan, C., Lambert, M. J., Harmon, C., Lars Nielsen, S., Smart, D. W., & Shimokawa, K. (2005). A lab test and algorithms for identifying clients at risk for treatment failure. *Journal of Clinical Psychology: In Session*, 61, 155–163.

Hatfield, D., McCullough, L., Frantz, S. H. B., & Krieger, K. (2010). Do we know when our clients get worse? An investigation of therapists' ability to detect negative client change. *Clinical Psychology and Psychotherapy*, 17, 25–32.

Hinshelwood, R. D. (2013). *Research on the couch: Single-case studies, subjectivity and psychoanalytic knowledge*. Hove, England: Routledge.

Hunter, V. (1994). *Psychoanalysts talk*. New York, NY: Guilford.

Ioannidis, J. P. A. (2005). Why most published research findings are false. *PLOS Medicine*, 2(8), e124. https://doi.org/10.1371/journal.pmed.0020124.

Jiménez, J. P. (2009). Grasping psychoanalysts' practice in its own merits. *The International Journal of Psychoanalysis*, 90, 231–248.

Kächele, H., Schachter, J., & Thomä, H. (2008). *From psychoanalytic narrative to empirical single case research: Implications for psychoanalytic practice*. New York, NY: Routledge.

Kahneman, D. (2011). *Thinking fast and slow*. New York, NY: Farrar, Straus and Giroux.

Leibovich de Duarte, A. (2000). Más allá de la información dada: cómo construimos nuestras hipótesis clínicas. *Revista de la Sociedad Argentina de Psicoanálisis*, 3, 97–114.

Leichsenring, F., Abbass, A., Hilsenroth, M. J., Leweke, F., Luyten, P., Keefe, J. R., … Steinert, C. (2017). Biases in research: Risk factors for non-replicability in psychotherapy and pharmacotherapy research. *Psychological Medicine*, 47(6), 1000–1011.

Leuzinger-Bohleber, M., & Fischmann, T. (2006). What is conceptual research in psychoanalysis? *The International Journal of Psychoanalysis*, 87, 1355–1396.

Leuzinger-Bohleber, M., Kallenbach, L., & Schoett, M. (2016). Pluralistic approaches to the study of process and outcome in psychoanalysis. The LAC depression study: a case in point. *Psychoanalytic Psychotherapy*, 30(1), 4–22.

Liberman, D. (1971). *Lingüística, interacción comunicativa y proceso psicoanalítico*. Buenos Aires, Argentina: Galerna/Nueva Visión.

Lingiardi, V., & McWilliams, N. (Eds.). (2017). *Psychodynamic diagnostic manual: PDM-2*. New York: Guilford.

Ogden, T. (1997). Reverie and metaphor: Some thoughts on how I work as a psychoanalyst. *The International Journal of Psychoanalysis*, 78, 719–732.

OPD Task Force. (2008). *Operationalized psychodynamic diagnosis OPD-2. Manual of diagnosis and treatment planning*. Cambridge, MA: Hogrefe & Huber Publishers.

Peirce, C. S. (1931–1958). *Collected papers of Charles Sanders Peirce* (C. Hartshorne, P. Weiss, & A. Burks, Eds.). Cambridge, MA: Harvard University Press.

P-E-P Web. (2017). Psychoanalytic electronic publishing. Website: http://www.pep-web.org/

Perry, S., Cooper, A. M., & Michels, R. (1987). The psychodynamic formulation: Its purpose, structure, and clinical application. *American Journal of Psychiatry*, 144, 543–550.

Pichon-Rivière, E. (1967). Introducción a una nueva problemática de la psiquiatría. *Acta Psiquiátrica y Psicológica de América Latina*, 13(4), 355–365.
Pichon-Rivière, E. (1998). *El proceso grupal. del psicoanálisis a la psicología social.* Buenos Aires, Argentina: Nueva Visión.
Ridderikhoff, J. (1993). Problem-solving in general practice. *Theoretical Medicine and Bioethics*, 14, 343–363.
Rodríguez Quiroga de Pereira, A., Borensztein, L., Corbella, V., & Marengo, J. C. (2018). The Lara case: A group analysis of initial psychoanalytic interviews using systematic clinical observation and empirical tools. *The International Journal of Psychoanalysis*, 99(6), 1327–1352.
Roussos, A. (2007). El diseño de caso único en investigación en psicología clínica. Un vínculo entre la investigación y la práctica clínica. *Revista Argentina de Clínica Psicológica*, 16(3), 261–270.
Sackett, D. L., Straus, S. E., Richardson, W. S., & Rosenberg, W. (1997). *Evidence-based medicine. How to practice & teach EBM*. New York, NY: Churchill Livingstone.
Sandler, J. (1983). Reflections on some relations between psychoanalytic concepts and psychoanalytic practice. *The International Journal of Psychoanalysis*, 64, 35–45.
Shedler, J., & Westen, D. (2006). Personality diagnosis with the Shedler-Westen Assessment Procedure (SWAP): Bridging the gulf between science and practice. In PDM Task Force (Ed.), *Psychodynamic diagnostic manual*. Silver Spring, MD: Alliance of Psychoanalytic Organizations.
van Eemeren, F. H., & Grooterndorst, R. (2004). *A systematic theory of argumentation: The pragma-dialectical approach*. Cambridge, England: Cambridge University Press.
Vinocur de Fischbein, S. (2018). Una propuesta de formalización del diagnóstico psicodinámico diseñado para casos únicos de psicoterapia psicoanalítica. In F. M. Gómez (Ed.), *Psicoanálisis latinoamericano contemporáneo*. Buenos Aires, Argentina: APA Editorial y Lugar Editorial.
World Health Organization. (2018). *International classification of diseases, 11th Revision (ICD-11)*. Retrieved from https://icd.who.int/

Chapter 7

Improving the interface

Comments on Bernardi: Moving from clinical inquiry to clinical research

Horst Kächele

Psychoanalytic therapy has many facets. Western society, mainly, but not exclusively, has shown a hundred-year-long enduring interest, critical and/or uncritical. Philosophers have written about it and displayed more or less competent insights (Grünbaum, 1984; Habermas, 1971; Wittgenstein, 1937/1984) and, last but not least, many artists have enriched our views.

The more immediate participants of this arena, the patients and their analysts, have inhabited quite diverse ecologies. Patients' views have no official standing, except in cartoons or in literary works, as heroes or victims of psychoanalytic therapies. The first substantial consumer-oriented study on how patients view their psychotherapy (Strupp, Wallach, & Wogan, 1964) has not found a replication with psychoanalytic patients as far as I know. What we have are a few reports from psychoanalysts on their experiences on the couch (Guntrip, 1975; Little, 1990; T. Moser, 1977) and quite a host of reports by former patients about negative experiences (Grundmann, 2009; Rey, 1989). One may wonder whether we could learn more from patients' experiences.

The psychoanalytic dialogue as the most immediate source of data was established only in the 1970s, when psychoanalysts like M. Gill and a small number of other academy-based clinicians (Dahl, Meyer, Thomä) presented their daily work using the tool of audio recording and thus established the basic scientific strategy of psychoanalytic process research (Dahl, Kächele, & Thomä, 1988):

> We hope that one unanticipated but happy result of this convergence and shift toward a basic science strategy will be that psychoanalysts and psychodynamic therapists more generally might accommodate to this fledgling science and to both the new research insights and the mini-theories designed to explain them. Ultimately (say in another quarter century) we might hope that research findings will share equal billing with published clinical reports. (p. VIII)

DOI: 10.4324/9780000000002-9

However, the dominating medium of presenting psychoanalytic work has been and is still the testimony of psychoanalysts following its founder's method of reporting. It has been demonstrated many times that analysts have had time to agree on reported clinical data. The consensus problem in psychoanalysis (Seitz, 1966) has remained a troublesome issue; replications such as the experiments by Pulver (1987) and Streeck (1994) confirmed the existence of the Achilles heel in psychoanalysis (Glover, 1952).

Bernardi's brilliant paper shows a way of moving from clinical inquiry to clinical research (Chapter 6, this book). He quotes Freud's (1923/1955) description of psychoanalysis as 'a procedure for the investigation of mental processes which are almost inaccessible in any other way' (p. 235).

The term *investigation* derives from the Latin *investigation,* meaning 'searching into'. Plants are receiving and processing information, as we now know; dogs and cats and babies are exploring their environment. Someone who is under investigation conveys an assumed criminal activity, and Wittgenstein (1953) titled his opus *Philosophical Investigations.*

This text treats philosophy as an activity, rather along the lines of Socrates' famous method of maieutic; he has the reader work through various problems, participating actively in the investigation.

So, the notion of investigation incorporates curiosity, an openness for the unknown, or what is not mapped out yet. It is indeed a wonderful description for the shared work by patient and analyst in the psychoanalytic session. It thus is no surprise that U. Moser's (1992) notion of the psychoanalyst's position as an 'online scientist' has been welcomed. However, U. Moser (1992) is quite stringent in also pointing out:

> Even if psychoanalytic therapists have been designed as 'on-line-scientists', they obviously also proceed off-line, namely, when they are occupied outside of the therapeutic hour with the therapy. They can reflect about the hour, they can – when the session has been videotaped – envision themselves along with the analyst and following a playback routine. In both cases, the research flows into the next therapy session. (p. 186)

From this it follows that the research activity of an analyst is working in two states of mind, one inside the session and the other when the patient leaves the consulting room. The one is a dyadic situation whereby both states of mind continuously influence each other; the other is a monologic situation with the virtual presence in the analyst's mind. Both activities can be subsumed as clinical research, but we certainly have to debate the issue of representation.

What is the relation of the analyst's mind in the online state to their mind in off-line state? How selective are our session notes – if there are any at all?

What kind of memory model are we assuming? Are analysts different in their digestion, or metabolization, of their in-session experiences?

In the context of a research project with Meyer and Thomä (Meyer, 1988), I reported an example of the impact of the physical separation on my feeling and thinking once the patient had left the session (Thomä & Kächele, 1992).

It would be naive not to reflect on the epistemological status of the analyst's report when considering the research qualities of the Three-Level Model. Bernardi's point is well taken; he indicates 'the proximity between clinical research and what has been called action research, since clinical observation takes place in the context of a therapeutic practice' (Chapter 6, this book, p. 000).

In action research, too – well-known examples about famous psychoanalytic ethnographers have been reported – the issue of what is taken home is at stake. The crucial point here is marked by what is called the 'significant clinical facts'. One may be reminded of the fate of dreams whose form and content often depend on to whom a dream is told. So, the very framing of a group discussion certainly has an impact on which 'clinical facts' are generated. Experimental studies varying in group compositions would help to check for such considerations.

The assumption that 'we have the best possible scanner conceivable for the apprehension of the unconscious' (Bernardi, Chapter 6, this book, p. 000) is – in my view – interesting, because it imports a metaphorical mechanical device that is very difficult 'to calibrate'. In my view, it is never possible to calibrate this tool, however long and arduous the training analysis may have been, due to the bi-personal nature of the clinical work. We always have to reflect on by whom and why a session report is made the object of further study, be it in a clinical discussion group or in the loneliness of writing a paper.

As a sobering experience, let us reconsider Kohut's famous second analysis of Mr. Z, published in the prestigious *International Journal of Psychoanalysis* (Kohut, 1979), that Kohut's biographer, Strozier (2001), qualified as a fiction. Time and again, Kohut (1979) used it to demonstrate the superiority of his new technique. For any clinical discussion groups delving into such material, it is useful to follow Bernardi's recommendation:

> It is necessary, therefore, for the analyst to be attentive to two poles. On the one hand, they have to be a participant in the process they are part of (the analytic field) and that later, in the second look, they can observe with a more objective attitude, which allows them to become aware of their own participation in it. (Chapter 6, this book, p. 000)

So, we agree that one of the challenges of clinical research is to combine the richness of the subjective participation with both the objectivity and the confirmation by third parties required. A second or even a third look as observers is not only useful but mandatory. In this regard, the triangulation of observers, data, methods, and theories as a strategy for reinforcing the validity of our hypotheses is a strong tool, as Bernardi points out (Chapter 6, this book).

Although the recommendation to implement formal single-case studies has been a topic for quite a while, starting with Wallerstein and Sampson (1971), it seems that such efforts have become more popular and do contribute to a reconciliation between clinical activity and formal research. Based on our experience with the specimen case of Amalia X (Kächele et al., 2006), we have experienced the value of transparency. By presenting a session to a fair number of colleagues at the New Orleans 2004 International Psychoanalytical Association Congress, 'Working at the Frontiers', we were enriched by learning about various modes of looking at the material (Akhtar, 2007). Therefore, I do wholeheartedly agree with Bernardi's conclusion:

> By doing so, theoretical or technical discrepancies become alternative hypotheses about the clinical material, each one of which has to show the clinical or extraclinical evidence on which it is supported. This results in an expansion and enrichment of the field of study. (Chapter 6, this book, p. 000)

One caveat might be timely. Hoping that aetiological assumptions, as Freud had hoped for, could be endorsed by clinical discussion groups using the Three-Level Model might be spurious. Eagle's (1984) comment on this issue is still pertinent: 'It seems to me ironic that psychoanalytic writers attempt to employ clinical data for just about every purpose but the one for which they are most appropriate – an evaluation and understanding of therapeutic change' (p. 163).

To achieve a more open critical discourse about what we can learn and understand about the psychoanalytic treatment is an important task.

References

Akhtar, S. (2007). Diversity without fanfare: Some reflections on contemporary psychoanalytic technique. *Psychoanalytic Inquiry*, 27, 690–704.

Dahl, H., Kächele, H., & Thomä, H. (Eds.). (1988). *Psychoanalytic process research strategies*. Berlin, Germany: Springer-Verlag.

Eagle, M. N. (1984). *Recent developments in psychoanalysis. A critical evaluation*. New York, NY: McGraw-Hill.

Freud, S. (1955). Two encyclopaedia articles. In J. Strachey (Ed.), *The standard edition of the complete psychological works of Sigmund Freud* (Vol. XVIII). London, England: The Hogarth Press. (Original work published 1923)

Glover, E. (1952). Research methods in psychoanalysis. *The International Journal of Psychoanalysis*, 33, 403–409.

Grünbaum, A. (1984). *The foundations of psychoanalysis. A philosophical critique.* Berkeley: University of California Press.

Grundmann, E. (2009). Berichte und erzählungen von patientinnen. Ein perspektivenwechsel. In H. Kächele & F. Pfäfflin (Eds.), *Behandlungsberichte und therapiegeschichten.* Giessen, Germany: Psychosozial-Verlag.

Guntrip, H. (1975). My experience of analysis with Fairbairn and Winnicott. *International Review of Psychoanalysis,* 2, 145–156.

Habermas, J. (1971). *Knowledge and human interests* (J. J. Shapiro, Trans.). Boston, MA: Beacon Press.

Kächele, H., Albani, C., Buchheim, A., Hölzer, M., Hohage, R., Mergenthaler, E., … Thomä, H. (2006). The German specimen case Amalia X: Empirical studies. *The International Journal of Psychoanalysis,* 87(3), 809–826.

Kohut, H. (1979). The two analyses of Mr. Z. *The International Journal of Psychoanalysis,* 60, 3–27.

Little, M. (1990). *Psychotic anxieties and containment. A personal record of an analysis with Winnicott.* Northvale, NJ: Jason Aronson.

Meyer, A. E. (1988) What makes psychoanalysts tick? In H. Dahl, H. Köhler, & H. Thomä (Eds.), *Psychoanalytic process research strategies.* Berlin, Germany: Springer.

Moser, T. (1977). *Years of apprenticeship on the couch.* New York, NY: Urizen Books.

Moser, U. (1992). On-line and off-line, practice and research: A balance. In M. Leuzinger-Bohleber, H.Schneider, & R. Pfeifer (Eds.), *'Two butterflies on my head …' Psychoanalysis in the interdisciplinary dialogue.* Berlin, Germany: Springer.

Pulver, S. E. (1987). How theory shapes technique: Perspectives on a clinical study. *Psychoanalytic Inquiry,* 7, 141–299.

Rey, P. (1989). *Une saison chez Lacan.* Paris, France: Laffont.

Seitz, P. (1966). The consensus problem in psychoanalysis. In L. A. Gottschalk & A. H. Auerbach (Eds.), *Methods of research in psychotherapy.* New York, NY: Appleton Century Crofts.

Streeck, U. (1994). Psychoanalytiker interpretieren „das Gespräch, in dem die psychoanalytische Behandlung besteht". In M. B. Buchholz & U. Streeck (Eds.), *Heilen, forschen, interaktion. psychotherapie und qualitative sozialforschung.* Opladen, Germany: Westdeutscher Verlag.

Strozier, C. B. (2001). *Heinz Kohut. The making of a psychoanalyst.* New York, NY: Farrar, Straus and Giroux.

Strupp, H. H., Wallach, M. S., & Wogan, M. (1964). Psychotherapy experience in retrospect: Questionnaire survey of former patients and their therapists. In G. A. Kimble (Ed.), *Psychological monographs general and applied. Psychological monographs, Whole No. 558.* Washington, DC: American Psychological Association.

Thomä, H., & Kächele, H. (1992). *Psychoanalytic practice: Vol. 2. Clinical studies.* Berlin, Germany: Springer-Verlag.

Wallerstein, R. S., & Sampson, H. (1971). Issues in research in the psychoanalytic process. *The International Journal of Psychoanalysis,* 52, 11–50.

Wittgenstein, L. (1953). *Philosophical investigations.* London, England: Macmillan.

Wittgenstein, L. (1984). *Culture and value* (H. von Wright, Ed.). Chicago, IL: University of Chicago Press. (Original work published 1937)

Chapter 8

What is 'clinical research'?

Historical, epistemological, and methodological remarks on the relevance of clinical research in times of theoretical and scientific pluralism

Marianne Leuzinger-Bohleber

Introduction

Ricardo Bernardi – in his contribution to this volume (Chapter 6) – gives an excellent overview of the current intensive struggles to capture characteristics of clinical research/clinical investigations in a new, innovative form, in contrast to extraclinical research. 'Psychoanalysis is essentially a clinical discipline that is supported by its own method, but it can and should resort to a variety of other methodologies when the questions it seeks to answer so demand it' (Chapter 6, this book). He formulates a plea for the integration of various forms of psychoanalytic research and emphasises the fertility and mutual enrichment of clinical and extraclinical research. As I have discussed in many papers: I strongly share his position.

Nevertheless, I would like to illustrate briefly, in the following, that such integration is anything but simple and inevitably leads the psychoanalytic researcher into a complex field of tension. As I can only briefly discuss in this context, these areas of tension have complex historical, social, and economic backgrounds, which, in my experience, cannot be resolved but can only be reflected upon and critically shaped again and again in our professional and scientific exchange.

I hope that this focus of my contribution will productively complement both Bernardi's chapter (Chapter 6, this book) and Hinshelwood's (Chapter 4, this book) differentiated epistemological considerations in this volume.

Clinical and extraclinical research in psychoanalysis: Chances and challenges. Some historical remarks

George Makari (2008) impressively traces back the origins of psychoanalysis and its research to the beginning of the 20th century and shows how much both are the product of European cultural and intellectual history.[1] In his understanding of psychoanalysis, Freud succeeded in integrating various

DOI: 10.4324/9780000000002-10

currents of biology, physiology, psychophysics, and psychology at the time; for instance, the controversies surrounding a new understanding of psychopathology around Charcot at the world-famous Salpetière Clinic in France, as well as the scientific study of human sexuality by Krafft-Ebing, Ehrenfels, Weinberger, Moll, Hirschfeld, and others into his theories of psychosexual development, the unconscious, and the psychodynamics of mental disorders (see Makari, 2008). Moreover, in this scientific orientation Freud was strongly influenced by Darwinism, which saw man as an organism driven by needs that he tries to satisfy under specific environmental conditions. Therefore, Freud defined, for example, *Triebe* (drives) at the border between the somatic and the psychic. He understood psychological qualities, the developmental stages of sexuality, and the ego functions as the product of a long evolutionary history in which man continuously adapted to inner and outer realities (Whitebook, 2010; Zaretsky, 2004).

One of the great achievements of Freud's discovery of psychoanalysis is, undisputedly, that he kept up with the natural sciences of his time but also integrated so-called humanities and cultural sciences. As a young man, Freud was very interested in philosophy and other humanities before he turned to the natural sciences, with a remarkably violent emotional reaction. In the laboratory at the Physiological Institute of Ernst Brücke, he got to know a strictly positivist understanding of science that attracted him throughout his life. Nevertheless, Freud later turned away from the neurology of his time, because he recognised the limits of the methods available in neuroscience of his time for researching the psyche. With the *Interpretation of Dreams* (Freud, 1900/1958), the birth certificate of psychoanalysis, he defined it as *pure psychology*. However, he continued to see himself as a physician who observed complex clinical phenomena like a natural scientist. According to Joel Whitebook (2010), his desire for a precise 'empirical' examination of hypotheses and theories protected Freud from his own inclination to wild speculation. As a 'philosophical physician' he was thus able to establish a new 'specific science of the unconscious' – psychoanalysis.

Makari (2008) and Zaretsky (2004) remarkably described how, even in the early days of psychoanalysis, Freud and his followers tried to find a way between, on the one hand, an open, innovative discussion, with constant questioning of the so-called truths – as they characterise a scientific discourse – and, on the other hand, the search for a common professional identity, the specific characteristics and beliefs of psychoanalysis.

According to Makari (2008), this understanding of psychoanalysis has been key to its success. In retrospect, it was a momentous decision for Freud to stick to his understanding of psychoanalysis in this area of content-related and institutional tension and to resist the danger of integrating psychoanalysis either into the world of medicine or into that of 'pure cultural sciences and humanities'. Psychoanalysis therefore retained its autonomy as a scientific discipline. Even in 1909 Freud considered integrating psychoanalysis into

August Forel's medical organisation Internationalen Verein für medizinische Psychologie und Psychotherapie or even into the Orden für Ethik und Kultur. On Sylvester Night 1910, he decided to found his own organisation, the International Psychoanalytical Association (IPA; see Falzeder, 2010). With this decision, the independence of psychoanalysis as a scientific discipline with its own research methodology and institution was protected. Afterwards, Freud always emphasised that psychoanalysis did not deserve to be 'swallowed up' by medicine. Instead he said, 'as a "deep-psychology", a theory of the mental unconscious, it can become indispensable to all the sciences which are concerned with the evolution of human civilization and its major institutions such as art, religion and the social order' (Freud, 1926/1959b).

However, as Michael Schröter (2019) argued, during the years 1918 to 1932, the Viennese group around Freud was characterised by a continuing openness towards the academic world, psychiatry, and other sciences.

> Unlike Berlin (or Germany in general), in Vienna there were major overlaps between the representatives of academic psychiatry and of psychoanalysis. This was largely due to the chair-holder Julius Wagner-Lauregg, who despite his negative attitude to psychoanalysis gave his academic staff the freedom to engage in research on it. (Schröter, 2019, p. 290, translated by author)

Schröter (2019) discussed three exponents of this concatenation: Otto Plötzl, Paul Schilder, and Heinz Hartmann. All three played a central part outside their therapeutic offices in working on empirical confirmation of psychoanalysis and encouraging further development. Other well-known psychoanalysts such as Helene Deutsch, Hermann Nunberg, and Erwin Stengel had positions in psychiatry or at the medical departments of the Viennese University. Felix Deutsch was a doctor of internal medicine, Josef Karl Freidjung worked with children and adolescents, Charlotte and Karl Bühler were famous professors of psychology. Hans Kelsen was into law, and August Aichhorn and Lili Roubiczek (Peller) were very much involved in social work. All of them were either psychoanalysts themselves or interested in the interdisciplinary dialogue with psychoanalysis, at that time the new, challenging science of the unconscious.

Schröter (2019) described the Association for Applied Psychopathology and Psychology, founded in 1920, as a forum for an unusual discussion. Erwin Stansky, professor at the Neurological Psychiatric University Clinic, was in charge of the discussion. The aim of the association was to promote the study and application of psychopathological and scientific–psychological knowledge to practical and social life, to cultural research and history. A series of lectures by psychoanalysts (Bernfeld, Ferenczi, Aichhorn, Schilder) and non-psychoanalysts (Allers, Kelsen, Stransky, etc.) was organised. Basic problems of psychoanalysis and its application in psychiatry, pedagogy, and cultural theory were discussed. The organisers of the lecture were very proud and described the events as the first serious academic discussion, at least in the German-speaking area, in which clinicians and psychoanalysts participated.

Within the framework of this chapter I can only mention that problems of empirical (clinical and extraclinical) research in psychoanalysis were raised during these early controversial discussions that are still relevant today. For example, Heinz Hartmann gave a lecture on Empirism in Psychoanalysis. His talk was followed by fierce controversies on the scientific understanding of psychoanalysis and tensions in the dialogue with the academic–scientific community (e.g., Hartmann, Pappenheim, & Stransky, 1931). For example, Allers (1922) criticised the psychoanalytical method because it presupposes in each of its parts the whole of the theory that it claims to justify. He argued that the demand that only those who make use of the psychoanalytical method can criticise it is a priori absurd. Further objections were directed against the quantitative–energetic approach – that it is not appropriate to the investigation of the human mind, etc. According to Schröter (2019), however, it became apparent that after some years there was no common ground on which the older generation of psychoanalytical practitioners, impressed by their therapeutic experience (and faithfully bound to Freud), could meet with methodically trained and methodically demanding academics and scientists.

Nevertheless, historically it is interesting that in Vienna in the 1920s many psychoanalysts and other researchers endeavoured to create a common ground with the non-psychoanalytical scientific world and – despite all of the difficulties just mentioned – and to not simply ignore academic and cultural discourses. In contrast, according to Schröter (2019), there were hardly any crossing borders in Berlin. There, the psychoanalytic community concentrated much more on internal education and theory development – and the 'internal differentiation' of psychoanalysis (*Binnendifferenzierung*), as Schröter (2019) called it.

We have discussed in detail in another paper (see Leuzinger-Bohleber & Plänkers, 2019) that, as a result of the traumatic history of psychoanalysis as a 'Jewish science' during the time of national socialism and the Holocaust – the 'breaking of civilisation in Auschwitz' – these discourses came to an abrupt end. The fruitful scientific debates of psychoanalysis as a specific, empirical science with the academic, non-psychoanalytical world in Europe broke down and led to institutional tensions, destructions, and ruptures that cast their shadows to this day.

For some decades the development of psychoanalysis thus mostly took place in the United States or other countries to which the Jewish psychoanalysts had emigrated (see, e.g., Young-Bruehl & Schwartz, 2011). In Germany and other European countries, the discourses on specific research questions of psychoanalysis were marginalised for decades.

The growing influence of 'evidence-based medicine' as a powerful *zeitgeist*

As mentioned, the relationship of psychoanalysis and medicine was complicated from the very beginning. In the United States, psychoanalysis was closely related to medicine and psychiatry for decades. Until the 1990s, for example, only physicians were allowed to receive full psychoanalytic training (see, e.g., Kernberg, 2006; Wallerstein, 2001; and many others). Psychoanalysis in the United States gained a unique political influence and an amazing social power: American psychiatry in the 1950s and 1960s was almost exclusively in the hands of psychoanalysts. Nonetheless, Zaretsky (2004) postulated that – seen retrospectively – this leaning of the American ego psychologists towards a positivist understanding of science in psychiatry created a paradoxical situation: 'The more they oriented themselves towards the model of medicine and sought protection there, the more loudly they were dismissed as "unscientific" by the medical–scientific side' (Zaretsky, 2004, p. 476, translated by author). This can be observed in various discourses; for example, about the *Diagnostic and Statistical Manual of Mental Disorders*, in which the influence of psychodynamic thinking continued to disappear from version to version, as well as in the emergence of the hegemonic 'evidence-based medicine'. The solely positivist understanding of research spread in connection with the rapid development of pharmacological treatment of mental disorders, which were perceived by society as 'cheaper', 'more efficient', and 'scientific'. This development increasingly pushed psychoanalysis out of psychiatry. Though in the 1980s a pluralistic approach to methods was still preferred – often a combination of pharmacological, psychodynamic, and psychosocial treatment – the fierce controversies triggered by Grünbaum and other 'Freud bashers' in the 1990s led to a complete denial of the scientific basis of psychoanalysis and to a predominance of cognitive–behavioural therapy in psychiatric clinics and universities, at least in the United States and many European countries.

To mention just one historical example from Europe: In Germany in the 1990s, the danger that psychoanalysis would lose its health insurance accreditation after Klaus Grawe, Donati, Bernauer, and Donati's attack in their book *From Confession to Profession* (1994) forced psychoanalysts to critically reconsider their rejection of empirical psychotherapy research. Studies of that kind are as old as psychoanalysis itself (see, e.g., Alexander & Wilson, 1935; Coriat, 1917; Fenichel, 1930) but have been barely noticed by mainstream psychoanalysis (cf. e.g., Fonagy, 2001a, 2001b; Leuzinger-Bohleber, Arnold, & Kächele, 2019; Wallerstein, 2001). Outcome research existed internationally but was an especially divisive issue in the German psychoanalytic community.

To counter the political threat, in the early 1990s the German Psychoanalytic Association (Deutsche Psychoanalytische Vereinigung, DPV) decided to conduct a large, representative, retrospective study to investigate the long-term effects of psychoanalysis and psychoanalytic long-term treatment – the so-called DPV follow-up study. Four hundred and two former patients were investigated using a combination of qualitative and qualitative methods. At that time, it was crucial for the acceptance of this first outcome study of a psychoanalytical society that the methods took into account the epistemological and sociological concerns outlined above and, for example, did not influence the ongoing treatments. Therefore, only a retrospective study was possible. With quantitative methods, we were able to show that more than 80% of former patients had improved in symptom load, quality of life, and social relationships at least 3 years after completion of long-term treatment. These results were important for the dialogue on the outcome of long-term psychoanalytic treatments in the context of mental health institutions. However, for the psychoanalysts involved, the results of the psychoanalytic follow-up interviews were far more interesting. Experienced psychoanalysts conducted three psychoanalytic follow-up interviews with more than 200 former patients, which led to new insights into the short- and long-term outcomes of psychoanalysis and sparked many controversial discussions within the DPV (see Leuzinger-Bohleber, Stuhr, Rüger, & Beutel, 2003). Therefore, this part of the study really proved to be 'research at the service of clinical work' (Bernardi, Chapter 6, this book). However, it was a bitter pill for many of the researchers and clinicians involved in the DPV follow-up study that this clinically fruitful and methodologically innovative study was hardly noticed by the world of evidence-based medicine mainly because it was a retrospective study.

This ignorance was apparently because the study did not meet some criteria of outcome research today, the so-called gold standard: the randomised controlled trial. These criteria – randomisation of patients, precisely described inclusion criteria, blind raters, standardised measuring instruments, manualised therapy procedures checked for their adherence, as well as the exact description of samples, dropouts, and applied statistical procedures – must be met in order for a study to be recognised both in the world of psychotherapy research and in health care systems. It is interesting from a historical and sociological point of view that in the DPV the study on long-term therapy of chronic depression (LAC depression study), which tried to meet all of these criteria mentioned, would not have been possible without the follow-up study in the 1990s. Only this concrete experience with empirical research convinced many clinicians of the DPV that an outcome study, which tries to satisfy the criteria of evidence-based medicine, does not lead to a nemesis of psychoanalytic treatments. In fact, it can open a space in which the outcome of psychoanalysis can be looked at from different (even epistemological) perspectives. This means that the associated demanding theoretical and epistemological questions must not be ignored even in a study meeting the criteria of evidence-based medicine, as foreign and unfavourable to psychoanalysis they might seem. Many of these questions and epistemological challenges can be critically discussed (at least in brief) even in the main publications of such studies (see, e.g., Leuzinger-Bohleber, Hautzinger et al., 2019; Leuzinger-Bohleber, Kaufhold et al., 2019).

Looking into some facets of the traumatic history of psychoanalysis may lead to the assessment that it is by no means guaranteed that good outcome research will save the future of psychoanalysis as a scientific discipline. Social and cultural processes that determine the position of psychoanalysis in health care systems, universities, and interdisciplinary research, as well as in the public and the media, are extremely complex and can only be influenced to a limited extent by research. We can only mention in this context that some of today's societal changes are worrying many of us and there might be more at stake than the future of psychoanalysis: the resurrection of right-wing extremism and nationalism, the growth of populist movements, and the associated splits in many countries – the global terrorism. This seems to be endangering the Enlightenment project of Western societies, which is so closely linked to psychoanalysis (see, e.g., Hampe, 2019). Psychoanalysis and its future indeed are embedded in these social changes. Nevertheless, many of us have the dream that the potential for Enlightenment, the unique understanding of unconscious meanings of individual (and societally driven) sufferings, conflicts, and fantasies, that lies within the realm of clinical research in psychoanalysis will be rediscovered in the near future. But is also on us to find our place and hold our ground.

On the other hand – and on a very different level – in the United States and Europe, psychoanalysis as a therapeutic offering in the health care system only has a future if we conduct comparative outcome studies and show, according to the criteria of evidence-based medicine, that its treatments lead to success measured by these very criteria. Many research groups and psychoanalytical institutions have devoted themselves to conducting and supporting empirical psychotherapy studies. For example, the Open Door Review (ODR) of the IPA (Leuzinger-Bohleber, Arnold, & Kächele, 2019) and Liliengren and Bräcke (2019) showed that a large number of empirical psychotherapy studies are now available and can be used as arguments.

To make a long story very short: In psychoanalysis it is always a central matter of protecting our *unique way of clinical research*; in other words, Freud's famous 'combination of research and therapy' (Freud, 1927/1959a, p. 256) – the *'Junktim von Heilen und Forschen'* – the conjunction between cure and research, the investigation of the idiosyncratic meanings of unconscious impulses, fantasies, and thoughts in our patients that can only take place in the safe, trusting setting of the professional, therapeutic relationship with the genuine psychoanalytic research method. Clinical psychoanalytic research can neither be accelerated, economized, nor medialised. At the same time, however – and this is a bitter pill that we all would like to deny – psychoanalysis, like every scientific discipline, must be accessible to criticism from outside and must be committed to extraclinical evaluation of its outcome if it is to remain a therapeutic treatment method in the health care system and to face up to academic discourses.

To summarise: On the one hand, psychoanalysis is in danger of adapting too much to a prevailing *Zeitgeist* of a narrow understanding of 'empirical research' and thus of losing its credibility, its authenticity as a 'science of the unconscious'. On the other hand, however, it must beware of the danger of withdrawing from communication with the non-psychoanalytical world, the public, and the interdisciplinary investigation of its outcome, as well as of burning social issues and denying existing dependencies on other scientific communities, politics, and the media. This would sooner or later lead to scientific and social marginalisation of psychoanalysis.

The richness of contemporary psychoanalytical research

I am still full of admiration for Freud's courageous, even radical, attitude towards research in the sense of an open mind towards new, unexpected experiences and discoveries, trying to endure 'not knowing', not understanding – and resisting denying the complexities of the conscious as well as the unconscious mental life.

In the first century of psychoanalysis many psychoanalysts have looked for their solutions to cope with different *Zeitgeists* and thus developed a rich spectrum of clinical and extraclinical research methods. We have collected a great number of studies, mainly outcome and process studies but also some investigations from other fields of psychoanalytical research (clinical, conceptual, developmental, and interdisciplinary research) in the third edition of *An Open Door Review of Clinical, Conceptual, Process and Outcome Studies in Psychoanalysis* (Leuzinger-Bohleber, Arnold, & Kächele, 2019; see also IPA, 2015). In the introduction of the ODR, several authors, such as Ricardo Bernardi, Dominique Scarfone, Peter Fonagy, and I, give short overviews on different epistemological positions of researchers within contemporary psychoanalysis.

I would like to briefly illustrate my own position by means of a diagram of clinical and extraclinical research in psychoanalysis, which I have developed in former papers (Leuzinger-Bohleber, 2010, 2015). To illustrate that research always takes place in certain historical, societal, and institutional contexts as well as not to flounder in abstraction, I refer in my plea for the creative use of a broad spectrum of current psychoanalytic research strategies to some concrete research examples (see Leuzinger-Bohleber & Plänkers, 2019).

Today we can differentiate between 2 different groups of psychoanalytic research, clinical and extraclinical. By *clinical research* we mean the genuine psychoanalytic research in the psychoanalytic situation itself. Ulrich Moser and von Zeppelin (2009) described it as online research, whereas extraclinical research (offline research) takes place after the psychoanalytic sessions and embraces a variety of different research strategies, as will be briefly described. As the feedback loops in Figure 8.1 illustrate, these two forms of research are connected in many ways and can complement and enrich each other in fruitful ways. In this respect, Bernardi (Chapter 6, this book) misunderstands this model slightly: Clinical and extraclinical research are not two completely different forms of research but always interconnected in some way or another. Both can enrich and complement each other.

Clinical research

In earlier papers on today's pluralism in sciences (see, e.g., Leuzinger-Bohleber, Dreher, & Canestri, 2003), we have discussed that the clinical research of psychoanalysis can be considered a specific research method for investigating unconscious fantasies and conflicts that follows its own specific quality criteria. It therefore not only has a hypothesis-generating, explorative function, as a 'feeder', so to speak, for extraclinical, hypothesis-testing studies, but is specific, irreplaceable, and independent in the sense of the plurality of sciences. It cannot be replaced by any other research method.

Clinical research takes place in the intimacy of the psychoanalytic situation and can be described as a circular process of discovery in which – together with the patient – idiosyncratic observations of unconscious fantasies and conflicts are successively visualised, symbolised, and finally put into words at different levels of abstraction, an understanding that moulds our processes of perception in subsequent clinical situations, even though we enter into each new session with the basic, genuine psychoanalytic attitude that has been described as 'not knowing' (see, e.g., Bion, 1962). The circular processes of discovery take place first, above all, unconsciously and in the realm of implicit private theories. Only a small part here is accessible to conscious reflection by the psychoanalyst.

The insights that are won in this clinical research are presented in and outside the psychoanalytic community for critical discussion. In agreement with many current psychoanalysts, as well as with Bernardi (Chapter 6, this book) and Hinshelwood (Chapter 4, this book) in this volume, clinical research is for me the central core of psychoanalytic research in general. It is connected with a characteristic psychoanalytic idea of experience and investigation and linked to epistemic values (*Erkenntniswerte*; see Guggenheim, Hampe, Schneider, & Strassberg, 2016; Toulmin, 1977/1983). Clinical psychoanalytic research deals with the understanding of unconscious construction of meaning, of personal and biographical uniqueness, as in the exact analysis of the complex weavings of various determinants in the microworld of the patient (Moser & Von Zeppelin, 2009), and for that reason can be characterised as *critical hermeneutics* (see, e.g., Leuzinger-Bohleber, 2010).

The psychoanalyst in the psychoanalytic situation applies specific clinical research methods (the detailed observation of free association/free-floating attention [*gleichschwebenden Aufmerksamkeit*], of transference/countertransference reactions, of 'embodied enactments' of the patient [see also Leuzinger-Bohleber, 2015]; Freudian slips, dreams, etc.). All of these clinical observations aim to investigate the actual unconscious psychodynamic of the analysand. The typical groping, psychoanalytic process of searching for 'unconscious truths' can only be carried out with the analysand and is regarded as one of the marked characteristics of psychoanalysis; for example, in opposition to the top-down procedure of behaviour therapy (see, e.g., research example by Hinshelwood, Chapter 4, this book). As Jonathan Lear (1995) so impressively described it, psychoanalysis is distinguished as the most democratic of current therapeutic procedures. Combined with this is the characteristic 'criterion of truth' of psychoanalytic interpretation: whether a certain interpretation of unconscious fantasies or conflicts is 'true' can only be decided *together* with the patient; that is, by the common observation of their (unconscious and conscious) reactions to an interpretation.

As is known, we owe to our specific psychoanalytic, clinical–empirical method of research, the intensive and detailed 'field observations' with single patients in the analytic situation, the most part of all insights that we have won in the last 100 years of our scientific history. Many authors also see in psychoanalytical clinical research the unique chance to recognise and critically reflect the deeper cultural changes by the ubiquitous exploitation mentality of global societal processes that influence the unconscious mental lives of modern man in the analytic relationship, which is not only highly relevant for the affected individual but also for an analysis of culture (see also Bohleber, 2011).

But still, let there be no misunderstandings: Peter Fonagy (2009) is right when he points out that not every clinician is automatically a researcher. A methodologically systematic procedure that – through exact description and lucid considerations – makes clinical observations accessible to the understanding and the critique of a third party is a precondition; a gain in knowledge in this form is not only a professional skill but also a clinical science. Psychoanalysis has at its disposal, as does hardly any other clinical discipline, a differentiated culture of intervision and supervision – closely modelled on psychoanalytic practice – in which the clinical processes of research and gains in insight can be critically discussed. However, there is much room for improvement. There are many well-known problems – for example, the chance selection of clinical case reports – that only *illustrate* theoretical concepts instead of *verifying* or *falsifying* them.

We urgently need good clinical research in order not only to hold our standing in the world of psychotherapy but also to continually develop our professional treatment skills (see Leuzinger-Bohleber, Arnold, & Kächele, 2019).

This was a goal of the Project Committee for Clinical Observation (Chair Marina Altmann) but also a Clinical Research Committee (Chair David

Taylor) to secure and improve the quality of clinical research in the IPA. As I have discussed in another paper, the Three-Level Model (3-LM) of clinical observation can be considered a first step in clinical research trying to systematise clinical observations in clinical research groups (Leuzinger-Bohleber, 2018). If the results of the investigations of transformations of the patients gained by the 3-LM are combined with any form of systematic, extraclinical research on a high level, then – in the best-case scenario – these results may contribute to outcome studies that find also acceptance in the non-psychoanalytic research world.

This was the aim of the application of the 3-LM in the frame of the LAC Study.[2] What we had developed was similar to the working parties of the European Psychoanalytic Federation or now also of the IPA: *our own form of clinical research*. In weekly 'clinical conferences', we discussed the treatment sessions that had been partially taped and systematically documented our discussion and applied the 3-LM. Based on this joint clinical research, narrative case reports have been 'expert-validated', and these belong to the most important results of this study (see, e.g., Leuzinger-Bohleber, Bahrke, & Negele, 2020). These case studies convey psychoanalytic insights about the specific psychodynamics of chronic depression, its complex individual and cultural determinants, and the details of treatment for the psychoanalytic and non-psychoanalytic community.

The method of expert validation was developed in the DPV follow-up study (see summary in the ODR; IPA, 2015). It is now integrated into the 3-LM, which we have developed in the Project Group for Clinical Observation since 2009 (see Bernardi, Chapter 6, this book; Altmann de Litvan, 2014). However, again, the bitter pill is that publications based on these parts of the LAC study only convince psychoanalysts and interested friendly colleagues (mostly in the field of humanities) but not researchers from other therapeutic orientations or representatives of mental health institutions or from the fields of medicine and academic psychology. These groups only accept the results of the quantitative parts of the LAC study following the criteria of evidence-based medicine in a very strict way (see Leuzinger-Bohleber, Hautzinger et al., 2019; Leuzinger-Bohleber, Kaufhold et al., 2019).

Psychoanalytic conceptual research

Some forms of clinical research are connected to research on concepts, a field of research that, likewise, is as old as psychoanalysis itself. The creative development and enhancement of concepts always distinguished the innovative minds of psychoanalysis and lends our discipline a great attraction for intellectuals, writers, artists, and researchers of other disciplines.

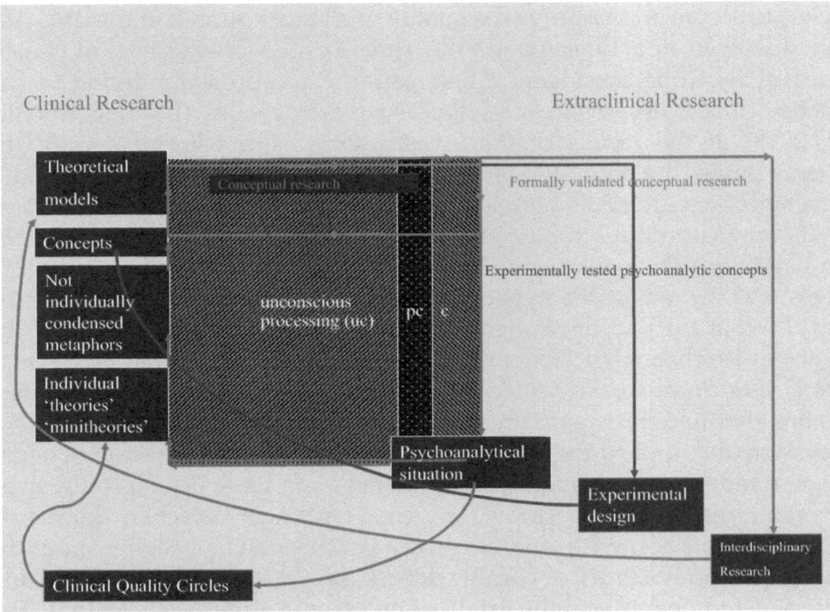

Figure 8.1. Psychoanalytical research.

A new characterisation of psychoanalytic conceptual research was finally laid out by Joseph Sandler and Anna Ursula Dreher in the 1990s (1996), setting themselves apart from other forms of psychoanalytic research. In the Research Subcommittee for Conceptual Research that was initiated by the then–IPA President Daniel Widlöcher in 2002, with the wish to build more bridges between the conceptual traditions in the different IPA regions, we attempted to further delineate and differentiate the research on concepts from 2002 to 2010, as well as to clarify criteria of quality for this specific psychoanalytic research and other involved epistemological questions (Figure 8.1; see also Leuzinger-Bohleber, Dreher, & Canestri, 2003).

Scarfone (2019) summarised another form of conceptual research mainly based on the French tradition (e.g., Laplanche's work) in his introduction to the ODR. He also mentioned conceptual research of the Project Committee for Conceptual Integration (see, e.g., Bohleber et al., 2013; Bohleber, Jiménez, Scarfone, Varvin, & Zysman, 2015).

Extraclinical research

The results of not only the clinical–psychoanalytic research but also the conceptual research can then in the next step become the subject of other extraclinical studies (see Figure 8.1). We distinguish between empirical, experimental, and interdisciplinary studies.

Extraclinical empirical studies

As an example of extraclinical empirical studies, I would like to mention psychoanalytic psychotherapy research because it is indispensable in the 'knowledge society' for political and public reasons, to prove the effectiveness of psychoanalytic treatment by the criteria of evidence-based medicine in the mental health systems of many Western countries. Therefore, outcome research is the main focus of the ODR.

Robert S. Wallerstein (2001) traced these attempts back to their beginnings in 1917 and defined different generations of psychotherapy researchers (for more details, see introductions to the ODR in Leuzinger-Bohleber, Arnold, & Kächele, 2019).

Perhaps it is too little known, above all, by clinicians of the IPA how many psychoanalytic research groups are currently involved in extraclinical studies. Fonagy (2009) spoke in a comprehensive survey of the worldwide psychotherapy bee-keepers who have verified with their industrious bee colonies the effectiveness of psychoanalytic short-term therapies (see Leuzinger-Bohleber, Arnold, & Kächele, 2019).

Careful extraclinical research requires enormous expenditures that can only be carried out in a research network that is correspondingly endowed and supported by a constant process of reflection of the accompanying dependencies – also among the generations of researchers involved.

May the LAC study serve as an illustration. In this multicentric study we were reacting to the threat that in Germany that health insurance companies may cancel their existing, generous support of psychoanalysis and of long-term psychoanalytic treatment if it is not possible in corresponding studies to verify its effectiveness, as measured by the criteria of the current health care system. We have therefore developed a design that, on the one hand, meets these criteria and have currently recruited 554 chronically depressed patients, a group of patients that has societal relevance because the large quota of recidivism resulting from all forms of short-term therapies can only attain lasting therapeutic change in long-term treatment. In addition, we attempt simultaneously to further clinical and conceptual research of psychoanalysis and thus to represent, in a self-critical but authentic manner, psychoanalysis as an independent, specific research method in the actual discourse concerning the politics of health care.

Another example is the Frankfurter attention deficit–hyperactivity disorder study. We compared the outcomes of psychoanalysis compared with behavioural/medical treatments of children suffering from a so-called attention deficit–hyperactivity disorder (see Laezer, Tischer, Gaertner, & Leuzinger-Bohleber, 2015).

Experimental psychoanalytic studies

It is self-evident that it is impossible to test psychoanalytic processes directly in a 'classical experimental design'. However, over the last decades, different research groups have been successfully working on an examination and, experimentally, on single psychoanalytic concepts; for example, on the preconscious and the unconscious processing of information in memory and in dreams, including the work group of Howard Shevrin; Steven Ellman and his group in New York; Wolfgang Leuschner, Stephan, Hau, and Fischmann at the Sigmund Freud Institute; Pfeifer and his research group in Zurich, working on the concept of embodied memory; Rainer Krause in Saarbrücken, working on studies of facial interaction with the help of the Facial Action Coding System; or Bradley Peterson and his group first in New York and now at the University of Southern California, focusing on interdisciplinary studies applying neuroscientific instruments (see Leuzinger-Bohleber, Arnold, & Kächele, 2019; Peterson et al., 2000).

In the Frankfurt-based fMRI/EEG Depression Study, we combined the extraclinical empirical Long-term therapy of chronic depression (LAC depression study) with an experimental investigation of chronically depressed patients in the sleep laboratory of the Sigmund Freud Institute and the brain imaging centre of the Max Planck Institute for Brain Research in Frankfurt (see Fischmann, Russ, & Leuzinger-Bohleber [2013] and summaries in the ODR: Leuzinger-Bohleber, Arnold & Kächele, 2019). In an ongoing replication study of the LAC study, the Multi-Level Outcome Study of Psychoanalytic Treatments of Chronically Depressed Patients with Early Trauma (MODE), we are taking up this tradition and combining psychological and neurobiological measures to investigate the influence of the frequency of weekly sessions on the outcome of psychoanalyses with early traumatised, chronically depressed patients (see Peterson et al., 2000).

Interdisciplinary research

The creative exchanges of, for example, attachment research, empirical developmental research, modern neurosciences, or embodied cognitive science are important fields of interdisciplinary research. Just as important is the interdisciplinary research in cooperation with literature and cultural studies, with social psychology, philosophy, the media, and communication sciences, as well as ethnopsychoanalysis.

In other papers I have am summarised our concept of 'outreaching psychoanalysis' in different ongoing projects of early prevention. These projects are connecting us with ongoing political debates and multidisciplinary discourses; for example, in the IDEA Center, in which around 120 scientists are studying children at risk in 50 different projects (see, e.g., Emde & Leuzinger-Bohleber, 2014). In the IDEA Center, psychoanalytic researchers have the unique chance to be in an interdisciplinary dialogue with colleagues from many different disciplines, including psychology, educational sciences, mathematics, linguistics, philosophy, and neuroscience (see www.sigmund-freud-institut.de, www.ideacenter.eu).

Finally, I might mention the pilot project Step-by-Step for supporting refugees in the first arrival institution Michaelisdorf in Darmstadt (2015–2017), based on psychoanalytical and interdisciplinary trauma research. This psychoanalytical research project now serves as a model for implementing four psychosocial centres for refugees in the state of Hessen. Psychoanalytic institutions and colleagues are engaged in all of these centres (see Leuzinger-Bohleber & Hettich, 2018).

Summary

1. Freud hoped that psychoanalysis and its clinical research, by means of 'objective research results', could win acceptance in the scientific community of medicine and natural sciences. On the other hand, it was only through the insistence on its own autonomy and specificity – as a method and institution – that psychoanalysis as a scientific discipline could secure its survival and its productive unfolding in the last 100 years.
2. In the first century of its history, psychoanalysis developed a differentiated, specific method of research for the examination of its own specific research object, of unconscious fantasies and conflicts, the so-called clinical research method (method of clinical investigation). It connected in diverse studies with a variety of forms of extraclinical research. The cooperation between experienced psychoanalytical clinicians, young academics, and senior psychoanalytical (extraclinical) researchers at universities has been fruitful and productive. As many large studies show, creative psychoanalytical research is an intergenerational endeavour.
3. Clinical research is considered by many analysts to be the heart of psychoanalytic research and has led to the vast majority of psychoanalytic insights into the effects of unconscious fantasies and conflicts in individuals and cultures. But it needs constant further development. The 3-LM can be considered, as such, an attempt to improve clinical investigations, a first step in the direction of clinical research trying to systematise clinical observations in clinical research groups (Leuzinger-Bohleber, 2018). If the results of the clinical investigations of transformations of patients gained by the 3-LM are combined with any form of systematic, extraclinical research on a high level, then – in the best-case scenario – these results may contribute to outcome

studies that also find acceptance in the non-psychoanalytic research world.

4 Contemporary psychoanalytic research takes place in an extreme field of tension. At one pole exists the danger of retreating to the psychoanalytic ivory tower and refuting the dialogue with the non-psychoanalytic community; at the other is the overadaptation to an inadequate understanding of science and therefore a loss of identity and independence for psychoanalysis. This field of tension cannot be resolved but can only be critically reflected upon and productively shaped again and again in an interdisciplinary and intergenerational dialogue. This critical reflection may also be seen as a safeguard against submission to the dominating *Zeitgeist*. As is well known, the gold of contemporary science may well be the iron of the future.

5 The future of psychoanalysis will be dependent on which innovative and creative insights can be found in its rich spectrum of different fields of research, including clinical, conceptual, empirical, experimental, and interdisciplinary research, and be transferred to scientific and non-scientific communities.

6 In today's politically, economically, and media-influenced knowledge society in which scientific experts compete at all levels for authenticity and credibility, it has in a new way become a question of survival for psychoanalysis – whether it can assert itself as an specific, irreplaceable, effective, and productive clinical research method of treatment and as a theory of culture. If it is publicly visible that psychoanalysis is still, through its specific research method, developing unique and effective forms of short-term and long-term treatments and has interesting and innovative explanations to offer for complex individual mental states or unconscious dimensions in societal conflicts, then it will time and again exert its attractiveness as a 'specific science of the unconscious'. *The* 'plurality of research' opens many new windows for psychoanalysis to many other contemporary scientific disciplines that could be productively used for an innovative future of psychoanalysis as a clinical practice and a specific clinical research method as well as a *wissenschaft*.

Notes

1 This section is a modified version of Leuzinger-Bohleber, Solms, and Arnold (2020).

2 LAC stands for the short and long-term results of psychoanalytic therapy as compared to cognitive-behavioural long-term therapy among sufferers of chronic depression: a prospective, multicentric therapy effectiveness study that is currently being conducted (project directors: M. Leuzinger-Bohleber, M. Beutel, M. Hautzinger, U. Stuhr, supported by the Deutsche Gesellschaft für Psychoanalyse, Psychotherapie, Psychosomatik und Tiefenpsychologie [DGPT], the Heidehofstiftung, and the Research Advisory Board of the IPA).

References

Alexander, F., & Wilson, G. W. (1935). Quantitative dream studies – A methodological attempt at a quantitative evaluation of psychoanalytic material. *The Psychoanalytic Quarterly*, 4, 371–407.

Allers, R. (1922). Über Psychoanalyse. In E. Stransky & B. Dattner (Eds.), *Über Psychoanalyse. Einleitender Vortrag von Rudolf Allers mit anschließender Aussprache im Verein für Angewandte Psychopathologie und Psychologie in Wien*. Berlin, Germany: Karger.

Altmann de Litvan, M. (Ed.). (2014). *Time for change, Tracking transformations in psychoanalysis: The Three-Level Model*. London, England: Karnac.

Bion, W. R. (1962). The psycho-analytic study of thinking. *The International Journal of Psychoanalysis*, 43, 306–310.

Bohleber, W. (2011). *Destructiveness, intersubjectivity and trauma: The identity crisis of modern psychoanalysis*. London, England: Karnac.

Bohleber, W., Fonagy, P., Jiménez, J. P., Scarfone, D., Varvin, S., & Zysman, S. (2013). Towards a better use of psychoanalytic concepts: A model illustrated using the concept of enactment. *The International Journal of Psychoanalysis*, 94, 501–530.

Bohleber, W., Jiménez, J. P., Scarfone, D., Varvin, S., & Zysman, S. (2015). Unconscious phantasy and its conceptualizations: An attempt at conceptual integration. *The International Journal of Psychoanalysis*, 96(3), 705–730.

Coriat, I. (1917). Some statistical results of the psychoanalytic treatment of the psychoneuroses. *Psychoanalytic Review*, 4, 208–216.

Emde, R. N., & Leuzinger-Bohleber, M. (Eds.). (2014). *Early parenting and prevention of disorder: Psychoanalytic research at interdisciplinary frontiers*. London, England: Karnac.

Falzeder, E. (2010, March). *Die Gründungsgeschichte der IPV und der Berliner Ortsgruppe*. Paper presented at DPG and DPV, '100 Years of the International Psychoanalytical Association (IPA) – 100 Years of the Institutionalized Psychoanalysis in Germany', Berlin, Germany.

Fenichel, O. (1930). Statistischer Bericht über die therapeutische Tätigkeit 1920–1930. In *Zehn Jahre Berliner Psychoanalytisches Institut*. Vienna, Austria: Internationale Psychoanalytische Verlag.

Fischmann, T., Russ, M., & Leuzinger-Bohleber, M. (2013). Trauma, dream, and psychic change in psychoanalyses: A dialog between psychoanalysis and the neurosciences. *Frontiers in Human Neuroscience*, 7(877).

Fonagy, P. (2001a). *An open door review of outcome studies in psychoanalysis*. London, England: International Psychoanalytical Association.

Fonagy, P. (2001b). The talking cure in the cross fire of empiricism – The struggle for the hearts and minds of psychoanalytic clinicians: Commentary on papers by Lester Luborsky and Hans H. Strupp. *Psychoanalytic Dialogues*, 11(4), 647–658.

Fonagy, P. (2009). *Psychoanalysis and other long-term dynamic psychotherapies*. London, England: Oxford University Press.

Freud, S. (1958). The interpretation of dreams. In J. Strachey (Ed.), *The standard edition of the complete psychological works of Sigmund Freud* (Vol. IV). London, England: The Hogarth Press. (Original work published 1900)

Freud, S. (1959a). Postscript to the question of lay analysis. In J. Strachey (Ed.), *The standard edition of the complete psychological works of Sigmund Freud* (Vol. XX). London, England: The Hogarth Press. (Original work published 1927)

Freud, S. (1959b). The question of lay analysis. In J. Strachey (Ed.), *The standard edition of the complete psychological works of Sigmund Freud* (Vol. XX). London, England: The Hogarth Press. (Original work published 1926)

Grawe, K., Donati, R., Bernauer, F., & Donati, R. (1994). *Psychotherapie im Wandel: von der konfession zur profession*. Göttingen, Germany: Hogrefe, Verlag für Psychologie.

Guggenheim, J. Z., Hampe, M., Schneider, P., & Strassberg, D. (2016). *Im Medium des Unbewussten: Zur Theorie der Psychoanalyse*. Stuttgart, Germany: Kohlhammer Verlag.

Hampe, M. (2019). *Die Dritte Aufklärung*. Berlin, Germany: Nicolai Publishing & Intelligence.

Hartmann, H., Pappenheim, M., & Stransky, E. (1931). *I. Internationale Tagung für Angewandte Psychopathologie und Psychologie. Wien 5.–7. Juni, 1930*. Berlin, Germany: Karger.

International Psychoanalytical Association. (2015). ODR III. Retrieved from https://www.ipa.world/IPA/en/Psychoanalytic_Theory/Research/open_door.aspx?WebsiteKey=cc9ea1bf-cec9-47a2-a143-7f12f1b8b0b4

Kernberg, O. F. (2006). The pressing need to increase research in and on psychoanalysis. *The International Journal of Psychoanalysis*, 87, 919–926.

Laezer, K. L., Tischer, I., Gaertner, B., & Leuzinger-Bohleber, M. (2015). Aufwendige Langzeit-Psychotherapie und kostengünstige medikamentengestützte Verhaltenstherapie im Vergleich. *Gesundheitsökonomie & Qualitätsmanagement*, 20(4), 178–185.

Lear, J. (1995). The shrink is in. *The New Republic*, 25, 18–25.

Leuzinger-Bohleber, M. (2010). Psychoanalysis as 'science of the unconscious' in the IPA centenary. *News of the International Psychoanalytical Association*, 18, 24–26.

Leuzinger-Bohleber, M. (2015). *Finding the body in the mind. Psychoanalysis, neurosciences and embodied cognitive science in dialogue*. London, England: Karnac.

Leuzinger-Bohleber, M. (2018). La ricchezza della ricerca psicoanalitica contemporanea. Osservazioni epistemologiche e metodologiche, alcuni esempi e il metodo di osservazione clinica a tre livelli (3LM). *Rivista di Psicoanalisi*, 64(2), 269–303.

Leuzinger-Bohleber, M., Arnold, S. E. A., & Kächele, H. (2019). *An open door review of clinical, conceptual, process and outcome studies*. Retrieved from https://www.opendoorreview.com/

Leuzinger-Bohleber, M., Bahrke, U., & Negele, A. (Eds.).(2020).*Was nur erzählt und nicht gemessen werden kann. Veränderungsprozesse in Psychoanalysen*. Giessen, Germany: Psychosozial Verlag.

Leuzinger-Bohleber, M., Dreher, A. U., & Canestri, J. (Eds.). (2003). *Pluralism and unity? Methods of research in psychoanalysis*. London, England: International Psychoanalytical Association.

Leuzinger-Bohleber, M., Hautzinger, M., Fiedler, G., Keller, W., Bahrke, U., Kallenbach, L., … Beutel, M. (2019). Outcome of psychoanalytic and cognitive–behavioural long-term therapy with chronically depressed patients: A controlled trial with preferential and randomized allocation. *The Canadian Journal of Psychiatry*, 64(1), 47–58. doi:10.1177/0706743718780340.

Leuzinger-Bohleber, M., & Hettich, N. (2018). What and how can psychoanalysis contribute in support of refugees? *International Journal of Applied Psychoanalytic Studies*. doi:10.1002/aps.1584.

Leuzinger-Bohleber, M., Kaufhold, J., Kallenbach, L., Negele, A., Ernst, M., Keller, W., … Beutel, M. (2019). How to measure sustained psychic transformations in long-term treatments of chronically depressed patients: Symptomatic and structural changes in the LAC depression study of the outcome of cognitive–behavioural and psychoanalytic long-term treatments. *The International Journal of Psychoanalysis*, 100 (1), 99–127. doi:10.1080/00207578.2018.1533377

Leuzinger-Bohleber, M., & Plänkers, T. (2019). The struggle for a psychoanalytic research institute: The evolution of Frankfurt's Sigmund Freud Institute. *International Journal of Psychoanalysis*, 100(5), 962–987. https://doi.org/10.1080/00207578.2019.1576528

Leuzinger-Bohleber, M., Solms, M., & Arnold, S. E. (Eds.). (2020). *Outcome research and the future of psychoanalysis. Clinicians and researchers in dialogue*. London, England: Routledge.

Leuzinger-Bohleber, M., Stuhr, U., Rüger, B., & Beutel, M. (2003). How to study the 'quality of psychoanalytic treatments' and their long-term effects on patient's well-being. A representative, multi-perspective follow-up study. *International Journal of Psychoanalysis*, 84, 263–290.

Liliengren, P., & Bräcke, E. S. (2019). *Comprehensive compilation of randomized controlled trials (RCTs) involving psychodynamic treatments and interventions*. Stockholm, Sweden: University College.

Makari, G. (2008). *Revolution in mind: The creation of psychoanalysis*. Melbourne, VIC, Australia: Melbourne University Publishing.

Moser, U., & Von Zeppelin, I. (2009). Implizite und explizite Formen der Reflexivität (am Beispiel von Traum, Wahn und psychoanalytischer Situation). *Psyche*, 63(12), 1181–1206.

Peterson, B., Leuzinger-Bohleber, M., et al. (2018). *Multi-level outcome study of psychoanalyses of chronically depressed patients with early trauma (MODE) – Initial phase*. Research Proposal to the ApsaA/IPA.

Peterson, B. S., Vohr, B., Staib, L. H., Cannistraci, C. J., Dolberg, A., Schneider, K. C., … Ment, L. R. (2000). Regional brain volume abnormalities and long-term cognitive outcome in preterm infants. *JAMA*, 284(15), 1939–1947.

Sandler, J., & Dreher, A. U. (1996). *What do psychoanalysts want? The problem of aims in psychoanalytic therapy*. London, England: Routledge.

Scarfone, D. (2019). Conceptual research in psychoanalysis. In Leuzinger-Bohleber, Arnold, & Kächele (Eds.), *An Open Door Review of clinical, conceptual, process and outcome studies*. Retrieved from https://www.opendoorreview.com/scarfone-conceptual-research-in-psychoanalysis

Schröter, M. (2019). Im Zwischenreich. Akademische Psychiatrie und Psychoanalyse in Wien 1918–1932. *Psyche*, 73(4), 264–290. doi:10.21o6/ps-73-4-264.

Toulmin, S. (1983). *Kritik der kollektiven Vernunft*. Frankfurt am Main, Germany: Suhrkamp. (Original work published 1977)

Wallerstein, R. S. (2001). The generations of psychotherapy research: An overview. *Psychoanalytic Psychology*, 18, 243–267.

Whitebook, J. (2010). *Sigmund Freud – A philosophical physician*. Lecture at the 11th Joseph Sandler Research Conference: Persisting Shadows of Early and Later Trauma, Frankfurt am Main, Germany.

Young-Bruehl, E., & Schwartz, M. (2011). Warum die Psychoanalyse keine Geschichte hat. *Psyche*, 65(2), 97–118.

Zaretsky, E. (2004). *Secrets of the soul: Psychoanalysis, modernity, and personal life*. New York, NY: Alfred A. Knopf.

Chapter 9

Discussion by Bradley S. Peterson

Scientific investigation in psychoanalysis

Bradley S. Peterson

The insightful and authoritative chapter by Professor Leuzinger-Bohleber (Chapter 8, this book) elaborates the distinctions and relations between clinical and extra-clinical research in psychoanalysis, and it positions these distinctions and relationships within their rich historical context. As Professor Leuzinger-Bohleber notes, this historical context includes the attempts by psychoanalysis, since its inception, to define and place itself within the larger scientific community.

Well-publicised debates about the scientific status of psychoanalysis have raged for a century (Allers, 1922; Grünbaum, 1977). Even longer and more broadly has been the debate over what precisely qualifies as science (Kuhn, 1970; Lakatos & Musgrave, 1970). The word *science* in English derives from the same word in Old French, meaning 'knowledge, learning, application, and a corpus of human knowledge'. That word derived in turn from the Latin term *scientia*, which means 'known and acquired by study; the assurance of knowledge and certainty; expertness' (Science, 2020). It is the present participle of the Latin word *scire* – 'to know', probably with an original meaning of 'to separate one thing from another, to distinguish', and relating to *scindere* – 'to cut or divide'. Certainty about how to divide and separate one thing in the world from another, acquired by study, seems to have been central to the meaning of science for ages. The term has also always included within it the meaning of being a socially embedded activity in which humans seek, systematise, and share knowledge. Science, in other words, is inherently a social activity, requiring the communication of knowledge between members of society in ways that convince and convey the certainty to others about how things in our world are systematically distinguished and related to one another. Plato may have been the first to recognise the social basis of science when he wrote, in *The Republic*, that knowledge is 'justified true belief' (Cornford, 1978; Santas, 1990), in the sense that justification is between one person and one or more others – a social activity. Indeed, this is a primary reason he wrote exclusively in dialogue form. Through the voice of Socrates, he furthermore praised the value of utterances that justify how things in our world are distinguished and then are related again to one another, as an aid to speech and thought:

DOI: 10.4324/9780000000002-11

> These utterances involve … dividing things again by classes, where the natural joints are, and not trying to break any part, after the manner of a bad carver. … Now I myself, Phaedrus, am a lover of these processes of division and bringing together, as aids to speech and thought; and if I think any other man is able to see things that can naturally be collected into one and divided into many, him I follow after and 'walk in his footsteps as if he were a god'. (Plato, ca. 370 BCE/1925, pp. 265b–266b)

The criteria that justify belief about the world – evidence or proof that a scientific theory and body of knowledge should be regarded as true – have also long been the subject of debate. Nevertheless, several criteria that justify belief in a scientific theory are generally accepted (Putnam, 1981) and include (a) the theory's *comprehensiveness* – the degree to which it accounts for observed phenomena in a given area of study; (b) its *instrumental efficacy* – the degree to which the theory provides a means to attain our desired ends, especially our capacity as individuals and as a species to survive and thrive; (c) its *functional simplicity or parsimony* – the extent to which the theory employs Occam's razor and avoids multiplying assumptions and hypotheses unnecessarily; and (d) its *consistency with tradition* and other accepted theory – the degree to which the proposed theory 'fits' with the rest of our body of knowledge. If belief in a new theory requires a radical break with traditional theory, then the new theory requires greater justification by being more comprehensive, having greater simplicity, or promising greater instrumental efficacy than the traditional theory. Relativity theory in physics, for instance, exhibited each of these characteristics and warranted the overthrow of Newtonian physics (Kuhn, 1970; Lakatos & Musgrave, 1970).

The activities that determine whether a scientific theory meets these criteria centre on the formulation and testing of hypotheses and predictions that flow from the theory. Contemporary society tends to view the testing of hypotheses and predictions in science as being inherently deductive – starting with a statement or hypothesis and then testing through observation to determine whether it is true: 'If my belief or understanding of this system is true, then when I probe the system in X way, Y is what I will observe in response'. Much of the day-to-day activity of science, however, is inductive, especially in fields that are relatively young and in which the subject matter is highly complex, as is the case in the brain and psychological sciences. Inductive reasoning starts with a series of observations and moves backward to formulate generalisations and theories. 'I notice that 10 of the Xs are red, and I predict that the 11th X will be red as well'. Inductive reasoning is largely descriptive, though, as this example shows, it still makes use of prediction. In between the generalisations that derive from induction and the probing of theories through deduction is the building of a model or theory for the inner workings of the system under study. Induction allows those models to be constructed, and the models allow predictions of the system's behaviour when probed – when one or more elements or variables in the model change or are manipulated.

As a neuroscientist who is also a psychoanalyst, I am convinced that the analytic process involves inductive reasoning about the patient's utterances and behaviours, the building of a model or theory about how the mental processes of the patient work, and the deductive testing of hypotheses that flow from that model for how the patient will respond or behave when 'probed'. In the earlier phases of an analysis, for example, I strive with my patient to inductively discern patterns in her thinking, emotional responses, and behaviours[1] and in the ways we relate to one another, creating names for, or classifying, those patterns as we go. We gain a mutual confidence in the predictability of the patient's patterns of thinking, relating, and behaving. Internally, I am constantly anticipating and predicting, in an inductive way, what the patient will say or do next. The patterns that the analyst discerns are undoubtedly heavily influenced by prior theoretical and technical orientation, which for me will bias patterns I identify and classify in terms of hopes, wishes, fears, fantasies, and especially defences – the myriad ways in which the patient avoids recognising, experiencing, and speaking about painful experiences and truths about herself – indeed, the ways in which the 'system' under our mutual study actively obfuscates its own observation, theory building, testing, understanding, and knowing. The same is true for scientists, of course: No one is a tabula rasa, and prior experience and expectation will bias and inform the observations one makes about the world or system under study. The analyst nevertheless strives to encounter the patient as a world unto herself, with her own unique features and laws that must be discovered anew. In fact, it is when the patient does not conform with her normal patterns of behaviour that we are compelled to re-examine our inductive classification and theories of the patient's inner world.

Throughout the analysis, but especially in its middle and later phases, the patient and I strive to make coherent sense of her patterns of behaviour by constructing models or theories about which hidden processes must exist to account not only for her behavioural patterns but also for how those patterns relate to one another. I acknowledge that this model-building seems to occur first and most prominently in my own inner world when trying to make sense of the inner world of my patient. I struggle constantly to discern how the elements of the evolving model (the patient's past formative experiences, hopes, wishes, fears, and both explicit and inferred fantasies) relate to one another, particularly how those elements conflict with one another; how the patient, usually unconsciously, mediates that conflict; and how these related elements and the ways in which their conflict is mediated can account for the patient's behavioural patterns that we have inductively classified. During this process of model-building, I am actively probing the model through use of various interventions, most commonly utterances that are intended to (a) empathically mirror my patient's emotional state and encourage development of her ongoing narrative; (b) pose clarifying questions that signal my desire and efforts to reduce ambiguity in the understanding of her meaning; (c) point out, or confront, her attempts to avoid or defend against facing painful material; and (d) interpret the reasons the patient tries to avoid facing that painful material, based on the emerging model we are actively constructing of her inner life (Peterson, 2002). When probing her inner life in this way, I always have in my mind, whether at a conscious or only preconscious level, a hypothesis and prediction of how the patient will respond. That response then either confirms or disconfirms my hypothesis. Though confirmation is certainly gratifying, it is the disconfirmations of my hypotheses that are most valuable to our work because they signal that not all is right with my evolving model of my patient's inner life and that further effort is needed to account for, or understand, these new observations and experiences with her. It is a true dialectic in the Platonic sense, one in which our dialogue evolves to an improved state of knowledge, of beliefs that are justified and that we regard as true.

The analytic process in the clinical situation, in my view, thus engages the same core activities of science that justify belief in our models or theories of how the physical world works. It instills the same degree of conviction in its truth as the best of our scientific theories. It is what allows us the conviction that I truly 'know' this person. The model or theory constructed in the case of psychoanalysis, however, is about a single patient who is a world unto herself, one with her own unique laws and principles that guide the workings of her inner life and behaviours. Whether the model or elements of the model will generalise to the workings of the inner world of another patient is an important but different question. Attempts to generalise across patients, to construct a model not of the psychology of a single individual, but a model and 'meta' psychology that extends across individuals, have historically been more difficult for psychoanalysts to justify to the rest of the scientific world as true belief. In part, I think this difficulty stems from the prodigious challenge of finding ways to codify, classify, and systematise observations in the clinical setting and of finding ways to formulate and test hypotheses and make predictions of observable behaviours that permit confirmation and – more important – disconfirmation (Grünbaum, 1977) of the hypotheses that flow from that metapsychological model. These difficulties particularly limit the instrumental efficacy of metapsychological models and undermine the ability of clinicians and researchers to adjudicate between competing models and theories to determine which of them is most justified to be believed as true.

These challenges have motivated efforts, such as the Three-Level Model (Altmann de Litvan, 2014), to systematise and codify clinical observations across patients that can support better inductive processes and that in turn inform the elaboration and testing of metapsychological theories and models. These efforts are laudable and in some ways heroic, though in my opinion they have suffered from the failure to include collaborating scientists from other disciplines who have essential expertise in designing technical procedures that yield psychometrically valid, informative, and reproducible measures of the system under study. Measures such as these would have the added advantage of being comprehensible to, and subject to critique by, researchers outside of psychoanalysis. They would have the potential to transform the perception of psychoanalysis as an esoteric, secular activity to one that provides clinical observations and builds metapsychological models that can be adjudicated as true or not. These scientific collaborators should include, among others, experts in study design, psychometrics, and biostatistics. Science is fundamentally a social activity, and the knowledge that science creates must be accessible to other disciplines and capable of adjudication if it is to extend beyond the deep and intimate knowledge created in the analytic situation with an individual patient. The real-world practical problem with this collaborative, social activity is how to financially support the time invested by the collaborative experts. The time and effort of these experts usually does not come free of charge, and it is an issue with which psychoanalytic research must grapple, though one that is beyond the scope of further discussion here.

A different approach to putting psychoanalysis on grounds where other scientists will understand and adjudicate its truth value is not to systematise and codify observations in terms that are specific to the analytic situation but instead to borrow the terms and experimental constructs of other scientific disciplines. This is what occurs when we test the efficacy of psychoanalysis to produce changes in measures of the patient that have been developed and used in other disciplines. These measures include, for instance, changes in the severity of depression or anxiety symptoms. These measures have great external validity – that is, they are valid to patients and researchers outside of psychoanalysis – but most analysts would agree that they have limited internal validity to the processes that matter most to analysts and their patients. Most analysts believe, for example, that what the analytic process changes most in patients is not the severity of specific symptoms but something much more fundamental, such as the recurrent maladaptive behavioural patterns that dominate a patient's life or the patient's basic personality organisation.

Finally, there is psychoanalytic research that is 'extra-clinical', research that is conducted outside and independent of the clinical situation. This research typically identifies theoretical constructs thought to be central to the psychoanalytic process and attempts to find, create, or adapt experimental models for that construct that can be studied in a laboratory setting. These kinds of models allow the control of many experimental variables and the systematic manipulation of one or a very small number of other variables regarded as critically important to testing of the model or to making predictions for what will be observed when those variables change. These models have the advantage of being immediately accessible to other scientists, and therefore their external validity is generally high. This kind of extra-clinical research is how I spend most of my professional life as a neuroscientist. I create and adapt experimental paradigms and models that I hope many analysts would regard as informing us about, or at least as being relevant to, core psychoanalytic constructs (Peterson, 2005). These include, for example, models to assess how the mind and brain resolve conflicting motives (Peterson et al., 1999, 2002); how the brain and mind control impulses (Peterson et al., 1998; Spessot, Plessen, & Peterson, 2004); the neural underpinnings of projection (Raz, Lamar, Buhle, Kane, & Peterson, 2007); the brain's processing of fear that is either within or outside of conscious awareness (Siegel et al., 2017); the neural correlates of pleasure and unpleasure (Colibazzi et al., 2010; Gerber et al., 2008; Landa et al., 2013; Posner et al., 2009; Tseng et al., 2016); and the brain basis for transference (Schwartz, 2015). How relevant and valid those models are internally to the field of psychoanalysis I leave to my analytic colleagues to judge. Nevertheless, the neuroscientific models as I implement them owe their existence entirely to my experience in, love for, and understanding of the analytic situation. Likewise, my understanding of my patients in the analytic situation owes something to my understanding of these constructs studied in the extra-analytic situation of my laboratory. I would say this latter debt involves a deeper understanding of and empathy for the extent to which we as human beings are constrained by constitution, biology, and the unfolding of our human maturational program and how extraordinarily potent and inexorable these forces are in driving our experience. I believe this is an appreciation Freud shared (Freud, 1905/1953). Professor Leuzinger-Bohleber (Chapter 8) is correct in saying that clinical and extra-clinical psychoanalytic research inform one another. They are, and should be, in constant dialogue – because scientific investigation fundamentally is, after all, a social discourse to justify which beliefs we should hold as true.

Note

1 Henceforth, as a shorthand, I will refer broadly to patterns of thinking, emoting, speaking, defending, and acting as patterns of 'behaviour'. I hope use of this term will not offend my psychoanalytic colleagues.

References

Allers, R. (1922). Über psychoanalyse. In E. Stransky & B. Dattner (Eds.), *Über psychoanalyse. Einleitender vortrag von Rudolf Allers mit anschließender Aussprache im Verein für angewandte Psychopathologie und Psychologie in Wien*. Berlin, Germany: Karger.

Altmann de Litvan, M. (Ed.). (2014). *Time for change, tracking transformations in psychoanalysis: The Three-Level Model*. London, England: Karnac.

Colibazzi, T., Posner, J., Wang, Z., Gorman, D., Gerber, A., Yu, S., ... Peterson, B. S. (2010). Neural systems subserving valence and arousal during the experience of induced emotions. *Emotion*, 10(3), 377–389.

Cornford, F. M. (1978). *The Republic of Plato*. Oxford, England: Oxford University Press.

Freud, S. (1953). Three essays on the theory of sexuality. In J. Strachey (Ed.), *The standard edition of the complete psychological works of Sigmund Freud* (Vol. VII). London, England: The Hogarth Press. (Original work published 1905)

Gerber, A. J., Posner, J., Gorman, D., Colibazzi, T., Yu, S., Wang, Z., ... Peterson, B. S. (2008). An affective circumplex model of neural systems subserving valence, arousal, and cognitive overlay during the appraisal of emotional faces. *Neuropsychologia*, 46, 2129–2139.

Grünbaum, A. (1977). Is psychoanalysis a pseudo-science? Karl Popper versus Sigmund Freud. *Zeitschrift für philosophische Forschung*, 31(3), 333–353.

Kuhn, T. (1970). *The structure of scientific revolutions* (2nd ed.). Chicago, IL: Chicago University Press.

Lakatos, I., & Musgrave, A. (1970). *Criticism and the growth of knowledge*. Cambridge, England: Cambridge University Press.

Landa, A., Wang, Z., Russell, J. A., Posner, J., Duan, Y., Kangarlu, A., ... Peterson, B. S. (2013). Distinct neural circuits subserve interpersonal and non-interpersonal emotions. *Social Neuroscience*, 8(5), 474–488.

Peterson, B. S. (2002). Indeterminacy & compromise formation: Implications for a psychoanalytic theory of mind. *The International Journal of Psychoanalysis*, 83(5), 1017–1035.

Peterson, B. S. (2005). Clinical neuroscience and imaging studies of core psychoanalytic constructs. *Clinical Neuroscience Research*, 4(5), 349–365.

Peterson, B. S., Kane, M. J., Alexander, G. M., Lacadie, C., Skudlarski, P., Leung, H. C., ... Gore, J. C. (2002). An event-related functional MRI study comparing interference effects in the Simon and Stroop tasks. *Cognitive Brain Research*, 13(3), 427–440.

Peterson, B. S., Skudlarski, P., Anderson, A. W., Zhang, H., Gatenby, J. C., Lacadie, C. M., ... Gore, J. C. (1998). A functional magnetic resonance imaging study of tic suppression in Tourette syndrome. *Archives of General Psychiatry*, 55, 326–333.

Peterson, B. S., Skudlarski, P., Gatenby, J. C., Zhang, H., Anderson, A. W., & Gore, J. C. (1999). An fMRI study of Stroop Word–Color interference: Evidence for cingulate subregions subserving multiple distributed attentional systems. *Biological Psychiatry*, 45(10), 1237–1258.

Plato. (1925). Phaedrus. In H. N. Fowler (Trans.), *Plato in twelve volumes* (Vol. 9). Cambridge, MA: Harvard University Press. (Original work published ca. 370 BCE)

Posner, J., Russell, J. A., Gerber, A., Gorman, D., Colibazzi, T., Yu, S., ... Peterson, B. S. (2009). The neurophysiological bases of emotion: An fMRI study of the affective circumplex using emotion-denoting words. *Human Brain Mapping*, 30, 883–895.

Putnam, H. (1981). *Reason, truth, and history*. Cambridge, England: Cambridge University Press.

Raz, A., Lamar, M., Buhle, J. T., Kane, M. J., & Peterson, B. S. (2007). Selective biasing of a specific bistable-figure percept involves fMRI signal changes in frontostriatal circuits: A step toward unlocking the neural correlates of top-down control and self-regulation. *American Journal of Clinical Hypnosis*, 50(2), 137–156.

Santas, G. (1990). Knowledge and belief in Plato's *Republic*. In P. Nicolacopoulos (Ed.), *Greek studies in the philosophy and history of science* (Vol. 121). Dordrecht, the Netherlands: Springer.

Schwartz, C. (2015,June 24). Tell it about your mother: Can brain-scanning help save Freudian psychoanalysis? *TheNew York Times Magazine*, 1–8.

Science. (n.d.). *Online etymology dictionary*. Retrieved from https://www.etymonline.com/word/science

Siegel, P., Warren, R., Wang, Z., Yang, J., Cohen, D., Anderson, J. F., ... Peterson, B. S. (2017). Less is more: Neural activity during very brief and clearly visible exposure to phobic stimuli. *Human Brain Mapping*, 38(5), 2466–2481.

Spessot, A. L., Plessen, K. J., & Peterson, B. S. (2004). Neuroimaging of developmental psychopathologies: The importance of self-regulatory and neuroplastic processes in adolescence. *Annals of the New York Academy of Sciences, 1021*, 86–104.

Tseng, A., Wang, Z., Huo, Y., Goh, S., Russell, J. A., & Peterson, B. S. (2016). Differences in neural activity when processing emotional arousal and valence in autism spectrum disorders. *Human Brain Mapping*, 37(2), 443–461.

Part III

Working with metaphors in psychoanalytic practice

Chapter 10

Clinical research

The role of metaphors in the analytic process

Ana-María Rizzuto

Clinical research

Psychoanalysis is a practice that involves prolonged exchanges between two people in the absolute privacy of the consulting room. Words are the prevailing medium of communication, but bodily expressions, the mode of being present, the manner of using the moments of their encounter, and many other factors contribute to the complex process of patient and analyst finding a way of starting and continuing what they have agreed to do together. The analysand seeks relief from suffering. The analyst intends to use the knowledge and skills obtained in training, reflecting, studying, and previous clinical work to find a way to assist the patient to uncover the sources of distress and, in the end, to live a better life. What happens between them can never be fully documented. Words, gestures, moods, and feelings are ephemeral manifestations of their exchanges and only a limited expression of the subjective and intersubjective experience and motives of each participants. How could we possibly research in the name of a scientific enough investigation transitory experiences that are unique to the pair and use them to create a significant piece of analytic knowledge that can be shared with colleagues and replicated in their analytic work? The difficulties seem to be insurmountable. Yet, I agree with Hinshelwood (2010) 'that clinical material [is] always the empirical basis of evidence in psychoanalysis' and that we need to 'rehabilitate the clinical material as an important evidence base for psychoanalysis' (p. 362). He adds: 'So psychoanalysis needs a formal method of critical discrimination – the authority of evidence, as opposed to the authority of experts' (Hinshelwood, 2010, p. 364). Comparing research in science and in psychoanalysis, Hinshelwood (2010) asserts: 'Whereas the physical sciences create meaningful generalizations about the objective world, psychoanalysis generalizes about meanings themselves' and 'that leads to the specific character of psychoanalytic research' and concludes, 'The nature of the field of study is subjective experience' (p. 365). Citing Ezriel (1956, p. 35), he proposes that 'psychoanalysis should focus more on the science-like causality of the here-and-now process *within* the session'. Ezriel points out that 'only such forces as exist at a

DOI: 10.4324/9780000000002-13

certain time can have effects at that time' (Ezriel, 1956, p. 35). This process can 'provide the basis for our justification process by assessing the immediate process of change around the interpretation' (Hinshelwood, 2010, p. 373). 'The meaning contained in the interpretation acts as a "cause" of a movement in the here-and-now process' (Hinshelwood, 2010, p. 375). I find these ideas cogent and very useful for a research that focuses on the causal temporal efficacy in the here and now of a moment of interpretation that effects change in the patient. The causal efficacy of an interpretation calls for a careful *observation* of what is happening at the moment and may extend to later moments dynamically linked to the interpretation.

'Assessing the process of change' places it at the level of what Waelder (1962) called the 'data of observation' (p. 619), the first step in making sense of what is happening in the analysis. The psychoanalyst learns not only about all such data but also about the configuration in which they appear (Waelder, 1962, p. 619). Linking many observations into some meaningful organisation, the analysts forms an interpretation in her mind and seeks the best way to communicate it to the patient. This is the level of clinical interpretation.

We must remember that observation is a subjective process on the analyst's part and that the data observed also originate in the subjective experience of the patient. In brief, these are two subjectivities attempting to obtain and recognise the more or less objective component of what is happening in the patient's experience after the interpretation has been presented to them, which again involves the level of the analyst's clinical observation *and* the patient's self-observation.

What happens with the metaphors that emerge during analysis, be they the patient's or the analyst's metaphors? Do they offer, in the here and now, a causality that brings about particular effects? And if they do, how do they do it?

A brief history of the conception of metaphor in psychoanalysis

Freud referred to metaphor in his exploration of the formation of jokes and in *Totem and Taboo* (Freud, 1913/1964). There are three references in *The Interpretation of Dreams* (Freud, 1900/1953) that use the term with its usual meaning, and once to interpret some dream component metaphorically. He said nothing about the formation of metaphor or its clinical significance. In 1950, Ella Freeman Sharpe wrote a classical paper that connected the formation of metaphor to the body, to early experiences, particularly pre-genital. Metaphors signal those experiences as the aspect of the analysand's preconscious knowledge that needs to be made explicit in analysis. Arlow (1979), a leader of ego psychology, concluded that

> Metaphors constitute *the only way* by which what was hitherto unknown may be organized and conceptualized in a novel way. Any

> new term for a set of relationships not previously discerned will ultimately have to be expressed in some form of metaphor because of the very nature of human thought and language. (p. 383, emphasis added)

He concluded that *the analytic process is metaphoric*. Many authors in the last 40 years wrote about the function and use of metaphor in analysis and, currently, a large number of analysts accept that psychoanalysis is a metaphoric process. Modell (2005) considered metaphor as essential for the functioning of the mind, based on its sensorial and relational experiences that facilitate the organisation and expression of *emotional memory*. For Modell (2005), there is an unconscious metaphoric process that organizes the affective memories of the past through which the present moment is interpreted. He concluded that metaphor is the fundamental cognitive tool of unconscious processing.

The notion of metaphoric process was greatly enhanced by the work of Lakoff and Johnson (1980), who demonstrated that language and even concepts are based on metaphoric processes. They affirmed that *human experiences* are the foundation of metaphoric processes: 'Metaphors allow us to understand one domain of experience in terms of another. This suggests that understanding takes place in terms of *entire domains* of experience and not in terms of isolated concepts' (Lakoff & Johnson, 1980, p. 117, emphasis added). A domain of experience

> is a structured whole within our experience that is conceptualized as … an *experiential gestalt*. Such gestalts are *experientially basic* because they characterize structured wholes within recurrent human experience. … They seem to us to be *natural kinds of experience*. (Lakoff & Johnson, 1980, p. 117)

The human body is at the core of those experiences. Lakoff and Johnson (1980) demonstrated that metaphor as a figure of speech finds its origin in the *experiences* of the person who creates it.

I have proposed in another paper (Rizzuto, 2009) that

> Metaphoric processes and verbal metaphors in analysis are at the service of *self-objectification* and activation of past affective experiences in the context of the transference in the present. The process of working through benefits from metaphorical processes capable of integrating in concise verbalizations complex somatic and sensory experiences past and present as *dynamically analogical affective experiences* while opening up new *affective* moments in the relationship with the analyst. The elaboration of the metaphors facilitates psychic transformation and leads to new metaphorical versions of who the patient is in relation to his past and present, himself and others. (p. 18)

The metaphor, whether it was already formed in the patient's mind or emerges for the first time at a particular analytic and transferential moment, has the dynamic function of capturing a particular type of complex experience between patient and analyst. Bodily experiences from the past and the present contribute to its formation but are not the source of the metaphor but rather a condition for its articulation. The creator of the metaphor is always the self as agent; that is, the total person as an indivisible unity (Meissner, 1993). Such unity is composed of a neural substratum, a mind, and a body immersed in an analytic moment that calls for the expression of a concrete analytic experience. Such experience can only be articulated in words by using a metaphor that integrates the subjective and the transferential state of the analysand. Quintanilla (1999) proposed that the function of the metaphor is not mainly to give a message but to provoke effects in the subjective experience of the listener (as cited in Beatriz de León de Bernardi, 2013, p. 248). In her paper, de León de Bernardi (2013) suggested a double function of metaphors: to 'transmit implicit meanings and produce unexpected effects in the patient or analyst, or in both, with the corresponding internal restructuration' (pp. 262–263). To this I add that the metaphor integrates, in concise verbalisations, past and present *dynamically analogical affective experiences* while at the same time they open a new affective moment with the analyst. Their elaboration leads to new metaphorical versions of who the analysand is in relation to his past and present, himself, the analyst, and others (Rizzuto, 2009).

Considering that metaphors reveal, in analysis, hidden aspects of ourselves, the analyst must resist the temptation of taking the metaphor at face value and rather interpret it based on its obvious verbal meaning. In analysis, metaphors are rarely obvious because they find their source in protracted creative dynamic processes aimed at articulating emerging states of self that have remained under repression or have never been articulated before (Rizzuto, 2009).

Brief theoretical considerations

The verbal expressions and actions of the patient are organised dynamically by the impact of the *context of the total analytic situation*: the frame, the transferential and actual relationship with the analyst, the emergence of preconscious memories with their affects, the sensing of past and present bodily experiences, the surging of desires in the context of habitual defences against them, and the analyst's task of exploring the patient's psychic life. The context also includes preexisting imagery of subjective experiences and of objects in reality, all of them loaded with affects from the past as well as the present affects experienced with the analyst as the person who, in listening to the patient, progressively opens to the patient the search within their own self. The analyst's aim is to help them to find themselves in their past and present experiences in a form that is tolerable and that makes it possible *to recognise themselves affectively and to accept being recognised by the analyst*.

I ask: What conditions and facilitates the dynamic formation or recollection of a metaphor in the patient's mind that the analysand decides to communicate to the analyst? Frequently, this metaphor becomes the organiser of an analytic moment and is significant in transforming the patient's self-experience. The analyst, in her work with the metaphor, needs to recall the concrete analytic situation before the metaphor was voiced by the analysand and document the progressive effects that that particular metaphor brings about in the patient's experience and the type of transformations that occur as a result of attending in depth to the different components of the metaphor. The analyst also *observes* the personal effects the metaphor has on her affects, bodily responses, and the understanding of the here-and-now experience, including the awareness of her countertransference and most specifically her spontaneous thoughts and imagery.

I will illustrate these points presenting the dynamic formation of a critical metaphor in the treatment of Mr. H. I have described this central metaphor in previous papers (Rizzuto, 2001, 2015) in which I did not examine the steps and circumstances leading to the formation of the metaphor in a man who described himself as living in a small room without windows in the remotest corner of a medieval castle with its entry bridge raised to prevent people from coming in.

The emergence of the metaphor in the analytic process

Mr. H was 45 years old and came to analysis due to his boss's encouragement, because he was having serious problems at work. His physical presence was pleasant but gave the impression of a wish to keep his distance from the analyst. In the initial interviews to consider analysis he revealed that he never had any friends, that his contact with his family was very limited, and that his emotional life was restricted to his work. He described his isolation in a flat, matter-of-fact way, somewhat implying that that was the way his life was and had always been. I sensed that implicit in his description was a message to me warning me to keep my distance from him. I reached the conclusion that he presented a grave case of a schizoid personality disorder and predicted that the treatment would be difficult and long. Mr. H accepted the conditions of the analytic frame and, from the start, he carefully respected them without any complaint but conveying the feeling that it was a major obligation imposed on him by his boss in his work situation. Following the agreement to talk, he began to speak, centring all of his attention and feelings on his fears in relation to me as a *new authority* that he had to face. He was afraid of bothering me, of being a burden to me. During the first year he had problems with the fear of having to submit himself to me as well as to others and the continuous dread of not being accepted and of being abandoned. He made no mention of other issues except a narration of his fears in relation to them, which he presented in an objective manner and in a monotone voice. His verbalisation of these concerns was emotionally flat and revealed little about him and much about his fear of me as a person who could overpower him.

I heard his communication as a continuous expression of a profound dread of people and of myself in particular, and I intervened mostly to assist him to articulate a bit more his feelings by attending more carefully to them. I consciously avoided any interpretations or even some clarifications that could seem intrusive to him. My intent was to help him *to start a process of self-observation* as a counterpart of his placing most of his attention to what I could do to him.

In the second year he was able to bring up some fantasies and a very painful memory. When he was 7 years old, while on a picnic with the family near a river, he tried to commit suicide by throwing himself into the river, hoping that he would drown. A relative saw him and, thinking that he had fallen accidentally, pulled him from the water. Nobody in the family paid any attention to the event. Nobody became aware of the child's desperation, leading him to feel acutely how deeply alone he was emotionally. I reflected that his presenting to me this memory signalled a change in the transference by revealing to me the very painful feeling that no one noticed his desperation. I commented with my best available empathy and a soft voice how difficult his childhood suffering had been by being so alone in the midst of his family. I did not, however, succeed in getting him to elaborate about the affective circumstances of his suicide attempt. I tried then to show him that, by talking with me about it, he was no longer alone. It was in this transferential context that he brought up the metaphor of living locked up in a castle. It was more a conviction than a fantasy. He was certain that he was secluded inside a medieval castle, surrounded by a moat whose bridge was always raised to prevent anyone from entering. He was never available to meet any visitor, supposing that someone might wish to visit with him. He saw himself sitting on the floor of a small fortified room located in one of the most remote corners of the castle. The room had no windows and he was sure that no one could find him. He said to me that he preferred to live there because he was convinced that 'he was not there' as a person, that there was 'nothing' in him that could be found. Anyone who could find him would be disappointed. I understood this fantasised and elaborate metaphor as a *message* and a *transferential warning* and as an obvious and indirect response to my empathic commentary that I was there with him in the analysis, that now he was not alone. The metaphor clearly signalled to me that any search on my part to find him would end in frustration, because he was not there, and that even if I found him physically I *would not find the person I was searching for*. I listen to the metaphor without making any interpretation but simply trying to understand how it had been formed. When he was a child he explored the family name and thought that they had some connection with European royalty, the people who lived in impressive castles. He became very interested in castles and collected pictures and images of them. Later on, travelling around Europe, he saw some of those castles.

Some changes began to occur at the end of the second year of analysis. He was able to make some superficial friends. In the analysis, he returned to describe himself in the castle but now he felt the *desperation* of his isolation and his deep fear of having 'nothing to offer'. We talked extensively about it and I noticed that his voice had a new affect and that the manner in which he described himself indicated an incipient wish to change. At that point I recalled that Mr. H had had a dream a few months before in which I had miraculously entered the castle and I was at its entrance, a place far removed from his hiding place. He only reported the dream briefly and made no comments about it. I did not try to analyse the dream because I felt that it could frighten him. I simply registered it in my mind as a major change that he was not yet able to make explicit and as a frightening wish for me to be with him. The dream *implied* that the bridge over the moat had been lowered and that I had passed through it to get to the castle's entrance. It also suggested a transferential opening in relation to my getting close to him. Immediately, I had a fantasy: I imagined myself walking towards his secluded room and placing myself in front of him saying softly, 'I found you'. Surprised, I carefully reflected for a couple of days about how I could use it and finally I decided to present it to him in the conditional mode: 'What would happen if I presented myself in your room and said to you, "I found you"?' He instantaneously responded with great vigour and a very unusual strong voice: 'I would run away as fast as possible'. We were both startled by the tone and the content of his answer. He continued with an unusual and new reflection about himself: 'I cannot let anyone find me; not even you'. This commentary introduced *a significant change in the analytic process*, the beginning of his and my exploration of how he has come 'to live' in such a remote room. The most significant point for the analysis consisted in the fact that Mr. H for the first time *consciously felt his conflict* between his infantile and adult desire to be known and accepted and his rigid defences that compelled him to reject any affective closeness with others.

Mr. H described that he never loved his family and did not want to be part of the life with them. Only occasionally he responded to his family invitations to join them in some family event or celebration. He reflected: 'I don't seem to have the capacity to connect with other people's lives. … My life is resisting anyone coming in'. I reminded him of the moment when I said to him imaginatively, 'I found you', and he responded: 'That is *the part of me* that doesn't want ever to be found, *not even by myself*'. When he said 'part of me', he indicated to me that he was considering other parts of himself, perhaps as alternatives to possible encounters.

Mr. H started progressively to search for a way to find himself and in a moment of analytic regression described graphically his deep conflict and psychic deficiency in relation to his internal dissociation. He said, 'I have no words … to speak [about it], not even in my mind for myself inside'. He reflected at that moment about his experience with me in relation to a previous session:

> It was a feeling that I didn't have a point of reference that I was there. I locate my body here, where I know my body is. But my identity, knowing myself, I couldn't find any connection. … *Not knowing what to do to search for myself,* no point of reference. … I was lost. I couldn't even know if it was me searching for myself, except for my physical exterior. … I felt it so clearly. … *I can't find a point of reference to say 'I'.* I knew I was physically here. *But I was not here.* That strong sense of dissociation. … I couldn't locate the I. … I have this feeling, … the word is *desperate,* … fear. … I disappeared from myself. If I am outside the frame, the usual, the expected, *even my body is the frame.* … When I asked, 'Where are you?', *I was surprised that the I wasn't there.* … My body couldn't respond to it. *I was searching for the internal I.* … The words came to me, 'Don't leave me'. It was myself talking to myself as I was lying here. … *My physical self wanted to find my other self.* … I had to talk to myself, tell my body to get up. …

This hour opened up a deep psychoanalytic investigation in which, with my constant participation, he became the active agent in searching for his 'I' in his psychic life. Slowly this led him to allow himself to have personal wishes for the first time in his life.

The genesis and dynamic function of Mr. H's metaphor

As I already said, verbal personal metaphors find their source in *dynamically analogical affective experiences* that have found in real objects or in images a manner of describing somatic, relational, and affective experiences that cannot be directly expressed in ordinary language. The fact that, as a child, Mr. H was dedicated to collecting images of medieval castles suggests that, even at that age, they offered him something *affectively analogical* of what he could not articulate about the dissociation between his bodily experiences and his experiences as a subject. The castle, with its impressive physical presence and its entrance controlled by a bridge over a moat, offered him an analogical *dynamic affective experience* similar to what he was able to articulate in analysis when he said, 'I knew I was physically here. *But I was not here*', revealing what was the dominant experience of his life. His body was like a castle that informed him about his existence without allowing him access to the person that he knew should be there but that he could not find.

Metaphorically speaking, his body was real but, like the stones of the castle, it lacked the affective capacity he needed to lead him to experience himself as himself in it. It was this experience that prompted him to form the desperate conviction that he should be *in* his body but that he could not find himself because he 'was not' in his body.

From the beginning of the analysis my technique consisted in using what Mr. H told me to assist him in paying attention to himself and to abstain from interpretations that could distract us from the task of helping him to become the explorer of his own psychic life. Any interpretation would have been *an incomprehensible and unacceptable invasion* to him. The metaphor that he presented to me in the analysis, describing him as located in the remotest room of the castle, suggested the integration of two experiences that he could not articulate verbally. The first is that, despite his convictions, he *was*, in fact, inside the castle and that when I told him that he was no longer alone but with me I not only frightened him but, simultaneously, offered him a certain hope. As for his side of the experience, the moment of sharing with me the component of the metaphor about his being in the remotest room of the castle was the equivalent of giving me the *address of his abode*; that is, an *indirect* invitation for me to visit with him. His dream about my being at the entrance of the castle as a new metaphoric component suggested that there had been a change in relation to me. It no longer frightened him that I had crossed the bridge that obviously had been lowered. I took it as a clear indication of the change in his defences and the surging of an explicit but fearful desire that I could move on and go to his hidden place. Shortly after, I had my own fantasy, in which I located myself inside the metaphor of the castle as if it really existed. In my fantasy I carefully advanced to the place where he was hiding and said to him with a moderated affect and a soft voice, 'I found you'. His instantaneous, vigorous, and defensive response was *simultaneously* a part of the metaphoric process *and* of the actual analytic moment between him and me. It clearly indicated to me that in the analysis, as well as in his metaphoric imagination, it terrified him that I could find him. Nonetheless, the prolonged analytic metaphoric process between us had already awakened, in the context of a technique that constantly invited him to listen to himself, his ego's capacity *to observe himself* in that dramatic moment and to be able to describe his psychic situation with sadness: '*I cannot let* anyone find me; not even you'. Here his response to my metaphoric participation succeeded in *awakening his agent self*: Mr. H assumed the *responsibility* that it was him who refused to be found and, in doing so, he transformed the metaphor of being trapped in a castle into the *recognition* of his deep and very old *psychic conflict* between his desire to be found and his fear that there was nothing to find.

At this point in my presentation, it is important to reflect about the profound dissociation between Mr. H's healthy and strong body and his subjectivity. He said it very clearly in a session that followed our metaphoric encounter: 'When I asked, "Where are you?", *I was surprised that the I wasn't there. ...* My body couldn't respond to it. *I was searching for the internal I'*. This description clearly illustrates my point about *dynamically analogical affective experiences* in the formation of metaphors during the analytic process: His body was and had always been similar to a medieval castle that cloistered a psychic self that he was unable to find – worse yet, that he was terrified to search for because he feared that it did not exist. It was during the analysis when I told him that he was no longer alone that he metaphorically located himself in the remotest room of the castle, as a first change resulting from our working together. In other words, the metaphor was articulated during the analysis as something he was communicating to me and *to himself*, as his attempt to describe his painful psychic situation. This occurred at the moment he *started to believe and fear* that I wanted to know him.

I find it obvious that, without this critical metaphor, it would have been very difficult to analyse Mr. H. As for the metaphor itself, we did not analyse it as such. Instead, he and I created, he with his dream and I with my fantasy, an imaginary *metaphoric dramatisation* that led him to recognise that his problem was not with others or with me but it involved his very profound *psychic conflict* between the wish to be found and his fear that he had nothing to offer because he was absent from himself. In this manner, with the castle metaphor and our dramatisation, Mr. H managed not only *to become a psychic object* for himself but to find himself as the 'I' that he in fact was; that is, *the active agent* of his psychic life. This very critical *insight* found its origin in a *metaphoric process*.

Technical reflections

Not all of the metaphors that a patient brings to analysis have such dynamic richness. There are dead metaphors, as the linguists call them. There are others that are banal, defensive, or provocative that may not deserve much attention or that have to be located in relation to the context of a particular analytic moment to decide how to use them. The metaphors in which the patient *describes themselves*, be it in a real or psychic context, must be listened to attentively to unveil all of their *dynamic richness* in the patient's experience as well as in the transference and countertransference of the analytic moment in which they appear. These are complex metaphors, based on somatic and relational experiences, and have a very intricate dynamic structure. They must be explored with careful attention in all of their components to gain access to the internal world of the patient who has created them and revealed them spontaneously in a particular dynamic moment. To take them literally and limiting their meaning to it is the equivalent to remaining with the manifest content of a dream. We must acknowledge that metaphors, as well as dreams, are multi-determined processes essentially constructed in the unconscious. The difference consists of the fact that the metaphor achieves a conscious verbal articulation that is *affectively* acceptable to the patient's ego and available to be communicated to the analyst at a particular moment of the analysis.

There is no special technique to work with metaphors. The analyst must accommodate her technique to the concrete circumstances of the metaphor's emergence in the analysis and her assessment of the analysand's readiness to delve into the personal experience that is articulated in the metaphor.

When I heard for the first time Mr. H's metaphor of the unapproachable castle and his locating himself in its remotest room, I spontaneously 'saw' the castle in my mind and 'felt' how far away from me and others he wanted to be. I felt that he was telling me that I could not reach him because I was, by definition, outside the castle and had no way to enter it. However, without thinking about techniques, I could not help but to feel that there was also a hidden invitation in it and, before I knew it, *I felt the need* to enter the metaphor as if there was a real castle in between us daring me to do something. It felt to me like I was invited in disguise to take some action without knowing what it could be, such as one does in some improvised game. At that point it was unimaginable for me to say anything that could be an interpretation of his words or situation. Besides, and this is key, I experienced within myself a ludic mood in the best sense of the term: a need to participate meaningfully in the dramatic moment that was happening between us.

So, before I myself knew it, my technique consisted in my entering a shared, ludic, enacted-in-fantasy metaphoric process in which the use of the conditional mode in my question during an imaginary scene placed the patient and myself in a hypothetic situation that was *affectively* very real and that demanded the participation of the patient in *a ludic and imaginary existential moment*. His dramatic and intense response shows that such unusual imaginary action on my part had the value of a *significant interpretation* that awakened his capacity for *self-observation and agency* ('I would run away as fast as possible') in relation to the defensive and conflictive act of not allowing himself to be found.

I want to insist on the profound dynamic richness of metaphors that refer to the patient as themselves, be they the ones the analysand brings to the analysis or the ones that the analyst creates, such as the case presented by Ricardo Bernardi at the International Psychoanalytical Association congress in Boston (Altmann de Litvan, 2015) in which he introduces the metaphor of the patient as a robot. The fact that metaphors describe *experiential gestalts* as Lakoff and Johnson (1980) suggested invites us to explore them in all of their component elements: their origin in bodily experiences, their relation to the term of comparison in actual life – medieval castle, robot – and what connects them at the experiential level, be it the fear of not existing as in the case of Mr. H or the absence of a living person in a robot or other *implications* of the verbal structure and of the image(s) that they evoke. It is important to recognise the *message* that the metaphor sends to the analyst and to the patient themselves at the moment of its use. The analyst must grasp the patient's implicit petition embedded in the metaphor to be able to decide how to use it at that particular moment of the analytic process. In my case *I felt*, as the Barangers describe (Baranger & Baranger, 2008), that I had to accept the implicit request present in the appearance of the metaphor to do something *to find* Mr. H in his metaphoric castle. My analytic preconscious created an imaginary scene within the structure of the metaphor that included the *invitation* that I felt he had made to me and *my own desire* to establish *affective contact* with him. This imaginary enactment brought to the open Mr. H's central conflict and allowed him to regress affectively in a dramatic way to *his very old corporeal experience of being unable to find himself as a living being by the mediation of his body*.

Concerning the different levels of metaphors, I believe that the descriptive and narrative levels are always *simultaneously* present in all of the metaphors that refer directly to the patient. The description *implies* a narrative that has to be made explicit in the course of analysis. How did the patient come to be like a robot? How did Mr. H place himself in the remotest room of the castle? The search for this narrative opens the personal history of the analysand with his primary objects and the type of interactions with them that, in the course of the analysis, return as memories or are replicated in the transference.

In brief, the essential value of the metaphors that describe the patient consists in helping them *to become a psychic object for themselves* and to focus their attention on their affective states and on their subtle and very complex experiences that cannot be articulated with ordinary words. The inexpressible *affective experiences* find in the components of the metaphor the instruments capable of integrating in verbal and imaginary forms, in the context of the dialogue with the analyst, what the patient has never been *able to name* in relation to himself. In this manner, as it happened with Mr. H, *self-referring metaphors open the analytic exploration to a depth that would be impossible without them*. Like dreams, personal metaphors are a royal road to open up unarticulated experiences that nevertheless are constantly active from the unconscious.

Metaphors and research

As I mentioned above, I agree with Hinshelwood (2010) 'that clinical material [is] always the empirical basis of evidence in psychoanalysis' (p. 362). Clinical research should be able to document a relation of cause and effect that could be used for comparison in the work of other analysts with their patients. To build a case for this assertion I will reflect on what happened with Mr. H's metaphor and the critical change it brought to him when we enacted together what the metaphor described as impossible: to find him.

As I mentioned earlier, Lakoff and Johnson (1980) described metaphors as understanding one domain of experience in terms of another experience, and they pointed to *entire domains* of experience and not in terms of isolated concepts; that is, they are *experiential gestalts*. Such gestalts are *experientially basic* because they characterise structured wholes within recurrent human experience. These experiential gestalts gather innumerable past and present experiences that *exceed by far the verbal articulation of the metaphor*. However, the great contribution of metaphors consists of gathering, in critically symbolic and brief meaningful terms, the essence of a particular domain of experience that does convey the subjective situation of the analysand while implying with its words and the evoked imagery in the patient and in the analyst that *the subjective experience exceeds with its complexity the words of the metaphor*. In fact, the etymology of the word itself indicates, with its Greek particle *meta*, that there is something beyond it. Mr. H's description of his desperate search for himself in his body points to the *dynamically analogical affective experience* of his actual body and the image of the castle. Interestingly enough, I came to realise later on that my preconscious imagery of the castle took it for granted that it was *an empty castle*, a preconscious matching on my part that, unknown to me, facilitated my 'walking' unimpeded to his remote room. In other words, my countertransference preconsciously perceived the depth of his isolation and, I believe, awakened in me, as an analyst and as a person, the conscious desire to establish emotional contact with him.

This description indicates that in analysis the communication of a personal metaphor initiates a complex process between the patient and analyst and their respective manner of responding to it in the context of a particular transferential and countertransferential moment.

How can we move from these considerations to the search for a reliable cause and effect clear enough to be offered to other analysts for them to see if they encounter similar patterns in their work? In the case of Mr. H, my imaginary action of finding him acted as a powerful cause whose *effect was a totally new response* on his part, which brought him to experience a new awareness of himself and of his participation in his isolation. I admit that my participation as an analyst was unusual. Nevertheless, I believe that analysts can and must carefully *observe and document* the type of causality our interventions have in relation to dealing with the metaphor in the analytic process. Attentive and *detailed clinical observation* on the analyst's part is necessary to *document the effect* that her use of the total metaphor or aspects of it has at the moment and later on, when the analysand grasps how the analyst is using the metaphor at that particular analytic moment. In the case of Mr. H, my imaginary enactment and his totally instantaneous reflex response became for us *a paradigmatic point of reference* to understand his emotional situation. He and I return to it many times at different levels of meaning, to progressively unveil how he had come to 'live' in that remote room.

The last statement suggests that the analyst's attention to a rich, self-descriptive metaphor that has been shared with her does not exhaust its effects in the immediate response to her first comments. What I am saying is that the effect of the analyst's intervention continues as long as the components of the metaphor reemerge during the analytic work. Frequently, each return of the metaphoric components reappears in other contexts, in which case a new moment of clinical observation is called forth, to document a new effect of the analytic use of the metaphor. The analyst's renewed attention to those components and the causality implicit or explicit in them lead us to see that there are other moments in which we must document the rich intertwining of the components of the metaphor to register the continuous effect brought about by them.

Personal metaphors collect many repeated experiences of a similar kind and emerge in analysis at the moment in which the analysand finds themselves in a particular dynamic situation in their relation to the analyst. It offers a description of their personal situation originating in different dynamic motives, be there a defensive move, a communication to the analyst, or both. In either case the articulation of the metaphor *objectifies* the patient to themselves and to the analyst. In other words, it offers a self-description that the patient wants the analyst to consider together with the message implicit or explicit in it or both. As I said earlier, Mr. H's metaphor sent me the message that I would not find him because I was obviously outside the castle but, simultaneously, it gave me the opposite message, the 'address' where he lived, just in case I could go there.

At the experiential level, as he and I discovered in returning to explore the metaphor, it became evident that the experience of his body and his inability to use it to find himself was a clear analogy with the impassable stones of the castle. There are other levels of our analytic use of the metaphor of the castle that I could describe, but I think what I have said is enough to make my point about research and metaphors.

I believe that my hypothesis that personal metaphors are an invaluable medium to help the patient find a way of objectifying their experiences and themselves as the psychic object who created them could be used to invite our colleagues to explore the issue to confirm my point or disregard it. We need analysts to observe and document, as carefully as possible, the effect or lack of it that the renewed exploration of different facets of the metaphor has in the progression of the analysand's self-discovery and the analyst's use of them to advance significant aspects of the analytic process. Then, after we have collected enough data, we may compare different cases in which a personal metaphor became a key organiser of the analytic process and confirm or discard the assertion that this type of metaphor has a continuous effect in the progressive articulation of the patient's pathology and psychic transformation.

References

Altmann de Litvan, M. (2015). Panel report, IPA Congress Boston 2015: Metaphors and the use of analyst as tools to improve our clinical practise panel and small discussion group. Organised by: IPA Project Committee on Clinical Observation. *The International Journal of Psychoanalysis*, 96(6), 1651–1654.

Arlow, J. A. (1979). Metaphor and the psychoanalytic situation. *The Psychoanalytic Quarterly*, 48, 363–385.

Baranger, M., & Baranger, W. (2008). The analytic situation as a dynamic field. *International Journal of Psychoanalysis*, 89(4), 795–826.

de León de Bernardi, B. (2013). Metaphor, analytic field, and spiral process. In S. M. Katz (Ed.), *Metaphor and fields: Common ground, common language, and the future of psychoanalysis*. New York, NY, and London, England: Routledge.

Ezriel, H. (1956). Experimentation within the psychoanalytic session. *British Journal of Philosophy of Science*, 7, 29–48.

Freud, S. (1953). The interpretation of dreams. In J. Strachey (Ed.), *The standard edition of the complete psychological works of Sigmund Freud* (Vol. IV). London, England: The Hogarth Press. (Original work published 1900)

Freud, S. (1964). Totem and taboo: Some points of agreement between the mental lives of savages and neurotics. In J. Strachey (Ed.), *The standard edition of the complete psychological works of Sigmund Freud* (Vol. XIII). London, England: The Hogarth Press. (Original work published 1913)

Hinshelwood, R. (2010). Psychoanalytic research: Is clinical material any use? *Psychoanalytic Psychotherapy*, 24(4), 362–379.

Lakoff, G., & Johnson, M. (1980). *Metaphors we live by*. Chicago, IL: University of Chicago Press.

Meissner, W. W. (1993). The self-as-agent. *Psychoanalysis and Contemporary Thought*, 15, 459–495.

Modell, A. H. (2005). Emotional memory, metaphor, and meaning. *Psychoanalytic Inquiry*, 25, 555–568.

Rizzuto, A. M. (2001). Metaphors of a bodily mind. *Journal of the American Psychoanalytic Association*, 49, 535–568.

Rizzuto, A. M. (2009). Metaphoric process and metaphor: The dialectics of shared analytic experience. *Pychoanalytic Inquiry*, 29(1), 18–29.

Rizzuto, A. M. (2015). Metáforas de una mente corporal. *Revista de psicoanálisis*, 72, 281–312.

Sharpe, E. F. (1950). Psycho-physical problems revealed in language: An examination of metaphor. In E. F. Sharpe, M. Brierley, & E. Jones (Eds.), *Collected papers on psycho-analysis*. London, England: Hogarth Press.

Waelder, R. (1962). Psychoanalysis, scientific method, and philosophy. *Journal of the American Psychoanalytic Association*, 10, 617–637.

Chapter 11

Metaphors for the patient's self as a multiple bridge for clinical research

Beatriz de León de Bernardi

In this chapter I will focus on the study of certain expressions that gain metaphorical meanings in the analytic communication. After a brief introduction on the subject of the metaphor from an interdisciplinary point of view, I will refer to certain expressions that emerge in the analytic field (Baranger & Baranger, 1961) and can be considered key metaphors for the patient's self. Questions about the genesis, dynamics, and functions of these key metaphors for the self are explored and described in a clinical vignette and in a clinical material studied in a working group with the methodology of the Three-Level Model (3-LM) for observing patient transformations. The clinical investigation carried out allows us to see how certain key metaphors set up bridges between different dimensions of the analytic communication: symbolic dimensions, images and words, and subsymbolic dimensions, feelings, and emotions. These metaphors for the self have a high figurative and dramatic impact on analyst and patient and can be considered 'embodied metaphors', because these expressions are anchored in the emotional and bodily experiences of the patient. They can also be considered useful interpretative tools insofar as the work on their latent aspects enhances the symbolisation process in the patient and also play an articulating role in the analyst's psychoanalytic conceptualisation, facilitating bridges between clinical experience and psychoanalytic theory, opening different paths to clinical inquiry and research. Finally, the limits of this approach are discussed.

Metaphor has been traditionally considered a figure of speech in literary criticism, a feature of poetic language. In *Poetics*, Aristotle (2004) defined it as an abbreviated comparison, by prioritising the conceptual similarity between the literal and the figurative sense. Aristotle gave emphasis to the transmission of meaning from one term to the other, causing the second term to acquire a new figurative sense that enlarges its original meaning. The word *metaphor* originates in Greek. It comes from the noun μεταφορά, μεταφορᾶσ (pr. *metafora, metaforas*), which comes from the verb μεταφέρω (pr. *metafero*), whose meaning is 'to transport'. This verb is formed by the prefix μετα- (pr. *meta-*), whose meaning is 'beyond, after'; and by the verb φέρω (pr. *fero*), whose meaning is

DOI: 10.4324/9780000000002-14

'to carry, to take, to bring'. Therefore, the etymological concept of this word is to move (the meaning of a word) beyond itself (to another meaning).

Linguists and philosophers have reflected on the characteristics of the metaphor. In 1962 the analytic philosopher Max Black highlighted in *Models and Metaphors* the conceptual aspects of metaphor and how these concepts operate with each other in an interactive system. The linguist George Lakoff and the philosopher Mark Johnson (1980, 1999) referred to the conceptual transmission of meaning that metaphor implies, from a concept's source domain to its target domain. However, their research went further by showing how metaphors are part of our cognitive processes, from the beginning of our lives, and this conceptual process is based on our embodied and sensual primitive experience being part of our cognitive unconscious.

Paul Ricoeur (1978), in his article 'The Metaphorical Process as Cognition, Imagination, and Feeling', emphasising the imagination and the feelings as indicators of truth in metaphorical construction, questioned the weight given to conceptual aspects by I. A. Richards and Max Black[1]: 'My thesis is that it is not only for theories which deny metaphors any informative value and any truth claim that images and feelings have a constitutive function' (Ricoeur, 1978, p. 143) and 'I claim that feeling as well as imagination are genuine components in the process described in an interaction theory of metaphor. They both achieve the semantic bearing of metaphor' (p. 155). Ricoeur (1978), taking up the rhetorical tradition, highlighted the pictorial aspect of the metaphor considered as a 'figure of language'. He agreed with linguists Roman Jakobson and Tzvetan Todorov, who defined *figure* as the visibility of discourse:

> The vividness of such good metaphors consists in their ability 'to set before the eyes' the sense that they display. What is suggested here is a kind of pictorial dimension, which can be called the picturing function of metaphorical meaning. … The very expression 'figure of speech' implies that in metaphor, as in the other tropes or turns, discourse assumes the nature of a body by displaying forms and traits which usually characterize the human face, man's 'figure'; it is as though the tropes gave to discourse a quasi-bodily externalization. (Ricoeur, 1978, p. 144)

Davidson (1978), in his article 'What Metaphors Mean', underlines the conceptual aspects but also the role of imagination and emotions as characteristics of the metaphor. To him the two terms of the metaphor retain their literal meaning and their conceptual weight.

> Whether or not metaphor depends on new or extended meanings, it certainly depends in some way on the original meanings; an adequate account of metaphor must allow that the primary or original meanings of words remain active in their metaphorical setting. (Davidson, 1978, p. 31)

To Davidson, the metaphor escapes the rules of language and its greatest value lies in the effects, including the emotions that it produces on the interpreter: 'Metaphor is the dreamwork of language and, like all dreamwork, its interpretation reflects as much on the interpreter as on the originator' (1978, p. 31).

Previous approaches, influenced by the cognitive or the rhetorical tradition, showed different characteristics of the metaphor: its conceptual, imaginative, and emotional aspects and the relevance of its 'picturing function'. These different contributions broaden the vision of metaphor, which is currently understood as a figure of speech but also as part of the general processes of human cognition, and the development of artistic, philosophical, and scientific thought and the different ways of communication and culture (Gibbs, 2008).

It is necessary to keep in mind that the subject of metaphor has been dealt with in psychoanalysis in a long tradition, and it has a place in the discussion of the metaphoric characteristics of metapsychological theories and the theoretical explanations of the unconscious functioning proper to different psychoanalytic approaches (Caspi, 2018), ideas to which I will refer later in the development of this chapter.

The subject of metaphors in psychoanalytic communication has been widely studied. Authors like J. A. Arlow (1979), T. Ogden (1997), A. H. Modell (2005, 2009), and A. M. Rizzuto (2001, 2009), among several others, have discussed the metaphoric character of analytic work and interpretative processes. In a general sense, we can say that psychoanalytic communication enables metaphoric processes between the manifest dimension of analytic interaction and its latent and unconscious dimensions (de León de Bernardi, 1999).[2] Nevertheless, in this chapter, I will briefly refer to certain key metaphors that emerge in the psychoanalytic communication specifically related to the patient's self.

The expression 'key metaphor' was proposed by Ellen Y. Siegelman (1990), who stated that certain metaphors are used to conceptualise the characteristics of an analytic encounter. In her work 'Metaphors of the Therapeutic Encounter', Siegelman (1990) showed how certain ideas appear as key metaphors, which are used to describe the characteristics and structure of the therapeutic space.

> These metaphors of the therapeutic process – the frame, the container, the holding environment – have wide currency. Each has a special flavor reflecting in some ways the life experience or personal myth of the theorist. And each should have certain consequences for the therapeutic process that differentiate one from another. (Siegelman, 1990, p. 175)

Siegelman (1990) shows how different theorists of psychoanalysis, such as Donald Winnicott, Robert Langs, William M. Milner, and Carl Jung, use different images to describe the characteristics of the frame and each image having a particular meaning. Winnicott, for example, gives importance to 'the creation of a "potential" or transitional space in the analytic setting as in the early mother–infant encounter: a third area of experience between fantasy and reality in which symbolic development is made possible' (Siegelman, 1990, p. 189).

Siegelman (1990) proposed a useful perspective to consider the role of metaphors in the construction of psychoanalytic theory of technique. However, in this chapter I will use the expression key metaphor to specifically characterise metaphors that refer to the patient's self, which are keys to open up different levels of a clinical investigation. The genesis, dynamics, characteristics, and functions of key metaphors for the self deserve to be investigated. In fact, how do they emerge and gain a relevant meaning in psychoanalytic communication? Where do their strength and dynamism come from? How are they characterised? Are they useful interpretative tools, or can they lead to misunderstandings? Finally, in what sense do they contribute to clinical research?

To answer these questions, I will refer in the first place to a previously published clinical vignette (de León de Bernardi, 2017) of Juan's case. This vignette is taken from a session of the second month of Juan's analysis, with a frequency of three weekly sessions.

> Juan is a 45-year-old man who consulted due to feelings of frustration in regard to the achievement of some aims in his life. His tendency to let aside valued goals calls my attention because this does not seem to fit with his capacities.
>
> Juan describes himself as someone who has suffered from severe shyness for a great part of his early childhood, having great difficulty integrating into the group. Others easily belonged and he felt left out. In one session of the analysis, he relives the painful feeling of being left out. Metaphors condense the infantile experience of self:
>
> I was considered a 'little bug'; I was a little bug; it was very hard for me to modify that.
>
> Besides, he was considered fragile because he was very thin and got ill very often. 'It was the allocated place'.
>
> Through the session, he shows another aspect of himself:
>
> They also called me 'little lion' because occasionally I seemed to be a 'furious lion', but they mocked me, and they didn't take me seriously.
>
> Juan also narrates how, in different moments of his life, it has been difficult for him to show his capacities.
>
> At the end of this session, he brings a brief transferential dream. 'In the dream you told me: "Now you can let go"', he said. To which I answered: 'Letting the lion go here?' (de León de Bernardi, 2017, p. 36). We smiled at the end of the session.

Genesis and dynamism

The way key metaphors arise in the analytic situation seems different from metaphors in literature. A classic example of 15th-century Spanish literature illustrates some of these differences. '*Nuestras vidas son los ríos que van a dar en la mar que es el morir*' (Our lives are the rivers that will give way to the sea that is death), verse by Jorge Manrique (1999) of his *Coplas a la muerte de su padre*, (Stanzas about the Death of his Father) shows us how the metaphorical poles life-river and sea-death condense conceptual similarities, imaginative processes, feelings, and visual aspects, as pointed out by the different authors I referred to in the introduction to this chapter. We can infer that in the *Coplas* the author elaborates his mourning process. But it is a personal experience that is shaped in the poem according to the aesthetics of that time, resounding in multiple interpreters over time.

In the vignette from Juan's analysis, we see how the images of 'little bug', 'little lion', and 'furious lion' appear as metaphors for the patient's self in the context of the analytic situation and relationship. These metaphors emerged in situ, in vivo, as a result of the immediacy of the personal contact established between patient and analyst, and both contribute to their genesis. In this case the patient is the one who introduces the sequence of images trying to explain various aspects of himself to his analyst: the insect, the little lion, and finally the lion are images to which the patient adds associations that enlighten their meanings. Images condense aspects of his vital experience, emotions, and the construction of his identity, opening up several meanings, conscious and unconscious, which are yet unknown to the analyst. As it has been stated, a metaphor 'provides a mode of apperception of otherwise disparate aspects of self-experience, and it creates a private mode of objectification of ineffable experience' (Rizzuto, 2001, p. 557).

As we seek to understand the genesis of the metaphorical construction, we see that psychoanalytic communication cannot be separated from understanding its dynamism. Images keep emerging through the session in a 'cascade' (Buchholtz, Spiekermann, & Kächele, 2015), one after the other and referring to one another. As in the classical definitions of metaphor, the different images of the patient's self gradually build polarities referring to the internal world of the patient, which overlap in a retrospective and prospective way, forming – like a dialectic spiral (Pichon-Rivière, 1998) – circuits of meanings that acquire experiential density referring to the patient's historical past and the analytic present. The image of the insect is resignified in the successive images of 'little lion' and 'lion', and this last image cannot be understood without its retrospective relation to the first ones. The metaphorical meaning of the images emerges from the patient's associations, but multiple meanings can also be inferred through the elaboration and intervention of the analyst. After the transferential dream of the patient, the analyst's contribution repositions a new polarity in the images brought by the patient, including the context of the transferential and countertransferential relationship. The analyst's intervention prioritises the role of inhibition of aggression, introducing the possibility of its modification in transference.

Characteristics

Key metaphors are characterised by their vivid figurative impact, which leads us to explore their conscious and unconscious determinants. The strength of this impact is determined by the emotions, the sensations, bodily representations, and the scenes of relational patterns that are embodied in the patient's subjective experience that, in Juan's case, the analyst seeks to evoke from his associations:

> The little bug metaphor evokes feelings of being diminished, feelings of abandonment, loneliness, suffering and stillness due to his infantile inhibitions, but also bodily representations of himself and ways of bodily contact with others, which are overlapped by the impulse to fight for his things and get expressed in the lion metaphor, which partly represents the wish to expand his emotions and aggression and bodily movements. (de León de Bernardi, 2017, p. 38)

Figurability in psychoanalysis is part of a broad reflection initiated by Sigmund Freud in his work on dreams and in his concept of thing-representation as characteristic of the unconscious system. 'Dreams, then, predominantly in visual images but not exclusively. They make use of auditory images as well, and, to a lesser extent, of impressions belonging to the other senses' (Freud, 1900/1953, p. 627). Piera Aulagnier's ideas about the pictogram (1979) return to this tradition. To her, figurative scenes that emerged in analysis, which she called pictograms, are pregnant with different emotions and are close to the thing-representations of unconscious and the drive or impulse life. E. L. da Rocha Barros (2000) conceived the pictogram as a translation of ideas into figurative scenes, as one of the first ways of representing emotional experience, which creates symbols through the figurations in dreams. Affective pictograms are not strictly thoughts, because they are expressed in images rather than verbal discourse, but they contain powerfully evocative elements that contain meanings in a state of suspension. 'In the process of being constituted and in their figuration, affective pictograms potentially contain hidden and absent meanings, kept in a suspended state' (da Rocha Barros, 2000, p. 1094). To Susan Isaacs (1948, p. 84), unconscious phantasies condense 'visual images; auditory, kinaesthetic, tactile, taste, olfactory sensations, etc.'

It has also been stated how the mind of the analyst in the session works with a mechanism that is similar to the formal regression described by Freud (1900/1953) regarding the mechanisms of dreaming. The analyst, based on their own emotional responses, establishes equivalences and correspondences among different registers of expression from the patient and themselves – feelings, bodily sensations, affects, and images – with the verbal expression in an analogical way. The metaphor in psychoanalysis is anchored in a transmodal process of emotional and biological basis (Modell, 1997; Wurmser, 2013), similar to what happens in the early infant–mother relationship (Stern, 1985; de León de Bernardi, 1993). 'Key metaphors for the self' build bridges for the analyst's inquiries and interventions selected from among different dimensions of the analytic communication: symbolic dimensions, images and words, and subsymbolic dimensions, feelings, emotions, and corporal sensations.

The analyst's response to Juan's transferential dream – in the previous vignette – shows how the analyst places herself in a regressive position, expressing herself in images, responding to the acoustic image of the patient's voice in the dream, and showing a concordant, countertransferential identification (Racker, 1957). Apparently, both patient and analyst move in unison in a shared, positive, emotional contact, which also includes representations of bodily gestures and voices. 'In the dream you told me: "Now you can let go"', said the patient. To which I answered: 'Letting the lion go here?' (de León de Bernardi, 2017, p. 36). We smiled at the end of the session.

It is necessary to consider key metaphors for the self the tip of an iceberg that cannot be seen in its entirety from the surface. The genesis and dynamism of these metaphors cannot be explained by considering their multidetermination, which escapes the analyst's first look. There is a shared substratum, a sequence in the analytic communications that is hidden and includes complex phenomena, the personal equation of patient and analyst, verbal and nonverbal communication, the conscious and unconscious dimensions of their communication, shared fantasies, etc. Key metaphors frequently are part of interactive dynamic knots (de León de Bernardi, 1993) in which images, affects, and words are established intricately between patient and analyst, having a figurative impact. A nucleus of interrelated meanings emerges as a neoformation in the analytic field, whose significance should be considered later, as the analytic process progresses. In the case of Juan, many questions remain about the effect of this intervention on the patient.

Until now I have referred to certain characteristics of the key metaphors for the self in a particular session as told by the analyst. I will now consider the role of key metaphors in a group discussion using the methodology of the 3-LM for observing patient transformations. I will refer to Ms. C's case (Altmann de Litvan, Fitzpatrick-Hanly, & White, 2021, pp. 34–59.) to consider to what extent the group of analysts working on clinical materials adds new perspectives and problems to the topic.

The work with the 3-LM (Bernardi, 2014, 2017) is focused on the investigation of transformations or absence of transformations that occurred in the patient over long periods of analysis. The work starts with listening to a clinical material presented by the analyst of the case. The group exchange is made in successive steps, which consider three levels of group reflection on the presented clinical material. In the first level, analysts highlight phenomena in the material associations, which evoke associations, observations, and emotional resonances in the participants, with respect to the patient's difficulties and changes or no changes in them. In a second level the group focuses its reflections on different dimensions of the changes that occurred in the patient and, finally, the group discusses the theoretical approaches that explain the mechanism of changes or absence of change that occurred in the analysis.

Ms. C's case

> Ms. C was a 36-year-old single woman, half Asian, half Jewish, who worked in a senior position as a social worker. The analyst spoke vividly about having to contain the anxiety during early years with Ms. C, given the very risky behaviours she engaged in on weekends, involving dangerous sex and drugs. During Ms. C's infancy and early childhood, her mother was depressed. The family had immigrated from Europe to the United States when she was 6 and moved within the country shortly after. Her mother was hospitalized several times when Ms. C was 10, as a result of medical problems (possibly following a hysterectomy). Some family members on the mother's side (not close) were killed in the Holocaust. The father and his extended family were from Asia; some still live there. Ms. C said her parents were 'distant' with her and often left her alone for weekends when she was a teenager, when she had wild parties. (Fitzpatrick-Hanly, de León de Bernardi & Leuzinger-Bohleber, 2021, pp. 60–76.)

In the first stage of the work with the 3-LM (Bernardi, 2014), the analysts participating are placed in a position in which they listen to the clinical material, open to their own emotional resonances and associations that may emerge, connecting with their own experiences of practice and training. The inferential processing is predominantly evocative, close to the oneiric model. The selection by the group of certain expressions as 'anchor points' or 'key metaphors', because of the density of their contents, seems to be guided (as in the clinical vignette) by the strong figurative impact that they generate in the participants. Selected words from verbatim passages, such as 'chill', 'naked lunch', and 'hide and seek' reverberated in the group's way of hearing the clinical material, becoming the basis of the group's reflection on the mechanism of change or absence of change in Ms. C's analysis. These expressions could be considered key metaphors for the patient's self, because they condensed significant aspects of the patient's subjective experience, emotions, bodily representations, and scenes that reveal patterns in her relationships, both current and from Ms. C's infancy, that were observed through the group discussion.

In the experience of the working group, the genesis of the metaphorical meaning of certain expressions comes from different sources: listening to the clinical material, the group's reflection on it, and the interventions of the analyst, who participated in the group exchange. The description of Ms. C's view of herself, emerging from the material, led the group to reflect on the metaphorical meaning of the expression 'chill', which condenses Ms. C being cold and having no feelings, as well as her grandiosity. 'She felt that she was "above normal needs and feelings"'; 'She liked to think of herself as self-sufficient, "on top"'. A second expression, 'naked lunch', condensed for the group scenes in which she lived a risky and promiscuous sexuality, disconnected from her feelings. The course of an 8-year analysis reveals the patient's central fear of being in deep contact with another and with her own femininity. The third expression, 'hide and seek', condensed her impulse to hide from emotional contact and at the same time her wish to be found. This unconscious relational pattern was enacted in transference and after 2 years of analysis could be interpreted.

The working group observed changes in the analyst–patient relationship that are expressed in the key metaphors for Ms. C's self. The meaning of 'chill' and 'naked lunch' acquired new retrospective and prospective dynamic meanings as the analysis progressed. The patient's unconscious patterns expressed in 'hide and seek' were enacted in the transference and could be interpreted. As the reflections on clinical material deepened, the group observed how the patient began to become retrospectively aware of the defensive aspects of her being 'chill', finally to accept being 'found' in the transference, in her relationships, and in her real life. In the advanced stages of analysis, Ms. C shows a greater capacity for emotional integration.

The 3-LM methodology contributes to deepening the psychoanalytic conceptualisation and understanding of the changes that occurred in the patient. As we have said, a free-floating listening to the clinical material is promoted in the first level of the 3-LM, and participants let themselves be immersed in the material. In a second stage, the work is focused on the observation of the transformations or absence of transformations that occurred in the patient over a long period of the analysis. The group highlights how Ms. C can better perceive her own internal states and conflicts, achieving better levels of integration of her affects and symbolisation. The careful observation of Ms. C's dialogue with her analyst in different moments of the analysis leads the group to infer unconscious fantasies, which are implicit in the expression 'hide and seek'. The patient's fears of contact, especially the fear of her own femininity, were linked to traumatic situations of her past. Ms. C wanted to escape from a feminine identification that meant contact with a depressive mother. In the third level of the group reflection theoretical explanatory hypotheses were linked to the feminine identifications of the patient and the notions of trauma and depression. The idea of the dead mother from André

Green was included in the discussion (Fitzpatrick-Hanly, de León de Bernardi & Leuzinger-Bohleber, 2021, pp. 60–76.).

Psychoanalytic conceptualisation

Metaphors are often the basis for psychoanalytic conceptualisation. Their role in articulating clinical experience and psychoanalytic theory is shown, as we have seen, in personal clinical practice and in the work of the 3-LM groups with clinical materials. This theme was developed especially by Leon Wurmser (1977, 2013), who refers to Robert Waelder's classification (1962) of five levels of abstraction in the theoretical construction to differentiate the level of data observation, considered as the empirical level on which the following levels are supported. The observational level is successively followed by the levels of interpretation, clinical generalisation, clinical theory, and metapsychology. In Wurmser's (1977, 2013) view,[3] the most creative metaphors and those that generate new meanings and theories grow out of the lower levels of abstraction, in contact with the special characteristics of each patient. Metaphors need 'the richness of the analysed individual case without the clichés of the high levels abstractions' (Wurmser, 1977, p. 493). But, in which sense can we say that metaphor in psychoanalysis is a construction of a lower degree in abstraction?

It has been pointed out as clinical inference (0 that it may mean the abduction process (Peirce, 1931–1935/1994); that is, selected clinical facts are integrated and lead to a new meaning and hypothesis. The process of abduction in psychoanalysis and in the emergence of key metaphors in analytic communication influence the analyst's implicit theorisation, their emotional experience with the patient, and their latent memories of the relationship and the analytic process.

The genesis of certain expressions like key metaphors for the self, as well as their elaboration and interpretation by the analyst, have their basis on their previous implicit theories, according to their life experience, personal analysis, and clinical practice. These aspects are integrated in their implicit theory (Bleger, 1969) and referential scheme (Pichon-Rivière, 1998), which implicitly directs the listening and interventions with a particular patient. The internalised implicit theories of the analyst imply deductive, internal processes from general theories, which lead to a selection process, always partial, as Sandler (1983) stated, where there is a predominance of phenomena from personal resonances as well as from unconscious motivations. This basis of implicit theorisation operates in a preconscious way, enabling abductive processes that spontaneously establish relations among different facets of clinical experience. But this also enables the analyst 'to establish bridges' to facilitate inductive reasoning, which includes more general theoretical hypotheses and the investigation of different clinical problems. In this sense, it is possible to establish a circularity among processes of deduction, abduction, and induction, which go from general to particular but also from particular to general. These processes are strongly determined in psychoanalysis by emotional aspects, in internal communication of the analyst with themselves, in the phenomena of resonance established in the communication with the patient, and also in the experiences of group in working on clinical materials with the 3-LM.

Interpretative tools for clinical research

There is one issue that we still have to discuss. Can key metaphors be considered useful interpretative tools? Do key metaphors have a status of truth, as Ricoeur (1978) pointed out when characterising metaphors? Or can they lead to misunderstandings?

The key metaphors for the self that emerged both in the clinical vignette and in the work of the group opened paths to interventions by the analyst that have the patient's emotional and conceptual transformations as their goal. But this is only true if the analyst's intervention can be critically evaluated in relation to the analytic process.

Let us return to the clinical vignette. The course of the analysis showed me that my intervention, as analyst, at the end of the session could be heard with a different meaning than the one I had in mind at that moment (Faimberg, 1996). It was true that the image of a lion represented the patient's desire to unfold aspects of himself, but at the same time it represented a refuge to hide his narcissistic grandiosity, because he wished 'not to feel small', and led him to deny his vulnerable aspects. Retrospectively, I could see how my intervention 'letting the lion go here' at the beginning of the analysis could have been heard as an invitation to reinforce his omnipotence and denying his difficulties. Sometimes his attitudes sought confrontation and were determined by paranoid fantasies that brought isolation as a result, as happened in his childhood memories. The later development of the analysis showed how images of the self were taken on some occasions as defensive bastions having a defensive fixation that limited the patient's internal changes and the process of emotional integration and symbolisation. To the contrary, in the analysis of Ms. C we can observe transformations in the meaning of key metaphors for herself during the analytic process. The clinical material showed the working group how Ms. C could discover her own defensive ways condensed in 'chill' and 'naked', expressions that allowed the working group to reflect on the unconscious determinants of these metaphors for herself.

Key metaphors constitute useful tools if they can be evaluated through the analyst's second look (Baranger, Baranger, & Mom, 1983). An analyst's second look after the session implies a change in the analyst's subjective position in which evocative inferential processes predominate, based on phenomena of emotional resonance, to a position where a critical reflexive inferential mode predominates (de León de Bernardi, 2018). These two positions of participant and observer imply different uses of the psychoanalytic theory. The implicit evocative theorisation of preconscious character is not guided by the principle of no contradiction and it is of partial character, as we could see in the selection of different key metaphors by the analyst and by the work of the group. The reflective theorisation seeks to specify the more general theoretical assumptions, looking for the coherent adjustment to the clinical material in a way that enables public dialogue with colleagues. It is guided by the principle of noncontradiction (Sandler, 1983). In Ms. C's case, notions of trauma and depression were discussed in the last steps of the group's work, evaluating how appropriate it was for particularity of the clinical case. Within current pluralism, the analytic work demands the dialectics of an evocative thought complemented by a critical thought that can evaluate the strengths and limitations of the analyst's perspective, enabling the discussion of different theoretical and technical approaches, considering their scope and limitations.

The investigation of the latent sense of certain key metaphors for the self in analytic communication built bridges towards different levels of clinical research on the characteristics of the psychoanalytic encounter and on the psychoanalytic conceptualisation of the transformation or lack of transformation which occurred in the analysis. In this chapter this perspective was nourished by the clinical practice of the analyst and the working group's reflections guided by the 3-LM. The experiences of working groups are in many ways like sounding boards for our individual experience, broadening our clinical and theoretical perspectives about unconscious transformation in the patient. The participation of a group of analysts reflecting on clinical practice also offers a broader foundation in the development of our personal experience and ideas. But much remains to be investigated about the differences and similarities between the experience of the session and the experience of the working group regarding emotional resonance, figurability, free-floating attention, and free association, aspects of particular significance in the emergence and description of key metaphors for the patient. The practice of observing and discussing clinical materials with different methodologies in groups of analysts from different psychoanalytic cultures offers new perspectives to enrich the lonely experience of the analyst with their patient and the ongoing training of analysts. Empirical systematic research indicated by individual or group experiences can provide new perspectives on the subject.

Notes

1 'I.A. Richards in *The Philosophy of Rhetoric*, Max Black in *Models and Metaphors*, Beardsley, Berggren, and others cannot achieve its own goal without including imagining and feeling, that is, without assigning a semantic function to what seems to be mere psychological features and without, therefore, concerning itself with some accompanying factors extrinsic to the informative kernel of metaphor' (Ricoeur, 1978, p. 143).

2 The conception of the analytical situation as a dynamic field (Baranger & Baranger, 1961) proposes the radical ambiguity of the analytical situation, whose latent dynamism is determined from unconscious fantasies shared by analyst and patient – conception based on ideas from Susan Isaacs and Wilfred Bion.
3 David Liberman, in Latin America, also developed the idea about the existence of different levels of abstraction in the use of psychoanalytic theory. He proposed the necessity of evaluating the phenomenological level and the theoretical hypotheses present in interpretations (Liberman, 1971), reformulate the theoretical constructions according to a 'coherent linking' (p. 394) with the observed data, attending to the empirical basis of the psychoanalytic session.

References

Altmann de Litvan, M., Fitzpatrick-Hanly, M. A., & White, R. (2021). Underlying clinical thinking on change and therapeutic action. In M. A. Fitzpatrick-Hanly, M. Altmann de Litvan, & R. Bernardi (Eds.), *Change through time in psychoanalysis: Transformations and interventions with the Three-Level Model*, pp. 34–59. London, England: Routledge.

Aristotle. (2004). *Poetics*. New York, NY: Dover.

Arlow, J. A. (1979). Metaphor and the psychoanalytic situation. *The Psychoanalytic Quarterly*, 48, 363–385.

Aulagnier, P. (1979). *Les destins du plaisir: Aliénation, amour, passion*. Paris: Presses Universitares de France.

Baranger, M., & Baranger, W. (1961). La situación analítica como campo dinámico. *Revista Uruguaya de Psicoanálisis*, 4(1), 3–54.

Baranger, M., Baranger, W., & Mom, J. (1983). Process and non-process in analytic work. *The International Journal of Psychoanalysis*, 64, 1–15.

Bernardi, R. (2014). The Three-Level Model (3-LM) for observing patient transformations. In M. Altmann de Litvan (Ed.), *Time for change: Tracking transformations in psychoanalysis – The Three-Level Model*. London, England: Karnac.

Bernardi, R. (2017). A common ground in clinical discussion groups: Intersubjective resonance and implicit operational theories. *The International Journal of Psychoanalysis*, 98(5), 1291–1309.

Black, M. (1962). *Models and metaphors: Studies in language and philosophy*. New York, NY: Cornell University Press.

Bleger, J. (1969). Teoría y práctica en psicoanálisis: La praxis psicoanalítica. *Revista Uruguaya de Psicoanálisis*, 11, 287–303.

Buchholtz, M. B., Spiekermann, J., & Kächele, H. (2015). Rhythm and blues – Amalie's 152nd session: From psychoanalysis to conversation and metaphor analysis – And back again. *The International Journal of Psychoanalysis*, 96(3), 877–910.

Caspi, T. (2018). Towards psychoanalytical contribution to linguistic metaphor theory. *The International Journal of Psychoanalysis*, 99(5), 1186–1211.

da Rocha Barros, E. L. (2000). Affect and pictographic image: The constitution of meaning in mental life. *The International Journal of Psychoanalysis*, 81, 1087–1099.

Davidson, D. (1978). What metaphors mean. *Critical Inquiry*, 5(1), 31–47.

de León de Bernardi, B. (1993). Presentation, IPA congress Amsterdam 1993: El sustrato compartido de la interpretación. Imágenes, afectos y palabras en la experiencia analítica. *Revista de psicoanálisis*, 50(4/5), 809–826.

de León de Bernardi, B. (1999). Attualità di una polemica: Le due dimensioni dell'interazione analitica. *Rivista di psicoanalisi*, 45(1), 131–152.
de León de Bernardi, B. (2017). Dialectics of transferential interpretation and analytic field. In S. M. Katz, R. Cassorla, & G. Citivarese (Eds.), *Advances in contemporary psychoanalytic field theory: Concept and future development*. London, England, and New York, NY: Routledge.
de León de Bernardi, B. (2018). Teoría del campo, segunda mirada y procesos inferenciales en el analista. In M. Gómez & J. M. Tauszik (Eds.), *Psicoanálisis latinoamericano contemporáneo*. Buenos Aires: Asociación Psicoanalítica Argentina.
Faimberg, H. (1996). 'Listening to listening'. *The International Journal of Psychoanalysis*, 77, 667–677.
Fitzpatrick-Hanly, M. A., de León de Bernardi, B., & de Leuzinger Bohleber, M. (2021). Bodily metaphors as anchor points in facilitating change. In M. A. Fitzpatrick-Hanly, M. Altmann de Litvan, & R. Bernardi (Eds.), *Change through time in psychoanalysis: Transformations and interventions with the Three-Level Model*, pp. 60–76. London, England: Routledge.
Freud, S. (1953). The interpretation of dreams. In J. Strachey (Ed.), *The standard edition of the complete psychological works of Sigmund Freud* (Vol. IV). London, England: The Hogarth Press. (Original work published 1900)
Gibbs, W. J. (2008). *The Cambridge handbook of metaphor and thought*. New York, NY: Cambridge University Press.
Isaacs, S. (1948). The nature and function of phantasy. *The International Journal of Psychoanalysis*, 29, 73–97.
Lakoff, G., & Johnson, M. (1980). *Metáforas de la vida cotidiana* [*Metaphors we live by*]. Madrid, Spain: Cátedra.
Lakoff, G., & Johnson, M. (1999). *Philosophy in the flesh. The embodied mind and its challenge to Western thought*. New York, NY: Basic Books.
Liberman, D. (1971). *Lingüística, interacción comunicativa y proceso psicoanalítico*. Buenos Aires, Argentina: Galerna/Nueva Visión.
Manrique, J. (1999). Coplas a la Muerte de su Padre. Losada, Spain.
Modell, A. H. (1997). Reflections on metaphor and affects. *The Annual of Psychoanalysis*, 25, 219–233.
Modell, A. H. (2005). Emotional memory, metaphor, and meaning. *Psychoanalytic Inquiry*, 25(4), 555–568.
Modell, A. H. (2009). Metaphor – The bridge between feelings and knowledge. *Psychoanalytic Inquiry*, 29, 6–11.
Ogden, T. (1997). Reverie and metaphor: Some thoughts on how I work as a psychoanalyst. *The International Journal of Psychoanalysis*, 78, 719–732.
Peirce, C. S. (1994). *The collected papers of Charles Sanders Peirce* (Vols. 1–6) (C. Hartshorne & P. Weiss, Eds.). Cambridge, MA: Harvard University Press. (Original work published 1931–1935)
Pichon-Rivière, E. (1998). *Teoría del vínculo* (Vol. 19). Buenos Aires, Argentina: Nueva Visión.
Racker, H. (1957). The meanings and uses of countertransference. *The Psychoanalytic Quarterly*, 26, 303–357.
Ricoeur, P. (1978). The metaphorical process as cognition, imagination, and feeling. *Critical Inquiry*, 5(1), 143–159.

Rizzuto, A. M. (2001). Metaphors of a bodily mind. *Journal of the American Psychoanalytic Association*, 49(2), 535–568.

Rizzuto, A. M. (2009). Metaphoric process and metaphor: The dialectics of shared analytic experience. *Psychoanalytic Inquiry*, 29, 18–29.

Sandler, J. (1983). Reflections on some relations between psychoanalytic concepts and psychoanalytic practice. *The International Journal of Psychoanalysis*, 64, 35–45.

Siegelman, E. Y. (1990). Metaphors of the therapeutic encounter. *Journal of Analytical Psychology*, 35(2), 175–191.

Stern, D. (1985). *The interpersonal world of the infant: A view from psychoanalysis and developmental psychology*. New York, NY: Basic Books.

Waelder, R. (1962). Psychoanalysis, scientific, and philosophy. *Journal of the American Psychoanalytic Association*, 10, 617–637.

Wurmser, L. (1977). A defense of the use of metaphor in analytic theory formation. *The Psychoanalytic Quarterly*, 46, 466–498.

Wurmser, L. (2013). Metaphor and conflict. In S. M. Katz (Ed.), *Metaphor and fields: Common ground, common language, and the future of psychoanalysis*. London, England, and New York, NY: Routledge.

Part IV

Working parties as research tools?

Chapter 12

Working parties as clinical research

William Glover and Bernard Reith

Background

The working parties (WPs) originated in the European Psychoanalytical Federation (EPF) in 2001 as a way to promote an investigative spirit into the fundamentals of our profession, in which all psychoanalysts could take an active part (Tuckett, 2002, 2003, 2004). One impetus behind the WP initiative was therefore the search for group discussion settings that could help analysts coming from different psychoanalytic traditions to create a more open shared 'meta' perspective, from which they might glean new insights into the clinical material, as well as a more third-person view of their own preferred theory, with its advantages and limitations. One aspect of the settings is a specific, ongoing investigative focus for each WP. From the outset, the WP effort thus combined a 'research' aspect (in the wide sense of the term) of deepening our knowledge of psychoanalysis, with an experiential aspect of individual value, highly appreciated by the participating psychoanalysts. Clinical WPs realise the 'inseparable bond (*Junktim*) between cure and research,' as Freud described in 'The Question of Lay Analysis' (1926/1959, p. 259). This *Junktim* is a conjunction of practice and research that bridges the divide between clinician and researcher.

Two models for clinical discussion groups that preceded and inspired these efforts are Faimberg's (1996) 'Listening to Listening' and Norman and Salomonsson's (2005) 'Weaving Thoughts' (2005). Faimberg developed her concept of 'listening to listening' into a method for studying clinical work in which the group listens to the patient's listening, and to their own listening, in a spiralling process, recognising assumptions and misunderstandings, leading to deepened understanding of the other. 'Weaving thoughts' is a model developed by Bjorn Salomonsson and the late Johan Norman (Norman & Salomonsson, 2005; Salomonsson (2012) cited Winnicott on the necessity of 'maintaining a symbolic gap between analyst and patient in order to reach a psychoanalytic attitude' (p. 930) and said,

DOI: 10.4324/9780000000002-16

> Weaving Thoughts presentation aims to establish the gap via a format in which the analyst reads out his text without interruptions. Meanwhile, the group listens with an attitude similar to the analyst's abstinence. ... Metaphorically speaking, presenter and patient are placed on an imaginary couch, 'behind' which every group member may reflect as he or she would during daily work. From the presenter's perspective, the group's associations are placed on a similar 'couch', behind which he or she becomes freer to look at the countertransference. (pp. 928-929)

In this way, the analytic session is 'copied' into the group for further psychoanalytic investigation. These processes of interanalytic peer group work form the background to which other complementary procedures were added as the WPs developed.

The WP model made a virtue of the diversity of traditions, theories, and languages in the EPF, to widen the net for listening to the unconscious. The new WP procedures significantly enhanced the openness, insightfulness, and depth of clinical and scientific dialogue in the EPF, and the resulting collegial atmosphere led to increased attendance at meetings. The model later migrated to Latin and North America, where variations and new initiatives have developed. One of these is the Clinical Observation Work Group (Altmann de Litvan, 2014; Bernardi, 2017), developed as a project of the International Psychoanalytical Association (IPA) that, although differently organised, works in a similar way. In the present overview, these various initiatives are seen as sharing similar and/or complementary objectives and methods and will be referred to collectively as 'WPs'. To coordinate these efforts going forward, the IPA formed a Working Parties Committee in 2017.

Working party methods

Though each of the WPs has its own features, they have three things in common: a *question*, a *method*, and a *setting*.

The question varies for each group and addresses a key aspect of psychoanalysis. For comparative clinical methods (CCM), this is the analyst's theory of technique, both implicit and explicit (Tuckett et al., 2008; Basile et al., 2010; Rudden & Bronstein, 2015). For end of training evaluation, the focus is on the supervisor's criteria for graduation (Junkers, Tuckett, & Zacharisson, 2008; Erlich-Ginor, 2010; Hinze, 2015). The Working Party on Initiating Psychoanalysis (WPIP) studied how analysis begins and how this is related to the unconscious dynamics of first interviews (Crick, 2014; Møller, 2014; Reith, 2015; Reith et al. 2018). Clinical Observation (CO) studies how patients change (Altmann de Litvan, 2014; Bernardi, 2017), and Specificity of Psychoanalytic Treatment Today (SPTT) examines analytic processes (Frish, Bleger, & Séchaud, 2010; Abram, 2018).

In most of these WPs, the methods combine the free associative group procedures outlined above, with semistructured protocols that invite thinking about the case more systematically, making sure that the group's findings are grounded in the case and beginning to categorise and formulate hypotheses for further investigation. This type of work promotes a more self-reflective and exploratory stance towards the group's experience of the case, resulting in what we will call here 'reflective elaboration'. It focuses on and contains the discussion, helping the group avoid supervision or sterile theoretical debate, and often enhances the psychoanalytic experience of the case. The results of such a semistructured procedure can also provide a basis for later stages of the research process. A palette of discussion methods has been developed, ranging from the strictly free-associative group work of SPTT, through the addition of a short set of discussion questions as practiced by the WPIP, to the more structured approach of CCM and the even more structured protocol of CO.

The overall setting is composed of three tiers; the *case*, the *clinical workshop* (CW), and the ongoing core WP, which can be called the *investigative team* (IT). The presence and interaction of all three levels are crucial, as with a three-legged stool; if you take away one leg, it does not work.

The starting point is the case. Experienced analysts are invited to present. Sessions from one case are studied in depth. The clinical workshop participants and the IT assume that the work is analysis, even if it may seem foreign to them, and strive to accept the work on its own terms. The emphasis is on close reading of verbatim material, although the analyst's selection and reading of the text are, of course, also very informative.

This work on the case is done at a clinical workshop, bringing together analysts who are preferably from diverse theoretical orientations. The CWs, which usually meet for a day and a half, are organised at IPA and regional conferences or at ad hoc seminars. Workshop discussions follow the procedures outlined above and are often audio-recorded for later study.

Like the CWs, the core, ongoing group, or IT, is a heterogeneous group of analysts from different societies and theoretical orientations who meet to develop the method of investigation, organise the workshops where they function as moderators or reporters, and study the data thus collected. The moderator or reporter, often both, brings the text of the sessions and a report on the workshop experience to the IT for further study. As a first step, the ITs of some WPs follow the same protocols as in the CWs. The results of the work on each case are then compared with other cases to look for common patterns. In some WPs, the core team's own proceedings are recorded for later review; some, like the WPIP, have developed systematic review procedures for these later steps (Reith et al., 2018).

The teams have been surprised by how the case also comes alive in their work, similar to what happens in the workshops, even without the presence of the presenting analyst (Reith, 2015; Reith et al., 2018). The unconscious is somehow transmitted through the text and the narration of the reporters. Because the IT continues to meet periodically to study data from the individual workshops, refine the method, check its evolving hypotheses against the cumulative material, and so generate findings that are returned to the psychoanalytic community through publications and presentations, it also submits itself to a form of ongoing analytic scrutiny. Returning to the weaving thoughts metaphor, we could say that the patient, presenter, workshop, and the IT's own proceedings are all placed on an imaginary couch behind which the IT can associate and reflect. Things that could not be thought about in the consulting room or in the workshop come into focus in the IT's 'third look'.

Institutional support has been essential in supporting the WPs through funding, space in conference programs, and, most important, the imprimatur of the host organisation. When the IPA, or the EPF, or the Federacao Psicanalítica da America Latina (Psychoanalytic Federation of Latin America, FEPAL) sponsors a WP, it indicates that this is a collective effort with a mandate to serve the psychoanalytic community, not a private group pursuing its own project. This mandate strengthens the WPs' containing function and broadens the appeal for members to participate.

As the WPs matured, the authors organised a series of 3 panels beginning at the IPA Congress in Prague in 2013, continuing at the EPF in Turin in 2014, and then again at the IPA in Boston in 2015 where leaders of the original clinical WPs, Comparative Clinical Methods, SPTT, End of Training Evaluation, Initiating Psychoanalysis, and their cousin, CO, met to discuss and compare their projects. (Such panels are now continued at IPA and regional conferences by the IPA Working Parties Committee.)

We identified three major themes that emerged in the panels:

1 Do WPs conduct valid research?
2 What are the respective contributions of free association and reflective elaboration?
3 How are the unconscious dynamics of the sessions communicated to the investigative groups?

Do working parties conduct valid research?

This is certainly not controlled empirical research but rather qualitative research similar to grounded theory in the social sciences where data are collected and coded to identify categories that can lead to new concepts and theories (Glaser & Strauss, 1967; Tuckett, 1994; Charmaz, 2006; Bryant & Charmaz, 2007).

We could say that each analyst attempts research from behind their couch in every session, or at least they should, but single-case studies are often dismissed as anecdotal in this era of empirical validation. A problem with Freud's *Junktim* thesis pointed out by Thomä and Kächele (1987) and others is that it can justify analysts' tendencies to find evidence for their theories without adequate means of testing their hypotheses. There are other traditions, however, such as grounded theory and what the historian of science John Forrester (2017) has called 'thinking in cases' that value the accumulation of knowledge from case studies. In such models, an insight arising from the study of one case can function as a paradigm (Agamben, 2009) illuminating or changing our understanding of other cases. Like qualitative research in the social sciences, psychoanalytic WP methods attempt to develop valid procedures for this approach.

One essential component is the psychoanalytic group work in the CWs and the core ITs. The WPs valorise and revitalise the traditional single case study method of psychoanalysis through what Marianne Leuzinger-Bohleber (2018) has called 'expert validation'. The subjectivity of the solo observer is augmented by the presence of other minds. One analyst's observation is an anecdote. When ten analysts agree, their intersubjective validation indicates something significant that they all recognise. When different groups study a case independent (or partially so) of each other, as happens when two or more CWs study the same case or when an IT studies sessions before comparing its own findings with those of the CW, and reach similar conclusions, the findings become even stronger.

Two core mechanisms that seem to be involved in such interanalytic group work across WPs and that have been described independently, but in interestingly similar terms, by CO (Bernardi, 2017) and the WPIP (Reith et al., 2018) are 'resonance' and 'triangulation'.

Resonance refers to the fact that different individual psychoanalysts will be sensitive to different aspects of the material being studied, drawing the attention of their colleagues to them and trying to find symbolic representation for them, setting off divergent but interweaving associative chains. This has also been described as a 'diffraction' effect (Kaës, 2005; Reith et al., 2018; Abram, 2018) allowing the group to capture different aspects of the material, much like a prism separating white light into its spectrum of colours.

The second mechanism, *triangulation*, describes how the prescribed group procedures help each participant to attain a more self-reflective perspective on their response to the clinical material. This operates on at least two different levels. One is triangulation between the group members, who, through observing each other's responses to the clinical material, can gain more insight into their own responses. The second level is triangulation with the method: Being asked to think about specific questions helps the participants to become conscious of aspects that they had only perceived preconsciously and to put words to them; it also helps the participants to become more aware of the differences between their own perceptions and formulations and those of other participants.

Some WPs introduce yet further levels of triangulation; for example, when IT takes a critical second look through systematic case reviews to test the validity of its earlier findings, as in the WPIP (Reith et al., 2018), or by encoding the CW's findings in complementary ways, including validated research instruments, as in CO (Bernardi, 2017). The psychoanalytic relevance of such procedures is debated but is best understood if they are seen as ways to encourage a reflective third-person or 'meta' perspective on the psychoanalytic findings of the individual participants or the group as a whole. This can include a heightened awareness of individual or group countertransference responses.

All of these procedures basically use something that psychoanalysts already know how to do well, namely, clinical case discussion groups, as a starting point for more disciplined and systematic forms of study: They turn clinical case discussions into a research tool. The individual case study is strengthened, and the collection of case studies enables the IT to derive more general observations for further investigation. Our psychoanalytic knowledge claims can be supported by this expert validation as well as by other forms of evidence.

The balance of free association and reflective elaboration

As described, each WP has a different emphasis on the balance between group processes promoting free-associative resonance and more structured procedures promoting triangulation and reflective elaboration. For example, SPTT emphasises free association and is the closest to the weaving thoughts method, whereas CCM and CO feature a more structured second phase of reflective elaboration.

The question that has been raised is whether free association, evenly suspended attention, insight, and interpretation can only occur in the consulting room or whether the investigative group of the CWs or core IT can also become part of the analytic field where these processes can take place, alongside reflective elaboration (which *also* occurs in the consulting room). The experience of those analysts who participate is that both free association and reflective elaboration take place in the groups and indeed that their combination is essential. Concerns have been raised, however, that one or the other modality may dominate and compromise the investigation.

On the one hand, there is concern that reflective elaboration can impose a theoretical lens, leading to arbitrary categorisation and compromising creativity. The WP methods in fact guard against imposing theory. Categorisation of the clinical material is a posteriori, not a priori. Participants are asked to avoid jargon and use descriptive language. They are encouraged to ground their observations in the text and to cite the specific passages that inform their thinking. When the group drifts into theoretical debate, the moderators bring them back to the text or ask what the debate may reflect about the case. The result of the semistructured procedures is often to stimulate a refreshed or sharpened approach to the material, producing a richer tapestry of free association.

On the other hand, there is concern that emphasising free association promotes group regression. Are the associations about the case and in the service of the investigation, or do they simply reflect the group's own internal dynamics? The group's preoccupations, like the analyst's, definitely influence things and must be taken into account, but even when these internal dynamics are manifestly present it does not mean that the group's associations are not related to the case. The mind of the analyst, or of a WP, is never an empty vessel. We can think of a topographic metaphor of the unconscious finding something on the surface of consciousness to attach itself to. One of the aims of the triangulation processes outlined above is to facilitate the detection of such regressive moments and the analysis of what they are responding to.

Thus, although at first sight there might seem to be a contradiction between the two modes of thinking, in practice this is not found to be the case. What is observed is more like a fruitful tension. Semistructured procedures and reflective elaboration do not necessarily hinder psychoanalytic exploratory work and can deepen it instead.

Unconscious communication in psychoanalytic investigation

Finally, there is the question of *how* the unconscious dynamics of the case are communicated by the analyst's account, through the CW, and all the way to the IT, in such a way that it can stimulate meaningful psychoanalytic work at all stages. (See flowchart in Figure 12.1 on the transmission of the unconscious in clinical working parties.) Exemplifying Freud's *Junktim*, the members of the CWs and ITs do not just study a case as a neutral object of research; they join the analytic field *as psychoanalysts*; they are moved by the clinical material and find that working through countertransference reactions is an essential part of their research. We may be tempted to take this phenomenon for granted, but if we want to justify the psychoanalytic nature of WP research, we must explain how this happens and why it works.

One clue may be found in the regressive group processes alluded to above. Most WPs have independently described enactment-like group processes that, when examined in the context of the sessions and the cumulative findings, can be understood to carry information about the session dynamics that had until then remained repressed, split-off or unsymbolised (Reith et al., 2018; Abram, 2018). They would thus correspond to an unconscious 'phoric'

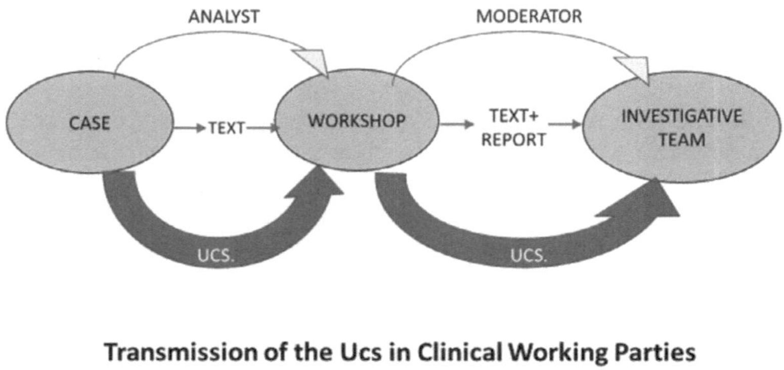

Figure 12.1. Transmission of the unconscious in clinical working parties. Ucs = unconscious communication.

function (Kaës, 2005), in which one or more group members act like 'messengers' for something embedded in the material that the group is trying to capture, represent, and understand. If so, they seem to reveal embodied unconscious thought processes or proto-thought processes, capturing poorly or unsymbolised phenomena that are conveyed by the analyst's presentation or by how the session material is written up. Concepts such as 'scenic' communication (Argelander, 2013), 'semiotic' communication (Bronstein, 2015), and embodied metaphor (Rizzuto, 2001, 2009) might be relevant here. These concepts and the mechanism of unconscious communication at different levels of investigation merit further study.

References

Abram, J. (2018). The inter-analytic mirror. *Bulletin of the European Psychoanalytical Federation*, 72, 203-209.

Agamben, G. (2009). *The signature of all things: On method*. New York, NY: Zone Books.

Altmann de Litvan, M. (Ed.). (2014). *Time for change: Tracking transformations in psychoanalysis – The Three-Level Model*. London, England: Karnac.

Argelander, H. (2013). The scenic function of the ego and its role in symptom and character formation. *The International Journal of Psychoanalysis*, 94, 337–354.

Basile, R., Birksted Breen, D., Bonard, O., Denis, P., Diercks, M., Ferro, A., … Tuckett, D. (2010). How do psychoanalysts work? The work of the EPF Working Party on Comparative Clinical Methods 2003–2009. *Psychoanalysis in Europe: Bulletin of the European Psychoanalytical Federation*, 64(Suppl.), 5–32.

Bernardi, R. (2017). A common ground in clinical discussion groups: Intersubjective resonance and implicit operational theories. *The International Journal of Psychoanalysis*, 98, 1291–1309.

Bronstein, C. (2015). Finding unconscious phantasy in the session: Recognizing form. *The International Journal of Psychoanalysis*, 96, 925–944.

Bryant, A., & Charmaz, K. (2007). Grounded theory in historical perspective: An epistemological account. In A. Bryant & K. Charmaz (Eds.), *The Sage handbook of grounded theory*. London, England: Sage.

Charmaz, K. (2006). *Constructing grounded theory: A practical guide through qualitative analysis*. London, England: Sage.

Crick, P. (2014). Selecting a patient or initiating a psychoanalytic process. *The International Journal of Psychoanalysis*, 95, 465–484.

Erlich-Ginor, M. (2010). The Working Party on Education. *Psychoanalysis in Europe: Bulletin of the European Psychoanalytical Federation*, 64(Suppl.), 33–56.

Faimberg, H. (1996). 'Listening to listening'. *The International Journal of Psychoanalysis*, 77, 667–677.

Forrester, J. (2017). *Thinking in cases*. Cambridge, England: Polity Press.

Freud, S. (1959). The question of lay analysis. In J. Strachey (Ed.), *The standard edition of the complete psychological works of Sigmund Freud* (Vol. XX). London, England: The Hogarth Press. (Original work published 1926)

Frish, S., Bleger, L., & Séchaud, E. (2010). The specificity of psychoanalytic treatment today (WPSPTT). *Psychoanalysis in Europe: Bulletin of the European Psychoanalytical Federation*, 64(Suppl.), 81–110.

Glaser, B., & Strauss, A. L. (1967). *The discovery of grounded theory: Strategies for qualitative research*. New York, NY: Aldine de Gruyter.

Hinze, E. (2015). What do we learn in psychoanalytic training? *The International Journal of Psychoanalysis*, 96, 755–771.

Junkers, G., Tuckett, D., & Zacharisson, A. (2008). To be or not to be a psychoanalyst – How do we know a candidate is ready to qualify? Difficulties and controversies in evaluating psychoanalytic competence. *Psychoanalytic Inquiry*, 28, 288–308.

Kaës, R. (2005). *La parole et le lien: Processus associatifs et travail psychique dans les groupes* (2nd ed.). Paris, France: Dunod.

Leuzinger-Bohleber, M. (2018). Depression and trauma: the psychoanalysis of a patient suffering from chronic depression. In M. Altmann de Litvan (Ed.), *Time for change: Tracking transformations in psychoanalysis – The Three-Level Model*. London, England: Karnac.

Møller, M. (2014). The analyst's anxieties in the first interview: Barriers against analytic presence. *The International Journal of Psychoanalysis*, 95, 485–503.

Norman, J., & Salomonsson, B. (2005). 'Weaving thoughts': A method for presenting and commenting psychoanalytic case material in a peer group. *The International Journal of Psychoanalysis*, 86, 1281–1298.

Reith, B. (2015). The first interview: Anxieties and research on initiating psychoanalysis. *The International Journal of Psychoanalysis*, 96, 637–657.

Reith, B., Møller, M., Boots, J., Crick, P., Gibeault, A., Jaffè, R., … Vermote, R. (2018). *Beginning analysis: On the processes of initiating psychoanalysis*. London, England: Routledge.

Rizzuto, A. M. (2001). Metaphors of a bodily mind. *Journal of the American Psychoanalytic Association*, 49, 535–568.

Rizzuto, A. M. (2009). Metaphoric process and metaphor: The dialectics of shared analytic experience. *Psychoanalytic Inquiry*, 29, 18–29.

Rudden, M. G., & Bronstein, A. (2015). Transference, relationship and the analyst as object: Findings from the North American Comparative Clinical Methods Working Party. *The International Journal of Psychoanalysis*, 96, 681–703.

Salomonsson, B. (2012). Psychoanalytic case presentations in a weaving thoughts group: On countertransference and group dynamics. *The International Journal of Psychoanalysis*, 93, 917–937.

Thomä, H., & Kächele, H. (1987). *Psychoanalytic practice: 1. Principles*. Heidelberg, Germany: Springer.

Tuckett, D. (1994). Developing a grounded hypothesis to understand a clinical process: The role of conceptualisation in validation. *The International Journal of Psychoanalysis*, 75, 1159–1180.

Tuckett, D. (2002). Presidential address: The new style conference and developing a peer culture in European psychoanalysis. *Bulletin of the European Psychoanalytical Federation*, 56, 32–46.

Tuckett, D. (2003). Presidential address: A ten year European scientific initiative. *Bulletin of the European Psychoanalytical Federation*, 57, 7–22.

Tuckett, D. (2004). Presidential address: Building a psychoanalysis based on confidence in what we do. *Bulletin of the European Psychoanalytical Federation*, 58, 5–20.

Tuckett, D., Basile, R., Birksted-Breen, D., Böhm, T., Denis, P., Ferro, A., … Schubert, J. (2008). *Psychoanalysis comparable and incomparable. The evolution of a method to describe and compare psychoanalytic approaches*. London, England: Routledge.

Chapter 13

Opening psychoanalytic space in first interviews

An overview of the aims and findings of the EPF Working Party on Initiating Psychoanalysis

Bernard Reith

Basic aims: Finding out how psychoanalysts really work

If psychoanalysis is the optimal treatment for many people, then why do not more of them enter it? What happens in preliminary interviews that leads the analyst to recommend psychoanalytic treatment and leads a potential patient to enter full analysis? What are the unconscious dynamics of such interviews, and how do psychoanalysts work with them? What skills are needed, and how can we develop and share them?

These questions were behind the creation of the Working Party on Initiating Psychoanalysis (WPIP) of the European Psychoanalytical Federation (EPF), as part of the EPF's Ten-Year European Scientific Initiative launched in 2001 under the presidency of David Tuckett.[2] The WPIP undertook an ambitious study of the dynamics of 'preliminary' or 'first' interviews.[3] More than 500 psychoanalysts from all over the world participated over a period of 8 years, in a total of 45 clinical workshops where case material from first interviews was presented. We wanted to use these presentations to look at how psychoanalysts *really* work – not how we would ideally like to *think* that they work – and attempt to understand the real-life psychoanalytic practice of experienced analysts. An international team of 12 psychoanalysts, composing the WPIP's core investigative team, worked together to pursue an in-depth study of 28 of these cases.

The clinical workshop and investigative team methods were those described in Chapter 12 on the working parties, with emphasis on the power of interanalytic group work as a tool for understanding the unconscious transference and countertransference dynamics, as well as on the use of case review procedures to make sure that the patterns described had paradigmatic value for a plurality of cases. The interested reader will find a full account of our methods together with rich clinical illustrations in our final publication (Reith et al., 2018).

DOI: 10.4324/9780000000002-17

A North American Working Party on Initiating Psychoanalysis was also set up to pursue similar work in its region and at International Psychoanalytical Association conferences. The scientific collaboration between the two groups was stimulating for both and led to the work described in Chapter 12.

The problem to explore: Moving from 'assessment' to the 'creation of a psychoanalytic couple'

The need to find new orientations and methods for clinical research in psychoanalysis was particularly relevant in the study of preliminary interviews. All empirical research that has tried to isolate patient characteristics that could inform the decision whether psychoanalysis should be initiated or not, or that could predict whether a psychoanalysis would succeed, has consistently failed to find any (Bachrach & Leaff, 1978; Bachrach, Galatzer-Levy, & Skolnikoff, 1991; Wallerstein, 1994; Caligor et al., 2009).

Several authors have suggested that the indication for analysis lies as much in the analyst as in the patient. Judith Kantrowitz's work (1986, 1993, 1996, 2002) was part of a shift away from the focus on analysability, first towards the compatibility of patient and analyst as individuals and later to their functioning as a unique, working analytic couple. Because of such work the focus has shifted towards the analyst and another question has arisen, namely, why analysts may be reluctant to take on analytic patients. Many authors (Ogden, 1992/2012; Rothstein, 1994/2012, 1998; Caper, 1997; Quinodoz, 2001/2012; Ehrlich, 2004/2012, 2013; Wille, 2012; Møller, 2014) have described different aspects of the possible resistances that analysts may experience about taking on new patients. Several have argued that psychoanalytic patients are not 'found' but are 'created' by analysts who are able to bear the dynamics of preliminary interviews (Rothstein, 1998; Levine, 2010; Crick 2014).[4]

This background suggests that the patient and analyst work together to co-create an *analytic couple* and that the analyst's role in this process is essential. It then becomes interesting to understand the developing dynamics of the analytic couple and how the analyst functions in this context.

One valuable characteristic of working party methods is that they allow us to picture the dynamics of the analytic couple in ways that respect the uniqueness of each case, while also allowing us to arrive at more generalisable hypotheses. The task is to identify and describe dynamic patterns that enable us to find psychoanalytically meaningful links between seemingly disparate phenomena in patient–analyst encounters, both within a given encounter and across different patient–analyst couples. Unless they capture such dynamic patterns, controlled quantitative studies may neglect core aspects of the psychoanalytic process. This may be one reason behind their failure to find factors that predict outcome.

First hypotheses: 'Initiating psychoanalysis' and 'switching the level'

Based on the literature and preliminary case studies, we expected first interviews leading to psychoanalysis to involve a relationship in which the analyst works to 'touch' the patient meaningfully (Quinodoz, 2001/2012, 2003) and so open their receptivity to what analytic work can be. The experience of this might be what gives the future analysand a sense of what psychoanalysis is about (Klauber, 1986/2012) and has to offer that is valuable and unique.

We tentatively subsumed these processes under the umbrella concept of 'initiating psychoanalysis', in the sense both of 'initiating the *process*' and of 'initiating the patient *to* the process'. *Assessment*, – for example, evaluating a potential analysand's ability to benefit from analysis – would be only one facet of what the analyst does and would largely be based on how the patient responds to it.

As one component of initiating psychoanalysis, we expected to see something we called 'switching the level', in which the analyst would help the patient to look at his problem or life story in a novel way. This would involve becoming aware of some central issue that was previously preconscious or unconscious. We thought that as the analyst and patient began working together there might be an upwelling of affective and representational derivatives of unconscious conflicts, increasing the overall intensity of the interview, until a point was reached where the analyst might be able to pick up something that touched or surprised the patient with a sense of discovering something emotionally significant, which they might be able to capture in a 'meaningful common formulation'.

Findings: 'Facing the unconscious storm' and 'opening psychoanalytic space'

Our findings were very different. Although we did see such 'switching the level' in some interviews leading to analysis, it was not present in all cases. When a 'switch' *did* take place, it was not always clear that it played a major a role in the outcome of the interview. Most important, we realised that whereas we had expected to see such a 'switch' predominantly in the patient, it fundamentally involved the *analyst*, who needed to switch the level internally to discover what the patient was trying to convey.

Indeed, in all cases we examined, the unconscious interview dynamics seemed to be even more intense than we had expected. There always seemed to be more going on in terms of unconscious conflicts and transference and countertransference dynamics than the analyst could possibly capture in the interview situation or when writing up the process notes. Contrary to the hypothesis that the analyst had to help the upwelling of unconscious affects and phantasies, these were powerfully present from the outset, including in manifestations appearing before the interview itself in the 'pre-analytic scene' (Reith et al., 2018; Wegner, 1992/2012).

Many of these phantasies seemed to be about the request for help and its consequences. The fear of what could happen was represented by the patient in unconscious phantasies referring to past experience and/or expressing recurrent object relationship patterns. This was communicated on varied levels of mental functioning, ranging from well-symbolised unconscious phantasies, through less well symbolised object relations phantasies with splitting and projective identification, to nearly raw experiences looking for a container.

These dynamics could strongly affect both members of the analytic couple, sometimes disturbing them or momentarily overwhelming them. This made it difficult to understand what was going on, let alone become aware of something new. 'Meaningful common formulations' were only rarely achieved. In many cases there did not seem to be work on a central conflictual issue but rather a general process where the analyst demonstrated ability and willingness to share the work of symbolisation, verbalisation, and elaboration, perhaps conveying a hope that something chaotic might find a container in an analytic relationship. Mutual enactments (Tuckett, 1997) were frequent, sometimes noticed and elaborated on by the analyst, sometimes not.

We adopted the concept of an 'unconscious storm' to describe this phenomenon, borrowing the notion of 'storm' from Bion's (1979/1987) paper, 'Making the Best of a Bad Job'. A new central hypothesis, that dealing with the 'storm' was the analyst's crucial task in first interviews, emerged. This involved striving to maintain an analytic position despite the intense dynamics, coping with the pressures of what could not be conceptualised on the spot to salvage the possibility of finding meaning. We came to think of this as 'facing the storm' and striving to 'open psychanalytic space' (Reith et al., 2018). The analyst's ability to tolerate the storm and to work within it might be what gives the patient some measure of trust and hope in psychoanalysis.

In retrospect, one can think of our hypothesis of switching the level, with its effect of surprise and 'meaningful common formulation', as a model of a preexisting psychoanalytic space ready to be discovered and entered, the analyst's work being to find a key to it. What we saw instead was that an analytic space must be *created*. To do so, the analyst needed to become aware of their participation in what was being played out in the interview dynamics. Sometimes this awareness arose spontaneously; at other times it was acquired through a struggle involving considerable internal work.

One might compare switching the level to the lifting of repression that becomes possible once mental conflict has achieved some degree of representation and facing the storm to the ego's ability to hold together and to function in the face of less well-represented drive derivatives or traumatic experiences. This seems similar to Levine's (2010) 'two-track' perspective on beginning or intensifying the psychoanalytic process: switching the level would correspond to his 'archaeological' model in which psychic contents are uncovered; facing the storm would correspond to his 'transformational' model in which the mind of the analyst has an essential function in the creation of psychic elements.

This was, however, a difficult task for the analyst, involving both conscious and unconscious work ranging from personal affective involvement to reference to theory. The interview dynamics had to be *experienced* before they could be symbolised and elaborated, confirming Bolognini's (2006/2012) contention that the analyst's 'concave' receptor and container is not some abstract function: it involves their whole person.

The vicissitudes of the analytic couple and different forms of analytic listening

The patient–analyst couples seemed to find many ways to deal with this transference and countertransference field. These ranged from more defensive, enacted, collusive, or narcissistic interview dynamics – for example through denial of a core issue and idealisation of psychoanalysis – to more open, creative, and triangulated situations where it was possible to take on board the issues and arrive at a thoughtful understanding of them.

However well the analytic couple seemed to deal with the storm, close examination showed that there were always aspects that they failed to notice or had warded off. The most reasonable assessment seemed to be that some combination of elaboration, defence, and enactment was always present, on both parts. What mattered was that they managed to use this combination to engage with the unconscious dynamics in a way they found tolerable, even if this involved an unconscious agreement to leave the most fraught issues for later.

As to the chronological development of the interviews, all of the encounters seemed to involve sequences with different qualities. There were fluctuations and breaks between moments of representation and elaboration, when analytic space was opened and switching the level became possible; moments that were more chaotic, when something unexpected broke through and the storm was manifested through enactment; and defensive moments, when one or both protagonists withdrew from analytic space. Such breaks and fluctuations should probably be thought of as an integral, inevitable, and perhaps necessary part of the process.

These 'vicissitudes of the analytic couple' resulted in different styles of analytic listening and different routes to recommending or not recommending psychoanalysis. There were cases in which a high-frequency psychoanalysis on the couch was decided upon, though it was not clear whether a psychoanalytic space had been opened, as well as other cases in which a sensitive, triangulated psychoanalytic process got started but where it was decided for good reasons to embark on psychoanalytic psychotherapy. The initiation of a psychoanalysis was sometimes based on a benign positive mutual idealisation where disturbing material was not consciously considered; this was not necessarily a problem, if the analytic couple could face the excluded dynamics at a later stage.

Our tentative conclusion from these observations is the opposite of what much accepted wisdom might lead us to expect: namely, that there was no discernible relationship between the kinds of processes that developed in the initial interviews and the treatment choice. Treatment recommendation seemed to be the outcome of a highly individual encounter. Both parties seemed to opt for the form of treatment that they thought would offer them the best possible conditions for dealing with the disturbing dynamics.

Support from the internal, external, and shared psychoanalytic frames

Many of the analysts described instances when they realised that they had temporarily lost their analytic position and had to struggle to regain it. Sometimes theory could help to regain a reflective position. Often, they would trust the analytic process (Wille, 2012), accepting not knowing and not understanding but believing that things would make sense in due course. There also seemed to be unconscious work, some of it more embodied than thought, corresponding perhaps to implicit specialised knowledge developed by the psychoanalyst over years of practice. We may describe this combination of internal processes through which the psychoanalyst strives to maintain and/or recover the psychoanalytic stance as the psychoanalyst's 'internal frame' (Møller, 2014; Reith, 2012).

The analysts could also find support in an *external frame*, particularly when working in institutional settings like psychoanalytic clinics with structuring procedures and the possibility of peer consultation between interviews. The institutional setting could sometimes take on a persecutory role in phantasy but could also have an important containing function.

The role of the psychoanalytic frame as a *shared frame* was evidenced by the impact of the analyst's interpretations. In general, the analysts were cautious about what they communicated back to the patient. What *was* said was usually formulated to take account of the patient's abilities and was followed by 'listening to listening' (Faimberg, 1996, 2005) to assess its impact. Some interventions communicated a tentative understanding to help the patient or to see how they would respond, but many aimed mostly to help the patients to tell their own story.

When analysts did say something of a more interpretative nature, this was often with the specific aim of exploring and/or facilitating the patient's use of the psychoanalytic process and setting. This could involve addressing the patient's anxieties about the request for help and the meaning or consequences of entering treatment. Such *interpretations of the transference to the process and setting* could usually be seen to further the process, decreasing anxiety and promoting new associations.

More direct *interpretations of the transference to the analyst* tended to be avoided. When they did occur, they could worsen the storm, increasing anxiety and confusion. In the turbulence of first interviews, unconscious wishes and phantasies are so strongly actualised that they tend to be experienced as really happening. This is amplified by the fact that there is not an established working setting yet. Interpretations of the transference to the analyst can then be experienced as a seduction, as opposed to an offer of a useful setting and process (Donnet, 1995, 2005).

Discussion: Describing both highly individual and very general phenomena

It seems that each patient–analyst couple must work together to find out whether a psychoanalytic dialogue is possible. It is the quality of the developing dialogue that determines whether they reach a belief that psychoanalysis can become beneficial. In this study we have seen a lively picture of real-life psychoanalytic work as a unique, highly individualised form of treatment in which psychoanalysts are willing to engage fully with another person's difficulties.

There seem to be, however, discernible patterns that these highly individualised indication processes have in common, such as the unconscious storm, the analyst's struggle to open and keep open a psychoanalytic space in which to receive the patient, and the development of a shareable frame adapted to their needs. Such patterns would merit further study to see whether they hold up under scrutiny, but meanwhile it is worth pointing out that the capacity to detect, explore, and test dynamic patterns like this is a core achievement of psychoanalytic clinical research.

The confrontation with so many real-life first interviews has broadened the WPIP members' understanding of competent psychoanalytic functioning and has helped us to overcome an idealised ambition as to what psychoanalytic work should look like. Our aims will have been reached if our study promotes further exploration and research in the psychoanalytic community, if it stimulates clinical reflection on our practice, and, especially, if it helps psychoanalysts in training to overcome their fears about beginning analyses.

Notes

1 This chapter is based on the work of many colleagues, members of the EPF Working Party on Initiating Psychoanalysis (WPIP) and especially the coauthors of the book *Beginning Analysis* (Reith et al., 2018): Mette Møller, John Boots, Penelope Crick, Alain Gibeault, Ronny Jaffe, Sven Lagerlöf, and Rudi Vermote. Exchanges with the members of the North American Initiating Psychoanalysis Working Party, Nancy Wolf (Chair), Bill Glover, and Maxine Anderson, have also been very useful.
2 We are grateful to the EPF for their support from 2004 to 2018 and to the Developing Psychoanalytic Practice and Training program of the International Psychoanalytical Association, which contributed until 2007.
3 For the purposes of this study we defined a 'first interview' as a formal consultation with an analyst, which can have a recommendation for psychoanalysis as one of the potential outcomes.
4 These and related views are discussed in Reith, Lagerlöf, Crick, Møller, and Skale (2012).

References

Bachrach, H. M., Galatzer-Levy, R., & Skolnikoff, A. (1991). On the efficacy of psychoanalysis. *Journal of the American Psychoanalytic Association*, 39, 871–916.

Bachrach, H. M., & Leaff, L. A. (1978). "Analyzability": A systematic review of the clinical and quantitative literature. *Journal of the American Psychoanalytic Association*, 26, 881–920.

Bion, W. R. (1987). Making the best of a bad job. In W. R. Bion & F. Bion (Eds.), *Clinical seminars and four papers*. Abingdon, England: Fleetwood Press. (Original work published 1979)

Bolognini, S. (2012). The profession of ferryman. In B. Reith, S. Lagerlöf, P. Crick, M. Møller, & E. Skale (Eds.), *Initiating psychoanalysis: Perspectives*. London, England: Routledge. (Original work published 2006)

Caligor, E., Stern, B. L., Hamilton, M., MacCormack, V., Winiger, L., Sneed, J., & Roose, S. P. (2009). Why we recommend analytic treatment for some patients and not for others. *Journal of the American Psychoanalytic Association*, 57, 677–694.

Caper, R. (1997). A mind of one's own. *The International Journal of Psychoanalysis*, 78, 265–278.

Crick, P. (2014). Selecting a patient or initiating a psychoanalytic process. *The International Journal of Psychoanalysis*, 95, 465–484.

Donnet, J. L. (1995). *Le divan bien tempéré*. Paris: Presses Universitaires de France.

Donnet, J. L. (2005). *La situation analysante* [*The analysing situation*]. Paris: Presses Universitaires de France.

Ehrlich, L. T. (2012). The analyst's reluctance to begin a new analysis. In B. Reith, S. Lagerlöf, P. Crick, M. Møller, & E. Skale (Eds.), *Initiating psychoanalysis: Perspectives*. London, England: Routledge. (Original work published 2004)

Ehrlich, L. T. (2013). Analysis begins in the analyst's mind: Conceptual and technical considerations on recommending analysis. *Journal of the American Psychoanalytic Association*, 61(6), 1077–1107.

Faimberg, H. (1996). 'Listening to listening'. *The International Journal of Psychoanalysis*, 77, 667–677.

Faimberg, H. (2005). *The telescoping of generations: Listening to the narcissistic links between generations*. London, England: Routledge.
Kantrowitz, J. L. (1986). The role of the patient–analyst 'match' in the outcome of psychoanalysis. *The Annual of Psychoanalysis*, 14, 273–297.
Kantrowitz, J. L. (1993). The uniqueness of the patient–analyst pair: Approaches for elucidating the analyst's role in the outcome of psychoanalysis. *The International Journal of Psychoanalysis*, 74, 893–904.
Kantrowitz, J. L. (1996). *The patient's impact on the analyst*. Hillsdale, NJ: The Analytic Press.
Kantrowitz, J. L. (2002). The external observer and the lens of the patient analyst match. *International Journal of Psychoanalysis*, 83, 339–350.
Klauber, J. (2012). Personal attitudes to psychoanalytic consultation. In B. Reith, S. Lagerlöf, P. Crick, M. Møller, & E. Skale (Eds.), *Initiating psychoanalysis: Perspectives*. London, England: Routledge. (Original work published 1986)
Levine, H. B. (2010). Creating analysts, creating analytic patients. *The International Journal of Psychoanalysis*, 91, 1385–1404.
Møller, M. (2014). The analyst's anxieties in the first interview: Barriers against analytic presence. *The International Journal of Psychoanalysis*, 95, 485–503.
Ogden, T. H. (2012). Comments on transference and countertransference in the initial analytic meeting. In B. Reith, S. Lagerlöf, P. Crick, M. Møller, & E. Skale (Eds.), *Initiating psychoanalysis: Perspectives*. London, England: Routledge. (Original work published 1992)
Quinodoz, D. (2003). *Words that touch: A psychoanalyst learns to speak*. London, England: Karnac.
Quinodoz, D. (2012). The psychoanalyst of the future: Wise enough to dare to be mad at times. In B. Reith, S. Lagerlöf, P. Crick, M. Møller, & E. Skale (Eds.), *Initiating psychoanalysis: Perspectives*. London, England: Routledge. (Original work published in 2001)
Reith, B. (2012). What interpsychic conditions lead to full analysis? Some findings from the Working Party on Initiating Psychoanalysis. Part 1: The analyst's internal frame. *Psychoanalysis in Europe: Bulletin of the European Psychoanalytical Federation*, 66, 94–102.
Reith, B., Lagerlöf, S., Crick, P., Møller, M., & Skale, E. (Eds.). (2012). *Initiating psychoanalysis: Perspectives*. London, England: Routledge.
Reith, B., Møller, M., Boots, J., Crick, P., Gibeault, A., Jaffè, R., … Vermote, R. (2018). *Beginning analysis: On the processes of initiating psychoanalysis*. London, England: Routledge.
Rothstein, A. (1998). *Psychoanalytic technique and the creation of analytic patients*. Madison, CT: International Universities Press.
Rothstein, A. (2012). A perspective on doing a consultation and making the recommendation of analysis to a prospective analysand. In B. Reith, S. Lagerlöf, P. Crick, M. Møller, & E. Skale (Eds.), *Initiating psychoanalysis: Perspectives*. London, England: Routledge. (Original work published 1994)
Tuckett, D. (1997). Mutual enactment in the psychoanalytic situation. In J. Ahumada, J. Olagaray, A. K. Richards, & A. D. Richards (Eds.), *The perverse transference and other matters: Essays in honor of R. Horacio Etchegoyen*. New York, NY: Jason Aronson.

Wallerstein, R. S. (1994). Psychotherapy research and its implications for a theory of therapeutic change: A forty-year overview. *The Psychoanalytic Study of the Child*, 49, 120–141.

Wegner, P. (2012). The opening scene and the importance of the counter-transference in the initial psychoanalytic interview. In B. Reith, S. Lagerlöf, P. Crick, M. Møller, & E. Skale (Eds.), *Initiating psychoanalysis: Perspectives*. London, England: Routledge. (Original work published 1992)

Wille, R. (2012). The analyst's trust in psychoanalysis and the communication of that trust in initial interviews. *The Psychoanalytic Quarterly*, 81(4), 875–904.

Chapter 14

Is the Three-Level Model a clinical research tool?

Marina Altmann de Litvan, Ricardo Bernardi and Margaret Ann Fitzpatrick-Hanly

The Three-Level Model (3-LM) for observing patient transformations has proven extremely useful in exploring the clinical materials presented by psychoanalysts to groups around the world. But can we say the 3-LM is a research tool?

This question is not easy to answer, but in the process of addressing the question, we hope to reach some conclusions and to shed light on the range of possibilities that the 3-LM offers to analysts as they seek to improve their analytic work with patients.

Research tool could be defined as something that becomes a means of collecting information for the clinical study of a patient. The term research tool is often reserved for standardised instruments whose results have well-known validity and reliability. Here we will use it in a broader sense because psychoanalytic clinical research requires methods that come from both the empirical and hermeneutical traditions.

The main purpose of research is to inform practice, to test a theory, and to improve preexisting knowledge or to build new knowledge in a field or study. The research process involves identifying, finding, assessing, and analysing the information necessary to answer a research question. A research tool needs to contribute to a research process; that is, to help better understand phenomena in that field of study. A research tool should help to compare results from different cases and have the potential to increase the professionals' knowledge concerning the object of their study.

The 3-LM is used to study changes and absence of changes in patients over the long term in psychoanalysis. The model's aim is to help with the development of clinical proficiency in the practice of psychoanalysis. (Bernardi, 2014b).

Summary of the Three-Level Model at work

Small groups of analysts gather for three sessions of 4 hours each to work together guided by the model, with a moderator and reporter. The

DOI: 10.4324/9780000000002-18

presenting analyst reads the six verbatim sessions of clinical material aloud (from the beginning, middle, and end or recent phase of the analysis). The group analyses the session material, through group discussion, from the three perspectives presented in the three levels of the model: phenomenological, dimensional, and theoretical analysis.

The first level studies the material from a phenomenological perspective, focusing on the presenting problems and attending to the resonances that the session material produces in the participants. Analysts exchange their views on the most significant difficulties, selecting these as 'anchor points' from the early sessions. The anchor points are written up by the reporter, revised by participants, and used as reference points in the discussion of later sessions on change and no change in the patient and analytic process. With this systematic second look at sessions over the years of analysis, the participants gain an awareness of the analyst at work, while developing their own perspectives. This group process corresponds to the Barangers' concept of the analyst as an observer-participant of the analytical process (W. Baranger, 1979; M. Baranger, Baranger, & Mom, 1983). The aims of the group discussion at level 1 are as follows:

> Listening as a group to the analytic session material read by the analyst and sorting out the main presenting problems and changes in the patient can help participants increase their sensitivity to unfamiliar clinical situations and make them more aware of blind spots and subtleties in the clinical material. (Fitzpatrick-Hanly, Altmann de Litvan, & Bernardi, 2021b, pp. 310-311)

The 3-LM tracks both intrapsychic and intersubjective elements of the patient's psychic functioning (Bernardi & de León de Bernardi, 2012), guided by questions at level 1. Participants track the patient's 'use of the analyst and use of the analyst's interventions', which reveal core dimensions of the intrapsychic functioning of the patient. Participants are asked whether it is possible to observe change in the life of the patient: in the capacity to love and sexuality, in the family and social relationships, in work and leisure, in interests and creativity, in symptoms and subjective well-being. Can the group observe the patient's perspective on changes he or she experiences? The model also asks members of the 3-LM group to consider whether these changes correspond with, and make sense given, changes in intrapsychic life of the patient, in the transference, countertransference.

The second level discussion explores operationalised diagnostic dimensions, taken from current psychodynamic diagnostic systems, the *Operationalized Psychodynamic Diagnosis-2* (OPD-2; OPD Task Force, 2008) and the *Psychodynamic Diagnostic Manual: PDM-2* (PDM-2; Lingiardi & McWilliams, 2017), among others. The aim is to refine the description of the transformations using the conceptual questions based on these 'dimensions' of psychic functioning, while continuing to refer to passages from the verbatim sessions selected at intervals over the course of the analysis. Participants discuss and assess both the nature and extent of the changes and the absence of change (Bernardi, 2014a).

> The following dimensions are considered indispensable for adequate understanding of psychic transformations: Patient's subjective experience of illness and concept and expectations of change; Patterns of interpersonal relationships in the external world and in the transference–counter-transference relationship; Main intrapsychic conflicts; Mental functioning and psychic structure: (a) capacity for self and other perception; (b) regulation (of impulses, affects, and self-esteem); (c) internal and external communication (including aspects related with bodily self); (d) attachment with internal and external objects; Type of personality disorder (if any); Therapeutic foci: analyst's view of the aspects that play a central role in the psychodynamics of the clinical picture, causing or maintaining the disturbances and that require treatment; Follow-up information about the evolution between and after the chosen points of reference. (Fitzpatrick-Hanly, Altmann de Litvan, & Bernardi, 2021b, p. 311)

The aims of the group discussion at level 2 are the following:

> First, to contextualize the transformations of the patient, finding a more comprehensive description of what is wrong in the patient. Second, to analyse changes in the patient according to diagnostic dimensions (using questions from Level 2 selected by the moderator) described in a language that is experience-near and theoretically unsaturated. Given the multiplicity of theories, it is a good idea to start the discussion using a phenomenological language based on words that comprise the smallest common denominator of the diverse existing theoretical versions of these concepts. (At Level 3 there will be the opportunity to reformulate and develop these theoretical aspects from multiple perspectives). (Fitzpatrick-Hanly, Altmann de Litvan, & Bernardi, 2021b)

The third level discussion explores the transformations as they appear to be brought about by interpretive strategies that come from various explanatory theoretical models and clinical approaches. Level 3 questions guide observations of which problems the analyst focused on in the clinical material and any changes in the focus of the interpretations over time. The questions ask participants to consider the session evidence available for assessing the effect on the patient of specific interventions. The aims of the group discussion at level 3 are 'to observe what the interpretations address in the clinical material, patterns of interpretations, and the effects on the patient of interpretations. To test and enhance the observational base of theoretical hypothesis about how the interpretations facilitate change' (Fitzpatrick-Hanly, Altmann de Litvan, & Bernardi, 2021b, p. 312).

The three levels of group discussion could properly be regarded as contributing an expert validation of clinical inferences concerning change and observations on how change happens (Fitzpatrick-Hanly, Altmann de Litvan, & Bernardi, 2021b).

Participants receive the clinical material in advance, following strict confidentiality norms. After reading the material and before the beginning of the group discussion, participants fill in a questionnaire to assess the degree of change globally and in specific dimensions of the patient's functioning. The group activity starts with the analyst reading the brief history and clinical material aloud. This reading allows participants to hear what is transmitted in the tone of voice of the analyst, which adds to the written words. At the end of the three discussion sessions, each participant fills in the same questionnaire again. The moderator then investigates the degree of consensus in the assessment of overall changes in the patient using the questions that the group answered as individuals. The moderator explores the degree of agreement among group members about the severity of the disturbance, using the PDM-2 form (Lingiardi & McWilliams, 2017) to compare the functioning of personality at the beginning and at the end of treatment.

The 3-LM as a research tool

Initially we will need to establish which kind of research questions this model would be useful to address. The 3-LM seeks to answer the following important questions about a psychoanalytic process: Did the patient change in the course of the analytic process? In which dimensions of psychic functioning did the patient change and in which dimensions did he or she not change?

The stronger the answers are to these questions, clarified through multiple references to the clinical text, the stronger the evidence for the positive changes in the analytical processes. The 3-LM improves psychoanalysts' observations of, and insights into, specific changes and absence of change in the patient over the course of a long-term analysis. This focused and differentiated set of observations provides a tool that nourishes analytic clinical research, based on participants.

The nature of the clinical material selected for presentation to the 3-LM groups is a central factor in 3-LM observational research. The presenting analyst brings a brief account of the patient, and verbatim material from five or six sessions, which are detailed transcriptions ('he said/she said') written by the analyst during and after the analytic sessions. The analyst's conceptual ideas are not included in the presented material and they are only shared with participants briefly in the last stage of the discussion. An important feature of the model is that the distinctions between observations, conceptualisations, and inferences are emphasised throughout the group process.

In contrast to a clinical material comprised of vignettes selected to illustrate theory, the presentation of detailed session material, from three phases of an analysis, offers the possibility of conducting a research that allows the group to draw conclusions based on the strength of the observations. A unique feature of the clinical material prepared for the 3-LM group discussion is that, though moment-to-moment characteristics of the process can be observed in a single session, the patient's central problems and repeating dynamics can also be observed over time as they change or do not change. The presenting problems of the initial sessions always repeat in various forms, become elaborated, and enter the transference if the process goes well. The problems change, or do not change, in ways that can be observed over a long period of time, a realistic timeline for change to occur in a psychoanalytic process.

Is it feasible for the 3-LM to be used by different analysts with different cultural or theoretical backgrounds? The 3-LM poses no special difficulties for the groups who have worked together in all regions of the International Psychoanalytical Association.

The 3-LM groups have usually included participants with cultural and theoretical differences. The gradual discovery during the 2 days of discussion of the existence of a common clinical ground in observations among the participants has offered a confirmation that the model is fruitful when used in different contexts.

Does the 3-LM offer a consistent procedure that can be repeated in different groups or contexts? This is one of the strengths of this model or method. The 3-LM consists of a full set of procedures. There is a systematisation of the group discussions, which are guided by a moderator through specific questions at the three levels of inquiry. The questions are selected to address core issues in an analysis that participants focus on as most pertinent for the clinical material under discussion.

Before advancing any further in describing the characteristics of the 3-LM, we would like to consider whether we, as psychoanalysts, need the same research tools that other sciences need and use. Because the object of our study is change or absence of change in psychoanalytic patients or psychotherapy patients over the course of a long therapy, we need research tools that shed light on the special characteristics of such processes. For example, we need tools that improve clinical observations of patient difficulties, inferential processes nourished by making links between changes in functioning and interpretations, also questioning the kinds and degrees of change. Because the model focuses on the patient, we need tools that do not depend on just one theoretical frame but rather tools that can be applied in observing psychoanalyses with a wide range of characteristics (frequency, length, theoretical background). Given the unique realities of our discipline, we need tools that apply specifically to psychoanalysis and psychotherapy. We will examine the model with these needs in mind.

The 3-LM is a method that improves clinical observations, improves reliability and validity of conceptual thinking, and offers clarity about inferential processes, interpretive and noninterpretive modes of intervention. The model offers a set of specific questions that enable the exploration of a clinical material from three complementary perspectives, which together offer a better understanding of the analytic process and of the gains for the patient. In these ways, the model is a useful tool for psychoanalysts.

Research in the analytic field cannot be conducted in the same way as it is conducted in other disciplines. Therefore, the authors of this model felt the need to design a new tool that would take into account the specific needs of our discipline.

The 3-LM fosters clinical thinking and also systematises it (see, for example, Altmann de Litvan, Fitzpatrick-Hanly, & White, 2021, pp. 34–59).

We could say that the 3-LM is a tool of action research. While the analysis with the 3-LM is taking place, the resulting exploration generates effects on the participants and on the analyst. The analyst acts on their patient and the participants of the group are likely to also act on their own practice and patients in the light of what they see and discuss in the 3-LM groups.

It has become clear to us over the years working with the 3-LM and observing other analysts working with it that the 3-LM enables psychoanalysts who have not been previously trained in research to improve their clinical formulations and observations through a more systematic methodology. It has become clear that better observation, as well as receptive participation, results in benefits for our patients and for the development of our analytic abilities and practices (see Fitzpatrick-Hanly, Altmann de Litvan, & Bernardi, 2021a).

This model promotes the participant-observer research attitude. We have also witnessed how participants develop a further sensitisation to expressions in the material that have unconscious meanings through the shared resonance with other group members and with the analyst. This can be clearly seen in level 1 as the group listens again and again to the verbatim passages of patient and analyst and hears the repetitions, variations, and changes in the couple's exchanges in the three phases of analysis.

Level 2 facilitates a critical conceptualisation of clinical phenomena and enables analysts to use the operationalised categories from current diagnostic systems (OPD, PDM, and others) in observing and discussing the session material.

At level 3, participants deliberate on possible change mechanisms or curative factors at work in the interventions in this analysis. The level 3 discussion also engages in an enquiry into aspects of the clinical material that were not addressed by the analyst. Hypotheses can then be made concerning alternative interpretations related to passages in the verbatim sessions that could have addressed problems observed in the patient or process (see Fitzpatrick-Hanly, Altmann de Litvan, & Bernardi, 2021b). The 3-LM facilitates observations of implicit, as well as explicit, theories (Sandler, 1983) generating critical clinical rethinking of personal working models. A natural combination of prospective and retrospective perspectives emerges in working with the 3-LM.

David Maldavsky (2001), in his paper on clinical research in psychoanalysis, proposed that in the process of self-rectification of the analyst, where he observed alternative proposals of intellection of a clinical situation, it is important that the analyst has at their disposal alternative ways of intellection of the psychic processes in a clinical moment of the patient. He considers that this self-rectification, which accesses consciousness, is more psychoanalytic than logical. (Maldavsky, 2001).

The third look of the 3-LM extends the process of inquiry, engaging in another level of discussion of change or no change and links with interventional strategies, after the report from the first 3-LM group. The participants of a second 3-LM group, who are expert in the model, reread the session material and reconsider the evidence for change and no change along several dimensions, some not explored in the first report. The various theories and clinical approaches with which the participants are familiar, as well as the long-term temporal dimension of the material, allows a multifaceted observation and a double perspective: progressive and après-coup or a posteriori.

Contributors to the third look, 3-LM participants ask new questions about change and mechanisms of change. They engage in heated debates about the evidence in the sessions for the severity and kind of difficulty in the patient, about the degree of change, and about areas of no change. The discussants consider links between changes observed and the interpretations of the analyst and ask the hypothetical questions about what other associations might have been addressed or addressed with a different interpretation. The participants prepare and revise a clinical narrative, rich in verbatim session material, demonstrating robust clinical thinking and tentative conclusions with data from sessions. Analysts engage in a discussion of the relevance of concepts, brought by analysts from different cultures and clarified by reference to the detailed session material.

The 3-LM entertains concepts from various theories but does not support the idea that a loose pluralism, or blurring of concepts, facilitates observation. The procedural steps of the model lead participants to discover which concepts and theories are most coherent and which have most explanatory power for a particular psychoanalytic process. A deeper understanding of a concept specific to a theory becomes possible when a member of a 3-LM group, who has been immersed in that concept for decades, shows its application to a set of clinical phenomena in the shared material.

In the expert 3-LM groups, participants have a unique opportunity to engage more systematically in this aspect of conceptual research. The group members from different analytic regions discuss what a concept means in the context of their joint observations of the session material. This detailed referential grounding provided by the unique 3-LM material allows participants to clarify, and to understand the bearing of, the concept in the clinical process. Scientific concepts are alive, and we can modify a concept (using Sandler's [1983] idea of the elasticity of a concept) to catch the clinical complexity we are observing to see whether a concept may need reformulation in order to create a better tool for clinical thinking.

The clinical narrative provides an assessment of the strength of evidence for observations and conclusions and notes areas in which the evidence is insufficient (Bernardi & Pérez Suquilvide, 2021, pp. 281–305). In addition, the common ground appears through the concepts of metaphors (Bernardi, 2017).

After months or years of analysis, analysts can check with the 3-LM whether the initial hypotheses of the analyst or the alternative hypotheses from the group proved to be useful or not.

The 3-LM, through its way of working, leads participants to seek evidence for their ideas about what is going on in the patient in analysis. The points made by members of the group must be linked to evidence in the clinical material.

This model naturally facilitates triangulation of data, in at least two ways:

Firstly, when participants discuss their ideas about the patient and the analytic process, they must always refer to the clinical material.
Secondly, participants regularly track how the significant facts selected from the material are viewed when explored at each level and how the clinical facts develop over the years of the analytic process.

To give an example, in one of the clinical materials discussed at the São Paulo conference we observed that, in the course of the analysis, the patient presented several representations of herself, expressed in dreams, in metaphors, and in images (for instance, as a house or hotel). The patient brought an abundance of dream images but was capable of very few other types of communication. The observations of the group in level 1 discussions were cross-referenced with observations at level 2, which triangulated the ways of observing the same phenomena. Level 2 questions allowed the structural problems in the patient to be clarified, reinforcing what had been observed at level 1. The phenomenological understanding of the patient's changes, acquired in analytic listening and observing at level 1, will be clarified, verified, or questioned with the conceptualisation of these transformations, using the dimensions of psychic functioning and mental capacities in the second level (see full example in Altmann de Litvan, 2021, pp. 79–101).

Another strength of the 3-LM is that it enables participants to bring their own theoretical approaches to the task of observing and understanding the patient's associations and enactments. For example, in the example above, Altmann and Bernardi prioritised different anchor points from those chosen by the 3-LM group. These approaches were in part complementary and in part divergent. Altmann selected the anchor point in the context of exploring changes and no change in the representation of self and others through images and metaphors, and Bernardi selected the anchor point of her panic attack symptoms and the lack of words.

Bernardi argued that in this study there is a selection bias in the choice of the aspects that are taken into account in the patient's dream images. In all dreams there are light and dark aspects. But Altmann's analysis highlights the gloomy aspects in the early dreams and the luminous ones in those of later periods, without explaining the reasons for that selection. In the same way, the meaning of dreams as a representation of the patient's self and bodily aspects is not sufficiently supported in patient's associations. The hypothesis that the house represents a refuge for the agoraphobic aspects of the patient is also possible.

As we can see, the 3-LM propels to explore these different hypotheses and to argue in favour and against each of them. This search for evidence for alternative hypotheses, and the conceptual and clinical analysis is contradictory or complementary and constitutes an important contribution to develop clinical research.

The 3-LM not only allows different perspectives but also motivates all participants to contribute to a many-faceted understanding of the patient and of their evolution in the analytic process. The participants are exposed to new ways of analysing clinical phenomena, linked to dimensions of psychic functioning and to theories of therapeutic action.

Strengths and limitations

We have underlined the strengths of the 3-LM as a research tool. It is important to also pay attention to its limitations, especially the possible biases and omissions when using it. These aspects are more extensively presented in the paper 'Assessing the Strengths and Limitations of Clinical Evidence in a Psychoanalytic Clinical Material' by Ricardo Bernardi and Luisa Pérez Suquilvide (2021). From these ideas we would like to develop some points here.

The 3-LM constitutes an observation of the analyst's observation. Therefore, although it also includes first-person and third-person observations, it has the strengths and limitations of second-person knowledge. The participants in the group observe through the analyst's listening and their narration. The group discussion helps to correct this observation through the comparison of multiple perspectives, seeking to find what is essential and most significant in the material. This is a different path than the one offered by other procedures such as audio or video recording (which can also be used in the 3-LM but without excluding the analyst's personal subjective report), randomised sample of sessions, etc.

The 3-LM helps to enrich the observation and to reduce some biases –for example, confirmatory biases based on theoretical preferences – because groups include analysts with different affiliations. However, it cannot avoid other biases. Group discussions are vulnerable to phenomena of groupthink, anchoring biases (i.e., giving more weight to the information that arrives first) and the 'halo effect' (which spreads initial impressions to the following material). It would be important to pay attention and study the presence of this and other kinds of biases.

Perhaps the most pervasive and difficult limitations are the omissions of information about the patient and the context of the treatment. The level of the evidence of a clinical material depends critically on the degree of contextualisation offered by the analyst's report – in the first place, by the possibility of observing the patient's reactions to the foci of interpretations and the degree to which they elicit unconscious reactions. It is also important to know to what degree crucial material for sustaining alternative hypotheses has been explored. For that reason, it is important to include a discussion session in clinical papers that confront different views and allow the reader to know which hypotheses have been explored and which were not and could constitute blind spots. The confluence of these diverse criteria for the quality of the clinical observation allows one to evaluate the degree of the evidence offered by a clinical material and therefore its strength to support theoretical and technical hypotheses (Bernardi & Pérez Suquilvide, 2021).

Conclusion

We propose that the 3-LM is a clinical research tool because it allows participants who use it to identify and to distinguish observations, concepts, interpretations, personal theories, and theoretical approaches. The 3-LM groups follow another path. Instead of taking a system of theoretical premises as a starting point, they move 'from the bottom up'; that is, from the patient's clinical problems to the participants' operating models and implicit personal theories. Clinical inferences predominantly use abductive reasoning, and deductive or inductive processes play a subsidiary role (Bernardi, 2017).

As Bernardi and Pérez Suquilvide (2021) stated,

> Perhaps the greater challenge we psychoanalysts face is to what extent we can advance in the observation of a patient's transformation using purely clinical tools; working to reduce the flaws in group validation

> and in the analyst's participation in the group process, our task is to advance as far as possible. However, in order to advance in clinical observation, we also need to advance in the conceptual analysis of the categories and dimensions of change and to be attentive to extra clinical evidence.

The 3-LM can also be used as part of single-case research, combining clinical and empirical systematic research. This work is done by a combination of diverse tools, including concurrent validity (Rodríguez Quiroga de Pereira, Borensztein, Corbella, & Marengo, 2018).

References

Altmann de Litvan, M. (2021). Changes and no change in the representation of self and others through images and metaphors. In M. A.Fitzpatrick-Hanly, M.Altmann de Litvan, & R. Bernardi (Eds.), *Change through time in psychoanalysis: Transformations and interventions with the Three-Level Model*, Chapter 4, pp. 79–101. London, England: Routledge.

Altmann de Litvan, M., Fitzpatrick-Hanly, M. A., & White, R. (2021). Underlying clinical thinking on change and therapeutic action. In M. A. Fitzpatrick-Hanly, M. Altmann de Litvan, & R. Bernardi (Eds.), *Change through time in psychoanalysis: Transformations and Interventions with the Three-Level Model*, Chapter 2, pp. 34–59. London, England: Routledge.

Baranger, M., Baranger, W., & Mom, J. M. (1983). Process and non-process in analytic work. *The International Journal of Psychoanalysis*, 64, 1–15.

Baranger, W. (1979). Proceso en espiral y 'campo dinámico'. *Revista Uruguaya de Psicoanálisis*, 59(17), 32.

Bernardi, R. (2014a). The assessment of changes: Diagnostic aspects. In M. Altmann de Litvan (Ed.), *Time for change: Tracking transformations in psychoanalysis – The Three-Level Model*. London, England: Karnac.

Bernardi, R. (2014b). The Three-Level Model (3-LM) for observing patient transformations. In M. Altmann de Litvan (Ed.), *Time for change: Tracking transformations in psychoanalysis – The Three-Level Model*. London, England: Karnac.

Bernardi, R. (2017). A common ground in clinical discussion groups: Intersubjective resonance and implicit operational theories. *The International Journal of Psychoanalysis*, 98(5), 1291–1309.

Bernardi, R., & de León de Bernardi, B. (2012). The concepts of *vínculo* and dialectical spiral: A bridge between intra- and intersubjectivity. *The Psychoanalytic Quarterly*, 81, 531–564.

Bernardi, R., & Pérez Suquilvide, L. (2021). Assessing the strengths and limitations of clinical evidence in a psychoanalytic clinical material. In M. A. Fitzpatrick-Hanly, M. Altmann de Litvan, & R. Bernardi (Eds.), *Change through time in psychoanalysis: Transformations and interventions with the Three-Level Model*, Chapter 14, pp. 281–305. London, England: Routledge.

Fitzpatrick-Hanly, M. A., Altmann de Litvan, M., & Bernardi, R. (2021a). A dialogue between 3-LM presenters and moderators. In M. A. Fitzpatrick-Hanly, M. Altmann de Litvan, & R. Bernardi (Eds.), *Change through time in psychoanalysis:*

Transformations and interventions with the Three-Level Model, Chapter 11, pp. 234–244. London, England: Routledge.

Fitzpatrick-Hanly, M. A., Altmann de Litvan, M., & Bernardi, R. (2021b). Guidelines. In M. A. Fitzpatrick-Hanly, M. Altmann de Litvan, & R. Bernardi (Eds.), *Change through time in psychoanalysis: Transformations and interventions with the Three-Level Model*, Chapter 15, pp. 309–334. London, England: Routledge.

Lingiardi, V., & McWilliams, N. (Eds.). (2017). *Psychodynamic diagnostic manual: PDM-2* (2nd ed.). New York, NY: Guilford.

Maldavsky, D. (2001). *Sobre la investigación clínica en psicoanálisis: deslinde de una perspectiva*. Retrieved from https://pdfs.semanticscholar.org/b440/1a8d6d384b0d423fa7278 604a1afe836f954.pdf

OPD Task Force. (2008). *Operationalized psychodynamic diagnosis OPD-2. Manual of diagnosis and treatment planning*. Cambridge, England: Hogrefe & Huber Publishers.

Rodríguez Quiroga de Pereira, A., Borensztein, L., Corbella, V., & Marengo, J. C. (2018). The Lara case: A group analysis of initial psychoanalytic interviews using systematic clinical observation and empirical tools. *The International Journal of Psychoanalysis*, 99(6), 1327–1352.

Sandler, J. (1983). Reflections on some relations between psychoanalytic concepts and psychoanalytic practice. *The International Journal of Psychoanalysis*, 64, 35–45.

Chapter 15

The Working Party on Comparative Clinical Methods (CCM) and the Investigation in Psychoanalysis

José Carlos Calich

The Working Party on Comparative Clinical Methods (CCM) has two main objectives: to facilitate communication among psychoanalysts (so, 'comparative') and to study how analysts actually work with patients. The three fundamental questions are: What do we really do? How do we do it? Why do we think what we do works?

The working method has been described in several publications and meetings (e.g., Tuckett et al., 2008, Rudden & Bronstein, 2015, Minninger, 2015 and Calich 2016). Just to guide this reflection, presenting it in an extremely synthetic way, it is based on the work of a group of colleagues (with its dynamics) that produces conjectures about the analyst's interventions, examined in two or three sessions. These assumptions are introduced by the participating members of the group, as descriptively as possible, to detail the material and its comprehension, to explain the phenomenon rather than the use of concepts (always problematic in groups of analysts from different orientations). The group must focus the task on these assumptions by reversing the 'I-would-do-it-in-this-other-way' model into the understanding of 'what-the-other-does', 'how-the-other-does-it', and 'how-this-other-thinks-it-works'.

Working with these questions leads to the construction of scenarios about the colleague-presenter's implicit model of the analytic process, which includes their type of listening, their model of psychic change, and their intervention technique that seeks this change.

The method here exposed in its foundations opens up the possibility of several axes of investigation. I will focus on four of these axes so that I can present them in some detail in this space. They are investigation in interventions; investigation in implicit models; investigation in communication among psychoanalysts, and investigation in psychoanalytic supervision.

Investigating the interventions

Because a core point of the method is the study of the analyst's interventions, continued work with them raises several investigation questions that the material obtained from working with the groups allows us to

DOI: 10.4324/9780000000002-19

develop. The one that most immediately caught our attention – and we tried to develop an investigative tool to expand its knowledge – was the transferential interpretation.

Although transferential interpretations are conceptually linked to the work of psychic change in the theory of technique of most models of the mind throughout the history of psychoanalysis, their definition and specificity tend to be vague, indiscriminate, and heterogeneous, affecting their transmission in communication and learning situations. Given its importance, the scarcity of publications on the subject in our literature is noteworthy.

An investigation could focus on several aspects: from its complexity and breadth level, through the impact on the patient (response to interpretation), extending to the transferential transformations perceived by the group, among several other possibilities. Our choice was to construct categories linked to the goal (purpose) of transferential interpretation. We created 17 categories that immediately helped us improve, with the group or in later studies of the material, the implicit model presented. The following are the categories developed, without being able, for space limitations, to go into detail and discussion. Please note that the last two categories refer to the analyst's acting-outs or enactments.

1 Interventions that use the patient–analyst relationship to build the analytical space, including the intersubjective link.
2 Interventions with the goal of maintaining the analytical space focused on the patient–analyst relationship.
3 Interventions that make use of the analytic relationship to suggest intrapsychic functioning.
4 Interpretations that make use of the relationship to make a wish, or its repression, conscious.
5 Interventions that use the analytic relationship to name or contain an unnamed or overwhelming emotional situation (meaning creation).
6 Interventions that use the analytic relationship to inscribe a representation in a symbolic chain.
7 Interventions that use the analytic relationship to promote the separation of self and object.
8 Interventions that use the analytic relationship to promote identity differentiation (tending to the recognition of sexual, temporal, and generational differences).
9 Interventions that use the analytic relationship to modulate superego anxieties.
10 Interventions that use the analytic relationship to suspend theories and beliefs.
11 Interventions that use the analytic relationship to promote subjectivity and the wish to know based on a life drive.

12 Interventions that use the analytic relationship to promote subjectivity departing from the recognition of the emergence of a true self.
13 Interventions that use the analytic relationship to work with crossing transferences.
14 Interventions that use the analytic relationship to promote spaces of symbolisation through negativity; absence in presence; search for a new object originated in a lack (e.g., André Green's [1983, 2001] negative hallucination or Lacan's [1951/1998] scansion).
15 Interventions that use the analytic relationship to communicate experiences of figurability of the analyst.
16 Interventions that use the analytic relationship to promote beliefs based on the ideology of the analyst.
17 Interventions that use the analytic relationship to promote an idealised relation with the persona of the analyst.

Another possible source of investigation in the CCM's field of work with the interventions would be the study of noninterpretative interventions and their relationship to the analyst's implicit working model. The same could be thought of for nontransferential (extratransferential) interpretations. There is a present tendency in the wide psychoanalytic actual work observable in clinical material both from international supervisions and debates in different societies to use predominantly extratransferential and noninterpretative interventions. It is possible to find in literature theoretical arguments for both trends, but it will be very useful and clarifying to study the implicit models of the mind and technique considered to better understand the 'why-do-we-think-what-we-do-works' item.

It would also be conducive and useful to investigate different types of interventions (transferential, nontransferential, noninterpretative interventions, etc.) and the frequency of sessions to help in this pervasive issue in the discipline.

Investigating the implicit models

On the implicit model axis, the CCM method and workshop groups could investigate, and have since its beginnings, the 'map' of implicit models in different regions and inside one region, identifying the constitution of these implicit models, as well as their relationship to time (for example, the evolution of implicit models in periods), with its cultural and theoretical changes. There is an a priori supposition that implicit theories change faster than (so to say) 'official' theories, influenced by general knowledge vicissitudes, cultural fluctuations, and partial theoretical developments.

In this axis, it would be very productive to study the participation of the non-psychoanalytic elements of these models and to compare them on an intraregional and interregional basis. Every implicit model is constituted by psychoanalytic and non-psychoanalytic components. It is possible to consider, in a very synthetic manner, that our psychism is formed by the transformation of our personal experiences by the activity of a 'meaning formation' element that will permit most of us human beings to know about ourselves, have a permanent potential of interpreting experiences, and have an intuition about others' intentions, pleasures, pains, and other feelings. The parcel of experiences that are not transformed in meaning throughout our lives will remain in a spectrum going from highly disturbing elements (psychotic and psychosomatic) to predominantly behavioural/adaptive ones, incapable of exerting a 'psychoanalytic function of the personality' (Bion, 1962/1991, p. 89) or a 'translating activity' (Laplanche, 2015, p. 194; see also Laplanche, 2011). Our personal analysis should expand this 'psychoanalytical function', but cognition, memory, logical thought, and our identifications (even those nonalienating) will contrapose the (so to say) meaning-searching drive and occupy a proportional space in the constitution of the implicit psychoanalytical model of each of us. The usefulness of this investigation would range from a better understanding of the effect of these 'non-psychoanalytical' constituents of our models and, consequently, in work with patients, to, occasionally, have a new hypothesis of why, in specific circumstances, our treatments do not work. I have already proposed some actions of these non-psychoanalytical elements in a comment to Jorge Canestri's paper in 'O conceito de processo analítico e o trabalho de transformação' (Calich, 2004).

Investigating communication among analysts

In the axis of communication among analysts, an instrument could be developed to assess how much the group (in principle, heterogeneous) can understand (not necessarily agree) with the other components of the group and how much the presenting analyst understood the group's considerations. Extending this issue, another instrument could be developed to identify what elements of communication facilitate or hinder this interaction, apart from trying to replace concepts with descriptions.

The communication among analysts is a highly relevant issue and a central motivation to the CCM working party. Even if we depart from some similar core concepts, like unconscious and transference, we must immediately face the big differences between each psychoanalytic model these concepts represent. It means going from the origins of the Unconscious, its constituents, dimensions, and dynamics to the repercussion of these differences in the goals of treatment, the theory of technique, concepts of psychic change, and every other small piece of our theories.

Investigating psychoanalytic supervision

Research involving psychoanalytic supervision would have to be more extensive than that of the previously mentioned groups, because it does not come from the working groups themselves but rather from the application of the method.

As previously exposed, adding to the 'I-would-do-it-in-this-other-way' model the understanding of 'what-the-other-does', 'how-the-other-does-it', and 'how-this-other-thinks-it-works' can add to the psychoanalytic supervision model by offering, in addition to understanding the patient material and the supervisor's suggestions, the understanding of the implicit model of the supervised. This knowledge allows the supervised colleague to understand which psychoanalytic and non-psychoanalytic elements are in their model, as well as what their model contemplates as psychic change, as an intervention of progress, and as the selection of interpretative material, among other components.

The investigative instrument could comparatively study the evolution of a group of supervisions with or without this change into focus, considering the transformation of the implicit model of the supervised in each situation. Of course, the instrument would have to consider other variables that potentially influence the transformation of the implicit model over time.

References

Bion, R. W. (1991). *Learning from experience*. London, England: Karnac. (Original work published 1962)

Calich, J. C. (2004). Comment on Jorge Canestri's article, 'O conceito de processo analítico e o trabalho de transformação'. *Revista de Psicanálise da Sociedade Psicanalítica de Porto Alegre*, 11, 2.

Calich, J. C. (2016,September). *Presentation about the CCM and current lines of research*. Report for the IPA Investigation Committee Meeting, São Paulo, Brazil.

Green, A.(1983). *Narcissisme de vie, narcissisme de mort*. Paris, France:de Minuit.

Green, A.(2001). *Life narcissism, death narcissism*. London, England:Free Association.

Lacan, J.(1998). *Escritos*. Rio de Janeiro, Brazil:J. Zahar. (Original work published 1951)

Laplanche, J.(2011). *Freud and the sexual*. New York, NY:Unconscious in Translation.

Laplanche, J.(2015). *Sexual*. Porto Alegre, Brazil:Dublinense.

Minninger, K. (2015). Panel report, IPA Congress Boston 2015: Working Parties Today III: Methods and findings from comparative clinical methods (CCM) and initiating psychoanalysis (WPIP). *The International Journal of Psychoanalysis*, 96(6), 1647–1650.

Rudden, M. G., & Bronstein, A. (2015). Transference, relationship and the analyst as object: Findings from the North American Comparative Clinical Methods Working Party. *The International Journal of Psychoanalysis*, 96(3), 681–703.

Tuckett, D., Basile, R., Birksted-Breen, D., Bohm, T., Denis, P., Ferro, A., … Schubert, J. (2008). *Psychoanalysis comparable and incomparable: The evolution of a method to describe and compare psychoanalytic approaches*. New York, NY: Routledge.

Chapter 16

Clinical groups on the specificity of psychoanalysis today

A new research method for clinical understanding

Ana María Chabalgoity, César Luís de Souza Brito and Ema Ponce de León

Introduction

The topic of today's meeting has been the focus of several discussions, because it has forced us to explore a new area that was not within our scope of work. Our impressions, combined with the analysis and the clinical exercise consisting of presenting clinical material to the work group for consideration, resulted in the initial observations shared in this study. We hope that it opens the floor for future discussions and studies with regard to the foundations of our field.

What is the role of metaphorical constructions in our group work?

In response to this question, we describe our working methodology, conceptual framework, and several hypotheses that developed during the course of our experience.

The group worked with free-floating attention and listened to the analyst, who read the clinical material out loud. Then the coordinators invited the group to do an exercise in free association, constructing different metaphors to account for a work that, although it is partially communicable in the secondary process, is determined by the infiltration of the primary process given the working frame of the Working Party (WP) on Specificity, which uses the analytical method for their clinical research.

With the group work and the coordinator's interventions, the metaphorical deconstruction takes place and allows us to unveil and perceive the invariants of the patient's sessions. The material was derived from the patient's conflict and modes of psychic functioning and the transferential modulations of the patient–analyst pair.

The deconstruction work that occurs along with the metaphorical deconstruction brings us closer to the metonymic form of expression, specific to the work of the unconscious, as well as to the different emotional experiences and their transformations in the analyst's mind.

DOI: 10.4324/9780000000002-20

During the analytical process, the material transformed by the alpha function of the analyst was offered to the patient within the framework of the peculiar setting of the patient–analyst encounter. Through the work of subjective appropriation, the patient can use and even reinforce their own alpha function, in order to later transform their own emotional experiences into psychic elements that could be meaning–re-meaning (Bion,1984) In other words, in the WP on Specificity, we came into contact with different aspects of the conflict and the patient's psychic functioning through metaphorical deconstruction and metonymy.

At the same time, we believe that the unconscious capturing of traumatic aspects or events of the patient's experiential history (some never disclosed before, not even in analysis) can be captured by the associative group work, because it constitutes an extended listening of the discourse of the patient and the analyst.

This allows us to explore further the iconic and indicial elements found in the verbal and paraverbal discourse of the material that the analyst shared that could be considered precursors of symbolisation work and that facilitate the work of *perlaboration* (or *Durcharbeitung*, or working through).

The path reminds us of Arminda Aberastury's (1962) classic concept that, during a patient's first interview, the main aspects of the patient's conflicts and mode of psychic operations are condensed and later unfold throughout the analytical treatment.

Theoretical–clinical research and psychoanalysis

Psychoanalytic theory emerges as the production of hypotheses and models of different levels of abstraction to understand the psychic phenomena observed in the clinic and from which the existence of the unconscious is inferred.

These models give way to a generalisation that is then applied to particular cases, keeping in mind that they are conceptual hypotheses with the aim of understanding what has been observed but also to be contrasted in every case, based on their operability for the purposes of diagnosis and treatment of psychic suffering. Clinic and theory nurture and transform each other into a permanent dynamic process throughout the therapeutic process and into the theory of psychoanalysis throughout history.

Since Freud, clinical reports have served to inspire and exemplify theories. They allow the exchange between different clinicians to advance in the production of shared knowledge with the aim of understanding the psychic subject.

A clinical story is not a true story. It is the product of a series of transformations around a core of unconscious subjective truths that surface during the experience that takes place between patient and analyst.

The patient transforms their psychic material to reveal it to the analyst and, in turn, they both produce transformations during their meeting. Similar transformations occur in the transmission to third parties, either an individual (colleague supervisor) or a group of colleagues who produce transformations during their exchange.

What matters is not the real event but the subjective experiences about the event. The psychic reality must be differentiated from the event. This produces an effect on each subjectivity that differs from the historical reality. The focus is not on the past but instead on what remains, making the past a perpetual present.

Freud's psychoanalytic method is a way to treat the patient's speech during sessions and to investigate the psychic processes observed during and after the sessions, while seeking the cure for or relief from suffering. It is also a theorisation restricted by its specificity and, at the same time, open to all disciplines focusing on mankind.

To Freud, it is impossible to separate the clinical research process from psychic disorder treatment and theories about the psychic functioning that psychoanalysis proposes.

Therefore, we believe that clinical group work has an enormous formative value as a transmission of psychoanalytic praxis and a group method of research in action.

Some psychoanalytic concepts are important tools for understanding the method that the specificity clinical groups use, such as transfer and countertransference, psychoanalytical field, psychic conflict, and the fundamental rule.

In the psychoanalytical technique, the patient is asked to speak spontaneously, to include details even if they consider them unimportant, and to say what comes to mind, not choosing words based on a previous rational judgement. Freud (1910/1962) called this technical approach free association, and he proposed to the analyst, the counterpart, to listen in a state of evenly floating attention; that is, not to focus on anything in particular, to take into account their own stream of thoughts, not to transmit them directly to the patient, and to keep them to themselves. In that mosaic of free associations and streams of thought, interpretation will emerge and take shape.

The working parties device on specificity clinical groups

1 The working parties device consists of work in small groups of between 8 and 15 participants, who form a circle.
2 At the beginning of the activity, the work methodology is explained to the participants, and questions are answered.
3 In Latin America, the group works 2 half days. Each 2-hour work period focuses on one of the patient's sessions.

4 The sessions are separated by a break, replicating, in some respects, the timing of the analytical process.
5 The international groups work one afternoon and the following day so that the participants have the night to do the dream work.
6 The group has two moderators, a presenter of the clinical material and a reporter to take notes. The exchange is also recorded digitally, and confidentiality is stressed in all cases. The psychoanalytic method model is applied based on what occurs in analysis as a result of free association. The work material consists not only of the story read out loud, but also its effects on the inter-analytical exchanges in the group. The result is an open situation; no one knows what is going to happen or what will be discovered, not even identifying in advance the predetermined goals. This forces the participants to suspend judgment, to let themselves be taken by the uncertainty, reproducing the conditions of the analytical session.
7 During the last 2 hours of work, time is set aside for the presenter and the observer to discuss their impressions about the group work and for the participants to exchange ideas (including the moderators, observer), as well as the presenter.
8 The work ends with comments by participants about their experience with the WP model of specificity.
9 The framework is as follows:

   a The presenter reads to the group a report of three or four sessions of an analytical process that they have conducted, leaving out the patient's biographical data and the history of the analytical process. The analyst is free to present the report in whatever manner they prefer, including the patient's verbal and nonverbal discourse and the analyst's interventions. Theoretical references or interpretations elaborated after the sessions are not presented to the group. It forces them to focus on the psychic reality and become more permeable to their own unconscious.
   b After the presentation of each session, participants are asked to do free association, reacting to the material presented, as spontaneously as possible, with the purpose of exploring their manifestations and working with them.
   c The presenter remains silent and does not answer any questions until the group activity ends. Then the analyst expresses their impressions of the group work. The interaction based on factual events is thus avoided, allowing unconscious elements to arise, materialise, and gain strength in the group.
   d The moderators do not interrupt the flow of thoughts (similar to working with dreams), so that the group remains in an associative mode of operation, avoiding rationalising processes and usual devices such as the collective supervision of clinical material and theoretical formulations.

Hypothesis and objectives of this methodology

1 The central hypothesis of this methodology is that the associative work of the group, which we call interanalytical work, becomes an amplifier of the analytical situation presented. The frame's aim is to reproduce aspects of the analytical session, so that the transferential and countertransferential phenomena stemming from the presented clinical material are displayed in the group's associations and its different aspects are expressed by the different participants.
2 The individual and group analytical device is in itself a facilitator for the emergence of different manifestations of the unconscious. In the transmitted sessions and in the group dynamics, dreams, reveries, occurrences, associative evocations, failed acts, displacements, transferential, and countertransferential phenomena occur, referring not only to the analytical pair but also to transfers between the group participants.

In the WP on Specificity, there are two objectives, one focused on the group experience in itself and the other on subsequent research.

1 During the group experience, the method is based on the analogy between the analysis session and its report to the group, who reacts to the listening with their associations.
2 As a research group, its aim is to work on the elements acting in psychoanalytic treatment as it is practiced today with the diversity of theories and practices. The material obtained serves as research material for another group of analysts that constitutes a research group.

The research objectives are to

1 Question the way in which the psyche treats and transforms perceptions, feelings, and thoughts.
2 Define the current conditions of the practice, what is done, how it is done, and why, leaving aside preconceived knowledge about the specificity of psychoanalysis stemming from clinical material
3 Understand multicultural aspects of current psychoanalysis by means of international conferences and meetings, so that the participants contribute with their original analytical culture.
4 Strongly mobilise psychic defences. Associating in a group is different from the associations that emerge during an analysis.

Observations about the groups

Different psychoanalytic theorists have studied the characteristics of group functioning: Bion (1961), Balint, Courtenay, Elder, Hull, and Julian (1993),

Anzieu (2009), Pichon-Rivière (1999), and Kaës (1995, 2000), among others, insist that the unconscious processes occur within groups. At the same time, the group mobilises specific aspects that are theirs.

Interanalytical exchanges produce material that is different from that of a dual discussion or group supervision (Kaës, 1995). The group is a specific psychic entity that cannot be broken down into individuals (Kaës, 2000).

Group communication occurs not only at the level of the conscious self but in the form of different conscious and unconscious group phenomena that develop between the different protagonists, producing between them transferential phenomena.

Kaës (1976) proposed the concept of a 'group psychic apparatus' that links and transforms psychic elements and cannot be reduced to individual psychic devices.

The group produces a particular intersubjectivity that is open to the multiple and, at the same time, is tied together by a creative associative thread that is unique and specific to each group in a given situation. This creative group process re-creates, in its operation, transference experiences and emotional climates, but at the same time it transforms the material into a new spiral of resignification.

It is important to keep in mind that a clinical report is already a transformation and what happens in the group is a new transformation-discovery of the report. The transferential elements of the analyst/patient pair were distributed between the different participants of the group

What is produced when working with this clinical method?

In the different experiences, the presenters observed that, surprisingly, the group associative chain (verbal discourse and nonverbal and paraverbal manifestations of the members) was able to reconstruct almost all of the elements of the presented cure and understand prospectively how the cure could continue.

Frequently, certain events not included in the analyst report and unknown to the analyst (not even represented) emerge, determining the transference–countertransference of the analytical pair.

This aspect, which always surprises us, is currently a focus of research. It is based on the question of how the group manages to reconstruct elements of the cure that do not appear in the explicit narrative, as well as why, in this kind of group work, certain aspects that are still unknown – referring to the unconscious traumatic, to aspects that the patient and analyst do not know – emerge through group associations in the form of images, similar to dreams, and redirect certain events in the patient's history, when the purpose is precisely to avoid presenting historical data.

Kaës (1995, 2000) described how the group is an activator of sensory experiences and of images, capable of intensely mobilising body and affections. As a group, the participants are able to transform and represent the affections of the other and transmit them to the 'group body'. We ask ourselves how it is possible that the psychic signs or marks that have not yet been translated by the patient's psyche take a posteriori significance in the production of the associative chain.

We hope that the ongoing research will further our understanding of individual and group psychism. Currently, we are focusing on many questions and challenges stemming from this way of working, mainly the emergence of group associations and their relationship with the material's nonmanifested aspects, some unknown even to the analyst. All of it brings to the centre of our discussions the work with the unconscious promoted by free association.

References

Aberastury, A. (1962). *Teoría y técnica del psicoanálisis de niños*. Buenos Aires, Argentina: Paidós.

Anzieu, D. (2009). *El grupo y lo inconsciente: Lo imaginario grupal*. Madrid, Spain: Biblioteca Nueva.

Balint, E., Courtenay, M., Elder, A., Hull, S., & Julian, P. (1993). *The doctor, the patient and the group: Balint revisited*. London, England, and New York, NY: Routledge.

Bion, W. R. (1961). *Experiences in groups*. London, England: Tavistock.

Bion, W. R. (1984). *Learning from experience*. London, England: Routledge.

Freud, S. (1962). Five lectures on psychoanalysis. In J. Strachey (Ed.), *The standard edition of the complete psychological works on Sigmund Freud* (Vol. XI). London, England: The Hogarth Press. (Original work published 1910)

Kaës, R. (1995). *El grupo y el sujeto del grupo. Elementos para una teoría psicoanalítica del grupo*. Madrid, Spain: Amorrortu.

Kaës, R. (1976). *L'appareil psychique groupal: Constructions du groupe*. Paris, France: Dunod.

Kaes, R. (1993). *Le groupe et le sujet du groupe. Elements pour une théorie psychanalytique du groupe*. Paris, France: Dunod.

Kaës, R. (2000). *Las teorías psicoanalíticas del grupo*. Madrid, Spain: Amorrortu.

Pichon, R. (1999). *El proceso grupal*. Buenos Aires, Argentina: Nueva Visión.

Chapter 17

Faimberg's Listening to Listening method

Haydée Faimberg

Introduction

We were asked by the editor of this book to provide a reflection about how the authors think that their method is a research tool, how they select clinical materials, where their emphasis is.

In our reading, these terms of reference imply the postulate that the methods of the working parties *are* a suitable tool for clinical research in psychoanalysis. To address these highly relevant questions, we need to adopt a decentred approach. The proposal asks not to speak of the method *as such*; they presuppose there are other places where to do it.

I was thus led to spell out the basic theoretical assumptions underlying our method (Faimberg, 2019) *and the means that we tested experientially in groups for that purpose*.

Ricardo Bernardi (Chapter 6, this book) states that the scientific conditions for clinical research (*Forschung* [Freud], translated as *recherche* [French]) require that what is studied should be reproducible so that it can be thus *verified that something is true*.

Because it is a scientific condition of the clinical research tool in psychoanalysis that what is studied should be reproducible, *reproducibility becomes at least in part an implicit organising principle* behind the questions and answers.

We concur with Bernardi (Chapter 6, this book) – *and this is also central to our method* – on thinking that *criteria of truth cannot be determined by the prestige of the person who enunciates them as such*. Idolatry (my term) and its authoritarian injunction effect need to be freely questioned. Through the concepts of traceability and reproducibility, Bernardi explores this essential issue. The place of traceability and reproducibility in our method is addressed below.

We have been able to distinguish two points (both important) in regard to our method:

First, it is our legitimate aspiration to have the existence of our method recognised as such by contributors to this esteemed publication, who have devoted a large part of their lives to clinical research, epistemology, and linguistics. In particular the editors of the book recognise that the method we

DOI: 10.4324/9780000000002-21

present in this chapter has its own existence without needing to subject us to a predetermined epistemological condition.

In the second place, on the basis of how we, at our working party, understand this recognition, we are free to think about the issue of clinical research and reproducibility exclusively insofar as it relates to our method. We shall do so by first spelling out the basic assumptions that guide our method and make it what it is. Our reasoning based on analysis of the logic framing our method allows the reader to see the traceability of how we have come to think as we do. I hope that the reader will share some of the curiosity that I felt while writing this chapter.

Questions in the light of our method

I asked myself what the basic assumptions underlying how we listen to, recognise, understand, and assess a clinical presentation were.

I recently wrote and published an article (Faimberg, 2019) as an answer I found for continuing to investigate new questions in psychoanalysis.

We invite the reader to read that article (Faimberg, 2019), which sets out an analysis of the basic assumptions underpinning our method, while bearing in mind these two questions:

1 Does our method allow what is to become intelligible (by virtue of the actual method) to be reproducible?
2 Would our method be capable of allowing such an operation of reproducibility in the future, in cases where we have not as yet considered it to be possible or even desirable?

Allowing the operation of reproducibility means allowing it *without* the method itself running any risk of being denatured (a) in its theoretical conception; (b) in *its way of functioning* in a discussion group; and (c) in the way that *the actual experience also becomes a tool for investigating the method itself*.

Basic assumptions

'Recognition of otherness' is one of the basic assumptions that help to shape this method. The goal of recognising differences is achieved through criteria that are developed experientially, in the actual practice of the method.

This means (a) that there are no criteria for *assigning preexisting content that might serve to anticipate* the dialogue that will emerge in a group, (b) nor are there criteria for *previously codified content whereby subsequently*, at any time in the dialogue, *the effects produced by the method* (in the practice of the dialogue) can be assessed.

The fact that the criteria for recognising differences are developed in the actual practice of the method does not mean that the method does not have clear goals in itself. The goal clearly set by the method is to discover the basic assumptions of a specific presenter that lead them to work as they do.

There is no content that had been previously singled out. This choice allows the possibility of what I have called an 'as yet situation' (Faimberg, 2013a). This is a clinical concept that I developed to refer to psychic temporality in psychoanalysis. It refers to a type of temporality that is *not* unilinear: it is a situation that has not happened ... yet.

When the situation 'happens', *the fact of its happening will be an effect of the actual practice of the method.*

We have four basic assumptions (Faimberg, 2019), initially only clinical concepts: (a) 'recognition of otherness'; (b) the 'as yet situation'; (c) 'listening to listening' (Faimberg, 1981/2005a, 1993/2005b, 2005d, 2007); and (d) 'misunderstanding' (Faimberg, 1995/2005c).

What are the characteristics of our method that make it what it is?

Our method meets a twofold requirement:

On the one hand, that of facilitating and preserving an acceptance of not knowing in advance the content of what we shall be listening to in the clinical presentation and in the discussion.
On the other hand, that of being curious and wanting to know when, 'in listening to ourselves listening' (which I call decentred listening), there are moments where we are able to deduce the presenter's basic assumptions and the basic assumptions of each participant.

This twofold requirement and the nonlinear temporality of the as yet situation constitute a *necessary condition* for our method.

Analytical listening

The importance we give to the ups and downs of analytical listening in our method is reflected in the very title: 'listening to listening'. It was initially conceptualised as a concept deriving from psychoanalytical listening in the session (Faimberg, 1981/2005a, 1993/2005b).

With this method of discussing clinical material in group (not to confuse with the psychoanalytical method in the session, which is the one Freud instaured), we listen to presentations and discussions by analysts from very different cultures, within a frame in which we all actively place ourselves in a *position of not knowing*. I have been guided not so much by the actual text written by Bion 'with neither memory nor desire' (1967) but, above all, by Bion's visit to Buenos Aires in 1968 (Faimberg, 1989, 2000).

I have called this entire dialectical complex the analyst's 'counter-transferential listening position' (Faimberg, 2013b): *Without theory there is no listening and without listening there can be no modification of any theory.* All analysts listen according to their own psychic life; the history of their transferential relationship with their own analyst; their relationship with their supervisors, seminars, and readings; their relationship with the institution to which they belong; etc. (Faimberg, 1989, 2013b).

We try to understand from what basic assumptions we are listening to the presenter and how we are trying to understand from what basic assumptions the presenter is listening to their patient and interpreting or not interpreting. We explore, in particular, the impact of each participant's basic assumptions on their own way of engaging in the discussion.

In listening to how each participant listens to each other participant, we try to detect, by listening, a sort of gap between the various ways of listening: *the sources of misunderstanding* can begin to reveal themselves. Potentially, then, we start being able to recognise what might be each participant's basic assumptions, which would be the source of the misunderstanding.

This form of misunderstanding that gives access to the basic assumptions in question is one of the ways of characterising the method.

Reviewing in the light of our method the two questions left in abeyance

1 Does our method allow what is discovered by the actual method to be reproducible?

To the extent that the method consists of *a process of discovery not foreseeable as such in advance (as yet situation) and is different in each experience, what is discovered by this method is not reproducible.*

How can we combine rigorous *thinking* with the method and the knowledge that each group meeting will map out through the psychoanalytical approach of free association paths that are specific to *that* group? Resolving this ticklish problem each time is a conscious goal of *this* method.

The Spanish poet Machado (2003, p. 16) put it well when he made us hear through the music of his poetry: '*Caminante, no hay camino / se hace camino al andar*' (Traveller, there is no road, but the road we make by walking).

2 Would our method be able, in the future, to allow the operation of reproducibility, without the method itself running any risks of being denatured in its basic way of functioning?

What would happen in the case of a *programmed decision, selecting something designed to produce some effect obtained by our very method* (whatever the effect to be reproduced)? The very attempt at such programming would bring about a qualitative modification of the actual method, since it would entail a change in its framing logic.

We believe that we have made it possible to *trace* the line of reasoning that leads us to maintain the method as such.

In the poem we have already quoted, Machado (2003, p. 17) also tells us: 'And when you look back, you see the path that you will never tread again'.

In the case of the International Psychoanalytical Association Working Parties on Clinical Research, the *frame* selected (in the sense that we understand the frame, following José Bleger; Faimberg, 2012) has its *own* life, which implies its *own necessity of evolution*, evolution that pertains to *the logic of its own frame*.

We are convinced that there are *different* ways of exploring psychoanalytical thinking.

As Bernardi (Chapter 6, this book) states, the German term *Untersuchung*, translatable as 'investigation' in both English and French, refers to an activity of exploration in the broad sense.

We may infer from this Freudian clarification that, in psychoanalytical investigation, the condition of a traceability that leads to reproducibility (a condition for research [*Forschung*]) *would not be*, from the perspective of our method, *a necessary condition*.

Genuine psychoanalytical investigation and genuine clinical research both start by bracketing (*epoche*) the principle of authority embodied in idols (often in psychoanalytical and other institutions).

Faimberg's Listening to Listening method may be classified as a method of psychoanalytical investigation (*Untersuchung*; Faimberg, 2019).

Like so many other analysts, we learned from José Bleger about the fundamental importance of the frame (Bleger, 1967). The question of the conditions under which each frame allows for a given goal to be explored is a whole topic in itself (Bernardi, 2009; Faimberg, 2012).

An opening rather than a conclusion

We choose not to subject our frame to any requirement other than that dictated by its own logic.

Our method focuses on fulfilling the requirement of mainly discovering the as yet situation; that is, the situation that has not happened … yet, and of being able to give a status to

1 the complex structure of misunderstanding;
2 the way of hearing misunderstanding through the 'listening to listening' function;

3 actively supporting the position of *not knowing in advance what type of misunderstanding would become relevant for our investigation* in the context of a *focused* discussion of one piece of clinical material;
4 detecting at what moment a situation *occurs* in which the basic assumptions in play in the dialogue can be perceived.

On this basis, wanting to know why the presenter works as he does becomes a genuine subject of investigation.

Without these basic assumptions, the method I have proposed could not continue to be the method that it is and that is designed for the 'hunting' of psychoanalytical thought, *including its unconscious dimension*.

What will 'reading of reading' make of this essay?

Note

1 See also Faimberg (2014). This method has been put into practice for more than 10 years on three continents, and an account of its implementation would require a separate paper. As an example, let us simply say that, in Latin America, this method has been and continues to be offered at congresses of the Federation of Psychoanalytic Societies of Latin America (FEPAL) and the Brazilian Federation of Psychoanalytic Societies (FEBRAPSI), with great attendance and interest. It is part of the regular activity or was present in meetings of psychoanalytic societies of São Paulo, Porto Alegre, Lima, Panama City, Montevideo, Buenos Aires, São José do Rio Preto, Uberlândia, Florianópolis, Ribeirão Preto, Fortaleza, and Marília. These activities are moderated by Cláudio Laks Eizirik and Sérgio Lekowicz and sometimes by Victoria Korin. If we add Dieter Bürgin, Antoine Corel, and Haydee Faimberg, we have the members who comprise our working party. Maybe we could add that the method is practised with a group of analysts belonging ideally to different psychoanalytical cultures (i.e., the European Psychoanalytical Federation, the International Psychoanalytical Association) and listening for the first time to a clinical presentation, or with a group consisting of analysts from the same culture (belonging, for example, to the same institution), where prime importance is given to *what distinguishes* each individual analyst. It is also practised by analysts in training belonging to different institutes (International Psychoanalytical Studies Organization, IPSO) or even to the same institute (i.e., in Australia, in Brazil).

References

Bernardi, R. (2009). Qué metapsicología necesitamos: Vigencia de J. Bleger. *Revista Uruguaya de Psicoanálisis*, 108, 223–248.

Bion, W. (1967). Notes on memory and desire. *The Psychoanalytic Forum*, 2(3), 272–280.

Bleger, J. (1967). *Simbiosis y ambigüedad* [*Symbiosis and ambiguity: A psychoanalytic study*]. Buenos Aires, Argentina: Paidós.

Faimberg, H. (1989). Sans mémoire et sans désir: à qui s'adressait Bion? *Revue française de psychanalyse*, 53(5), 1453–1461.

Faimberg, H. (2000). Whom was Bion addressing? In P. Bion Talamo, F. Borgogno, & S. S. Merciai (Eds.), *W.R. Bion between past and future*. London, England: Karnac.

Faimberg, H. (2005a). 'Listening to listening': A contribution to the study of narcissistic resistances. In D. Birskted-Breen (Ed.), *The telescoping of generations: Listening to the narcissistic links between generations*. London, England, and New York, NY: Routledge. (Original work published 1981)

Faimberg, H. (2005b). *'Listening to listening' and the telescoping of generations: Listening to the narcissistic links between generations*. London, England, and New York, NY: Routledge. (Original work published 1993)

Faimberg, H. (2005c). Misunderstanding and psychic truths. In D. Birskted-Breen (Ed.), *The telescoping of generations: Listening to the narcissistic links between generations*. London, England, and New York, NY: Routledge. (Original work published 1995)

Faimberg, H. (2005d). *The telescoping of generations: Listening to the narcissistic links between generations*. London, England, and New York, NY: Routledge.

Faimberg, H. (2007). Plea for a broader concept of Nachträglichkeit. *Psychoanalytic Quarterly*, 76(4), 1221–1240.

Faimberg, H. (2012). José Bleger's dialectical thinking. *The International Journal of Psychoanalysis*, 93, 981–992.

Faimberg, H. (2013a). The as yet situation in Winnicott's Fragment of an Analysis (1955): Your father 'never did you the honor of' ... yet. *The Psychoanalytic Quarterly*, 82(4), 849–875.

Faimberg, H. (2013b). 'Well, you better ask them': The countertransference position at the crossroad. In R. Oelsner (Ed.), *Transference and countertransference today*. London, England, and New York, NY: Routledge.

Faimberg, H. (2014). Método Faimberg 'escucha de la escucha', [entry *'método'*, 'method']. In C. Borensztein (Ed.), *Diccionario del psicoanálisis Argentino*. Buenos Aires, Argentina: Editorial APA.

Faimberg, H. (2019). Basic theoretical assumptions underpinning 'Faimberg's method listening to listening'. *The International Journal of Psychoanalysis*, 100(3), 447–462.

Machado, A. (2003). Cantar XXIX. In *Proverbios y cantares*. Madrid, Spain: Diario El País.

Chapter 18

Developing the capacity for clinical investigation

The Working Party Microscopy of the Analytic Session

Roosevelt M.S Cassorla, Ana Clara Duarte Gavião and Cláudia Aparecida Carneiro

'If you want to be universal start by painting your own village'.
(Leo Tolstoy, 1828-1910)

Since the 1990s, two of the authors of this text have been seeking methods to improve the analytic capacity of the candidates of the Brazilian Psychoanalytic Society of São Paulo. Years later, now knowing the various working parties (WPs) of the European Federation, these experiences have broadened. From tests conducted with groups of candidates and colleagues, technical procedures have gradually arisen to suit the objectives and preferences of the coordinating team. With a defined methodology, it came to be offered as an elective course to São Paulo candidates. The course has been running since 2008, with high demand. In 2009, it was adapted to become the WP Microscopy of the Analytic Session, which came to be held, by invitation, in societies of Latin America and in all of the Latin American and Brazilian psychoanalysis congresses. In this text we will give a summary of how it functions.

The principal objective of the WP is to develop the capacity to practise and think about the psychoanalytic clinic.

The specific objectives are to

1 develop the intuitive capacity of the participants.
2 develop the capacity for thinking about the phenomena experienced.
3 develop the capacity for constructing interventions/interpretations, including the paths that lead to this.
4 identify and understand implicit and explicit theories that guide the analytic work.
5 develop the capacity for validation of the clinical work.
6 develop the capacity for clinical investigation.

The WP permits the investigation of other specific objectives depending on the ways in which the material is studied.

DOI: 10.4324/9780000000002-22

The coordinators use theoretical assumptions and hypothetic models that guide their observation:

1 The WP members' ensemble constitutes a group in which there is the installation of a field (Baranger & Baranger, 1961–1962/2008), the WP field, in which group members influence each other. The clinical material and the analyst who presents the material also influence the members. In the WP field nothing occurs with any member that does not reverberate in the others.
2 Each intervention made by a group member is seen as an emergent field that reveals its dynamics in that exact moment.
3 The WP field functioning is considered analogous to the mind functioning. The adopted model of the mind implies unpredictable connection possibilities between aspects with varying degrees of symbolisation and nonsymbolisation. It also involves attacks on both the possibilities of connection and the connections already established. The symbolic and nonsymbolic facts include affective aspects that involve and are surrounded by them. These aspects express and evoke feelings and emotions. In this model, the mind is the outcome of the fertilisation of other minds and they are also fertilised by that one.
4 The phenomena occurring in the WP field are transitory and constantly changing. The observer influences them, and they modify the observer as well. Their apprehension, which occurs whenever they move, is punctual, and while they are apprehended they have already changed.
5 The WP field is considered a 'dream's' field (Cassorla, 2016). This model considers that the emotional experiences occurring in the WP seek transformation into images – like waking dreams – which, in turn, are connected to words. The field will reveal both the dreams symbolised by words but also facts seeking symbolisation (non-dream) that are revealed by emotions, discharges, acts, and other forms of non-thought.
6 The analyst's interventions result from the negotiation between intuited aspects and thought about these aspects; the analyst working with the patient does this task consciously and unconsciously. The interventions are the culmination of this negotiation that includes the dreams being dreamed and non-dreams that are looking for dreamers. The same occurs in the WP field: a conscious and unconscious negotiation between the intuitions that arise in the field (that is, this field constituted by the interaction among the WP members and other field products).
7 The factors of the interventions refer to dreams and non-dreams in interaction that manifest themselves in the field before the interventions done. The intervention is, therefore, a function of these factors.

The technical procedures are based on the detailed study of clinical material presented by a colleague.

1 The colleague in charge presents part of a session. The part is interrupted before the analyst intervenes.
2 The group, invited to 'dream' the clinical material, discusses freely.
3 Based on the discussion, the 'selected facts' of the group are identified, which are the bases for hypothetical interventions that are proposed to deal with the material presented.
4 The group seeks to identify the implicit theories that have determined the proposed hypothetical interventions.
5 The group listens to the intervention done by the analyst and the sequence of the clinical material. Possible implicit theories that have determined the analyst's intervention are discussed.
6 The group compares the analyst's intervention, the interventions proposed by the group, and the dynamics of the psychic change (or its absence) in both observation fields (the session and the WP). At this point, facts related to the scientific validation are discussed.
7 Another part of the session is presented, and so on …
8 During the activity, at the discretion of the coordinators, the group is encouraged to observe and discuss the group dynamic when faced with the material presented.
9 At the end, the presenting analyst takes the floor and discusses the material and their impressions of the group work.
10 Next, the group evaluates, in detail, the work that has been done. Two weeks later each member responds in writing to questions set by the coordinators.

Each group was composed of approximately 15 psychoanalysts or candidates. Work was conducted for 8 to 12 hours. There was a coordinator and one or two co-coordinators, whose functions were defined.

The meetings were recorded and the co-coordinators took notes as they listened. The record was transcribed and complemented by these notes.

The data were analysed using technical procedures of qualitative research applied to psychoanalytical facts (Cassorla, 2011; Turato, 2011). In this method, as occurs in the psychoanalytic clinic, the researchers make hypotheses that are linked to new hypotheses, and so on, reaching provisional conclusions that open up to new hypotheses, etc. The investigator tries to identify factors that expand (or not) the known universe.

Researchers know that the edition of the original material of the WP containing the comments of the members of the group, and the hypotheses formulated by the investigators are influenced by conscious and unconscious assumptions about them. As occurs with the psychoanalyst in their practical activity, the task of both the psychoanalyst and the investigator is to transform into objective their subjective apprehension. The reader, having access to the material, will be able to formulate their own assumptions.

The type of research proposed requires lengthy texts that make their presentation difficult. The transcripts of the meetings with the researchers' comments would take around 100 to 120 pages.

This text will present, only as an illustration, small excerpts from a WP conducted as part of a congress, with candidates and members from various societies. In addition to the teaching objectives, we use the original material to discuss the paths taken by the group to arrive at the interpretations. The same material was presented to another group and the results were compared. We will not have room in this text to address these aspects.

Illustrative excerpts from the work in the working party

ANALYST: It's the first session of the week, Monday, 7:30 in the morning. I open the door of the consulting room and find him standing outside, wailing, hugging his briefcase. He comes in and stays standing, crying; he seems not to know what to do. I ask him if he wants to lie down on the couch; he lies down on his stomach and remains in this position for some time, until he turns to me and says: 'Good morning. I'm sorry to present myself in this way, I can't be like this with anyone, not even with you. I almost called to say I wouldn't be able to come, but I came, because I need help. Either I come here, or I throw myself out of the fifth-story window! Because I'm feeling really bad [he cries a lot]. I feel like I can't do anything, I don't know how to live a happy life being who I am, there's just no way to fix it!'.

COORDINATOR: You're all free to express your own experiences, communicate your fantasies, dreams, waking dreams.

Intervention

1: The first thing that occurs to me is the emotional impact, the feeling of helplessness, despair, desolation, these emotions.

2: I thought he was like someone standing on the edge of a precipice, where the ledge is the analyst.

3: I thought about the briefcase he's holding. He's standing there hugging it and he was also lying down hugging the couch.

4: I was wondering whether this person only lives with a sense of urgency, whether this situation also applies to life. I felt very called upon, very summoned to be there beside him in this precipice, and to see what might be done.

5: I also went down this line of thinking, this impact of 'what can I do?' It's part of this impulse to protect, to secure, to support.

6: I noticed something beyond the impact, something to do with disorientation, as though he had lost his sense of direction.

7: I heard something more like: 'I thought about not coming, but I came; I thought I could cope, but I need someone, because it's not working on my own'.

8: I started thinking about ambivalence, when he says he needs help and at the same time ends by saying, 'there's no way to fix it, but I need help'. So, if he needs help, then there is a way to fix it. …

9: After the impact, I see the beginning, the preoccupation with the fact that he 'can't be like this with anyone' and 'can't be like this even with you'. This thing of 'not being able', of 'I can't' also made me think of one of my patients, who was a strong, manly guy. He was my first patient who lay down on his stomach and stayed there defending the most fragile part of his body, and still watching me, because I think there's this whole idea of helplessness. …

10: It also had an impact on me, and I felt really moved. But, at the same time, when he apologised, I felt a certain estrangement. It's not really estrangement, but I'm going to use a word that might sound exaggerated: it's almost a certain aversion, when he talks about being sorry; things seem to be all mixed up; I feel really moved and concerned, and, at the same time, very little, when he talks about being sorry, saying he couldn't come.

11: It's funny how, as we're listening, the ideas are being reorganised in our heads. Without really understanding, I latched onto the second part of the phrase, 'I can't be like this with anyone, not even with you', but he is being like this! It's almost like a question, 'can I' or 'can't I be like this with you?' 'Am I being paranoid?' or 'am I not?' Then there's the other phrase: 'either I come here, or I throw myself out of the fifth-story window', which also, in a sense, contains something distancing and, at the same time, very despairing, but also a certain threat.

12: I had the impression that his speech was highly manipulative, an attempt to induce the analyst into an emotional state. … I have the impression … of a very old form of functioning. …

13: I felt anxious, a little unsettled, imagining if this were to happen with me during an initial contact, how would I behave?

14: I had the sense of someone who is overwhelmed, unable to cope, in despair, and almost drowning, reaching out their hand: 'if you don't give me your hand, I will drown', and in a hopeful, more established, relationship.

15: I was thinking about the subject of hope, because this is someone who says he can't do anything. He doesn't feel he can do anything; he has no hope. So, something is changing, something said like this, 'I'll throw myself out of the fifth-story window' is a line from a song by the band Legião Urbana, and there's another line, 'nothing's easy to understand'. I think he's going through a really hard time, he's distrustful.

COORDINATOR: Could you please repeat the song lyrics. …

15: 'She threw herself out of the fifth-story window. Nothing's easy to understand. I want you to hold me. I'll run away from home. Can I sleep here with you? I'm scared, I had a nightmare. …'

16: I remembered a phrase by Machado de Assis (a writer), 'it is better to fall from the clouds than from a third-story window'. Then I got thinking … why would this patient be so distressed and hugging the briefcase, as though he was holding a teddy bear or his favourite blanket?

17: He believes that he couldn't be happy. He also has an idea of happiness and believes it can be fixed. Fixing is used to refer to a thing, an inanimate object.

18: I'm thinking about something else. It seems that this short excerpt has two parts. The first is when he presents himself without saying anything, non-verbally. There he is in despair, clutching his briefcase; you used the word 'hugging', but I just see him clutching the briefcase; and there he is, wailing with someone at 7:30 in the morning; he's bursting into tears, clutching the briefcase, and he seems to be lost, disorientated, and when the analyst asks if he wants to lie down on the couch, I thought it was very strange that he said, 'good morning'. What's that about? You burst into tears here; what kind of despair is this? And then you come here, what's all this 'good morning' about? It strikes me as false; the day already began in one way and now you're trying to organise it; I don't know. It doesn't fit!

19: And something else that caught my attention was when the analyst suggested that he lie down, and this made me feel a certain estrangement, because there he was crying, clutching the briefcase, and the analyst asked if he wanted to lie down. It seemed to me to be a little out of place given what was happening with him. So, I don't know what this reveals about the analyst's dreaming at this point, about perception. …

COORDINATOR: Could you tell us your dream of the analyst's dream?

19: It seemed a little out of place to me, … maybe I would have given him a handkerchief, a tissue I had at hand, something like that. I would've done that, but someone who apologises too much, who's very self-conscious like that, makes me react with estrangement, like 'why are you apologizing so much?' Another feeling comes over me again that distances me from the initial feeling of being moved.

COORDINATOR: There are lots of people wanting to speak. But we must carry on. Who's missing?

20: I think this person hadn't slept. They were in such a state of insomnia and despair in the early hours of the morning, I have the impression that he's very regressed, like when we're in the middle of a nightmare. For me, the image that came to mind was that of someone filled with crows of the night.

21: What also made me feel a little estrangement was 'do you want to lie down on the couch?' I saw the analyst's posture, of asking if he wanted to lie down on the couch, as a call to action from the other in the face of this sense of urgency.

22: I imagined someone like certain executives, wearing their suits like armours, with a tie and a briefcase; a false bottom, which is the only thing he has to hold on to, because the real one is gelatinous and comes apart, has no backbone, and he needs a backbone, yours or that of the couch.

23: In any case, I think he feels he is experiencing great danger. I don't know what, and he doesn't want to say that it's bad; it mobilises an intense fear in him, in his way of life. I was reminded of a joke: the groom arrived with the bride at the entrance to the hotel and said, 'I want a room with a high window and a strong latch, because it's the wedding night!' Fear can make someone want to throw themselves out of the window – so the latch is strong, and the window is high so that the patient can't run away or throw himself from the fifth floor.

COORDINATOR: I shall try to sum up what has occurred within the group. Then you can add to it. Initially, there was a very strong emotional impact, a sensation of shock, anxiety, fear; the initial statements from the group were in relation to the helplessness, the patient's despair and disorientation, his plea for help. Then, a certain distrust began to emerge on the part of the group, as though feeling an aversion; the middle group recoiled in the face of helplessness; from this, emerged the suspicion of manipulation and questions such as: 'Good morning!' 'What's that about?' 'Is it false?' 'What is true and what is false?' Then, the group started to get annoyed: 'can't do anything', 'not moving forward' I think this is the reflex of impotence. Then, there were a few jokes in relation to the third and fifth floors, memories of songs, questioning of the meaning of lying on one's stomach, looking, despair, manipulation, protection, wariness, regression. But it's manipulative, and we arrive at the carapace of the executive.

You've seen how the impact has been changing as the group has been thinking. We've had half an hour here, but in the session the psychoanalyst has only a few seconds. A lot can happen in these seconds. We're going to hear one more section, starting with the analyst's interpretation.

A: What do you think needs to be fixed and what seems to be irreparable? [Silence].

PATIENT: I'd like to be content with myself. I'm not content in the relationships I have, mainly with my family, and this weekend I spoke to my mom, dad, sister. ... Why are some people happy and they don't know it? Because I think so much about existence, and the more I think, the more I ask myself, 'what's happening?'. [He interrupts himself and says]: I don't like the couch! Can I sit in the chair? [He waits for my reaction, and I suggest that he sits wherever he prefers.]

***

The group continued reading and stopped before an intervention was made by the analyst. The process described above is repeated. Then:

COORDINATOR: The next step: you are going to try to imagine what you would say to this patient now. What intervention would you make? Some of you are perhaps thinking, 'I wouldn't say anything; I'd wait a bit longer'. But as part of our exercise, you must tell us what is going through your minds, even if you don't speak to the patient. [Silence]

58: [After hesitating over what words to use, concludes]: So-and-so, thinking is no substitute for the experience of contact with the other.

59: I'd talk about changing chairs and I'd talk about what he's looking for, that he can't seem to find a place where he feels comfortable. I don't know ... [hesitation].

COORDINATOR: Try to put it into words. ... Let's carry on and we'll come back afterwards.

60: I think I would say something along the lines of: 'What is happiness, what place is this? Who invented this concept of happiness?' I wouldn't say it in a clinical meeting, but I would say to the patient, 'Where do people find this kind of happiness?' [laughter].

61: I thought about how important the modulation of the voice would be for this patient. ... There's terrible pain. I think words are secondary, but the content would be that I'm seeing how he's suffering. ... 'I'm seeing how you are suffering, but I can also see that you've come here to share this suffering, this pain, with me'.

62: I have an intervention. I don't know. ... 'So you nearly called me to say you weren't going to come, but you came, and you spoke to your mother, your father, and your sister, but I don't know if you feel you were helped by them. You wondered what's happening to you and you came here. You almost didn't come, but you came, and I think that you imagine that, by talking with me, we might be able to understand what's happening to you'. And when he asks: 'can I sit in the chair?' I think he's looking for a place too, in such a way that the analyst might be able to help and clarify what is happening.The analyst and the group think this intervention is very long, addressing different aspects at the same time. With the help of the group and the coordinator, the intervention is reworked.

62: Now I can put it better: 'I think you want me to help you to understand what's happening to you'.

59: [Resuming]: 'I see that you're suffering, but you are in great suffering and have come to see me so that I can help you feel better'.

COORDINATOR: Based on this material and the group work, five hypothetical suggestions have emerged. There are more that could emerge, but we're going to stop here.

64: I'd like to make a new suggestion that has only just occurred to me: 'Are you trying to be happy here?'

COORDINATOR: Now we're going to work on the third step, we're going to leave the clinical part momentarily, and we're going to try to discover which theories have influenced these interpretations, primarily the implicit theories. You are not prohibited from talking about explicit theories … according to Lacan, according to Klein or Bion, … but what will interest us most are the ideas that the analyst used, consciously and unconsciously, which led him to make this intervention. The first interpretation was: 'Thinking is no substitute for the experience of contact with the other'.

65: I thought the analyst could be thinking about the emotional contact present in the session, between him and the analyst.

66: I see three points of focus in the interpretation. Thinking is no substitute for the experience of some kind of contact: one focus is thinking, thought; another focus is the experience; and maybe the third focus is the other, so it's just one speech that encompasses three points.

COORDINATOR: And what are the theories behind this? What factors have led them to favour these three aspects, and in this way? You don't have to respond, it's for all of us to think together. …

67: The experience of contact with the other.

68: I understood that the analyst is trying to think about her own experience, that things are dispersed. How can this be dealt with through thinking? And what is the experience of being with someone in this way? I think she wasn't just saying this to the analyst, and she was saying this to herself. …

69: I think there is an invitation for an emotional experience, but I'm asking myself whether it's clear to the patient that it's an invitation. Thinking about the analyst, she speaks 'of the emotional experience'. I'm wondering whether the patient felt more the question of no, of defensiveness, or whether he picked up on the invitation; the invitation is subtler.

COORDINATOR: How are we going to know what the patient has picked up on?

70: In the next step. …

COORDINATOR: Exactly, this would be the fourth step, a stage we will be encountering shortly, which is validation. We are going to see what the patient did with the intervention, only the patient is not here. From this point on, we will do it with the analyst's intervention. Right now, we are going to continue with our own. But let's observe that there is no interpretation that disagrees with the others, all of them more or less complement each other. This leads us to think that they're all following a close path, which may be right or may be totally wrong, but if it's totally wrong, then the patient will show us, and then we'll see whether the analyst is also following our suggestions ... [laughter].

***

The group continues the discussion, addressing the other interpretation proposals. Next, it will focus on the analyst's interpretation, and so on. Once this stage is finished, they continue reading the material, returning at each stage.

When the discussion of the material is finished, the analyst who presented the material takes the floor. The analyst talks about what they want, about the patient, what they observed in the group work, about their feelings, etc. Then the group joins in to add to what the analyst has said, with the participation of the analyst and the coordinating team.

Finally, an evaluation of the activity is conducted, with each member of the group contributing in the way they want to. Two weeks later, each member sends an evaluation in writing.

Individual evaluation of the group work

What follows is an example of one of the individual evaluations, very similar to the rest:

> (...) the WP enabled transformations in the way I worked. The ability to exchange experiences and being able to see how colleagues from different places and at different stages of training think has been very productive. It is difficult to put into words, but I think that what best represents my sensation is a broadening of the thinking capacity. Listening, recounting, exercising my clinical comprehension, honing my listening skills. Feeling, within the group, something close to what the patient is bringing, but which must be worked through in the group mind for some time before emerging in the sequence of the session, this was one of the great lessons. The attitudes of colleagues, the most varied, the unidealised, the different levels of comprehension, the plurality of possibilities for understanding are all, in my view, examples of learning. The observation and comprehension of the unconscious phenomena, the patient, colleagues in the group, the group itself, and my own unconscious working enabled the

expansion of knowledge and emotional experiences. Another aspect refers to what has been learnt about various theories and technical aspects, indirectly. I took advantage of our theoretical differences, adding to them, which can and should be developed in this type of work.

Another interesting point was the question you raised: 'How could we talk to the patient about this or that?' producing an exercise in reflection, seeking to transform the 'dreaming-in-group' into 'psychoanalytic language'. I don't feel I'm able to describe the learning very well, but I can assert that the WP is a fundamental activity in the construction and maintenance of the analytic identity.

Conclusions

Our method does not reach final conclusions. We travel paths, we verify the alternatives that made these paths covered in the way they were, and we are aware that other possibilities exist. We reflect on the factors that led us to certain choices. We identify expansions and retreats of the analytic field and discuss them.

When we review all of the material, from the beginning, we see how the various facts involved (out of session, in the inner world, in the analytical field, in the WP field) were 'dreamed'. The group chooses to interpret these aspects. Certainly, the reader can travel other paths, and it is this fact that characterises the psychoanalytic clinical research. The paths taken by other researchers will be more or less similar or quite different. But they will always be additional. Otherwise, we would not be facing a field of knowledge.

We are referring to the investigations that every psychoanalyst performs, in their daily clinical work, as a highly involved observer in the investigation process with their patient. The analyst is encouraged to observe closely what they do, increasing their ability of participating, observing, feeling, appraising, discussing, reflecting, validating, and invalidating clinical facts; that is, dreaming and thinking them.

The psychoanalytic method shows us that 'as we walk, we make our path' (*se hace el camino al andar*). The WP investigative method makes us take some distance and observe how this walk is being done while we walk. It is what a psychoanalyst does in their clinical work. But when this is done in the WP field, there are many visions, various vertices of observation and understanding, performing that 'second look' (not always possible in their lonely work), enriched by 'many eyes'.

The investigation continues. The very analyst, in reviewing what happened during the WP, in reading the transcripts, in rethinking the experiences, will find other vertices that will expand their thinking capacity. They will find new readings and vertices. The reunion with the patient, new interactions, other discussions, other WPs, and the analyst will increasingly know themselves. This is the desired outcome of investigation – to expand the professional self-knowledge.

The same occurs with the WP participants. Each new experience will be linked to the previous experiences of the participant analysts, increasing dreams and the ability to dream that will be available when working with their patients.

In recent years, we have been investigating what happens when, after detailed discussion of the material, we return to it again from the beginning. Other forms of second looks, as we have seen, involve the same material being studied by different groups. Themes such as 'the construction of interpretation' (Cassorla et al., 2016), 'unconscious communication', 'development of the symbolisation capacity', 'transformations in the analyst's way of working', 'comparisons in the psychoanalytic work with analysts from different theoretical fields', etc., may form various outlines that determine specific objectives in the investigation. There is nothing to prevent the metrics of certain aspects also being used.

References

Baranger, M., & Baranger, W. (2008). The analytic situation as a dynamic field. *International Journal of Psychoanalysis*, 89, 795–826. (Reprinted from *Revista Uruguaya de Psicoanálisis* 1961–1962)

Cassorla, R. M. S. (2011). Introdução. In E. R. Turato (Ed.), *Tratado de metodologia da pesquisa clínico-qualitativa* (5th ed.). Petrópolis, Brazil: Vozes.

Cassorla, R. M. S. (2016). Dreams and non-dreams: A study on the field of dreaming. In S. M. Katz, R. M. S. Cassorla, & G. Civitarese (Eds.), *Advances in contemporary psychoanalytic field theory: Concept and future development*. London, England: Karnac.

Cassorla, R. M. S., Gavião, A. C. D., Carneiro, C., Galvani, M. R. P., Silva, M. P., & Carvalho, R. M. L. L. (2016, October). *The construction of interpretation: Investigation performed during the Working Party 'Microscopy of the Analytic Session'*. Paper presented at IPA Clinical Research Meeting, São Paulo, Brazil.

Turato, E. R. (2011). *Tratado de metodologia da pesquisa clínico-qualitativa* (5th ed.). Petrópolis, Brazil: Vozes.

Part V

Working parties in action

Chapter 19

Zoe

Luisa Pérez Suquilvide

Zoe was in her mid-20s when she contacted me for the first time through WhatsApp. She was a beautiful, smart girl with a childish air and a very neat and fashionable look. She lived alone and had a stable job. She described her suffering as a 'depersonalization syndrome', an unusual expression for everyday speech, which surprised me. There was a remarkable contrast between the coldness of this term, her prosody, and the images that she used to describe how she felt: the feeling of detachment from her body; looking at life from behind a glass; seeing others live and not being connected; opening an invisible door toward another dimension; being displayed on a window. In those early days, crying often interrupted her story.

Her childhood was marked by the divorce of her parents when she was 9; the mood swings of her mother, mostly depressions; and her mother's death in a car accident when she was 11 years old. Afterwards, she went to live with her father and his new wife until she was 18, becoming the only one among her schoolmates to live by herself at that age. Although she had suffered when her mother died, it was at 17, under the influence of a large dose of cocaine, that she faced a sinister suffering and a real horror that burst out like a volcano, along with a huge and unbearable fear that she could only handle through her depersonalization syndrome.

The first year of analysis, getting closer to her memories and in contact with her pain was a way to feel and understand what the depression and death of her mother had left like inside her, as scattered pieces of a puzzle or as an enigma. Getting in touch with her emotions and breaking through the blockade maintained for so long enabled the symbolization of the horror of her mother's death, her own finitude, and the fear of madness. Narcissistic aspects and identifications were also at stake. After the death of her mother, who was the only one who had made her feel valuable, confident, and strong, she started feeling like a number, something without special value.

After 2 years of analysis, transference began to change, and anger took the scene. At that time, it was related to frustration or feeling excluded by her boyfriend, or ignored by her father, or bullied by her friends when she was a little girl. Lived as an internal enemy, anger could be controlled by splitting

DOI: 10.4324/9780000000002-24

and isolation and was expressed through different metaphors, such as living on autopilot and getting inside an egg or a capsule. A common metaphor built independently, but at the same time by the two of us, came as a surprise to me: spinning in a hamster wheel. Creating routines, spinning things around kept her feet on the ground, making her feel that everything flowed but nothing happened, an opposite feeling to depersonalization. Routines were a way to deal with her daily life and to modulate the intensity of anger, perceived as a big and nasty monster asleep inside her. The monster metaphor condensed the aggressive aspects of her mother, the threat of her illness and death, and her own hatred. But, still, it was a way of keeping her alive. Zoe feared leaving her past behind and identifying with her mother. She felt as if she did not know who she was and wondered whether she could be someone without her, as if she were trapped in a bubble between the world of the living and the world of the dead. Slowly, she began to catch a glimpse of how badly she had to disconnect back then from the feeling that she could die without her mother, while connecting with the intense emotions that were blocked at that time, moving forward on grieving.

In the third year of analysis, she moved in with her boyfriend and started a degree in social work. Conflicts with him were growing along with a pent-up anger that she felt she had to block and smile instead. Feeling unhappy, she started to think she had to leave him. It was hard to face that there was something inside her that tended to provoke him to leave her, instead acknowledging some sort of pleasure in breaking up, in detaching herself from the burdens she felt she had in her life.

News from Aleppo were breaking stories those days, and Zoe was horrified by the bombs exploding on people. Even if she could be happy, she felt something self-destructive, disturbing, and macabre inside, like a missile that could be activated and detonated by any argument with her boyfriend. At that moment, spinning in the hamster's wheel took on another meaning, a way of not getting in touch with those feelings. A dream came up: a dog barking with its body split apart, detached from it, but unknowing of being dead. Her associations brought the identifications and lack of discrimination of her mother. She felt that there was a side of her that was living without a part and would die, because nobody can survive without a part of their bodies.

Sometime later, after having had a presentation at the university, though she felt terribly nervous prior to the talk, she was very confident and calm when she started speaking and very happy afterwards, feeling that she was in a wheel spinning and going somewhere. Two things struck her those days: realizing the importance of the bond that had grown between us and how a breakup would hurt and how much she loved her boyfriend and how painful it was to think about losing him, becoming aware that the more she loved him, the weaker she felt. Her career, a creative personal project, showed her that there are surprises in life that are not completely negative, giving her hope when she was feeling stuck. Separation was no longer like death, nor was her inner world full of death and destruction. The hamster wheel, which spun in the same place without moving forward, was now a spinning wheel to spin somewhere new.

Chapter 20

Panel

How are metaphors identified and elaborated by the different working parties?

Elizabeth Lima da Rocha Barros

The aim of this presentation is to show how the working party known as Comparative Clinical Methods (CCM) identifies and works with metaphors, although this was not part of our initial approach.

I believe this discussion aims at making the work of the many working parties potentially comparable, and the theme of the metaphors has been selected as a possible source for comparison.

Modell (1997, p. 219) suggested that metaphors are 'the currency of the mind', an idea that I agree with. It almost goes without saying that metaphors, as a currency of the mind, vary in significance and comprehend a number of possibilities, because they include several dimensions of the human emotional experiences.

Our aim in the CCM is to try to identify and unravel what is guiding the analyst's interventions; in other words, the implicit theories and beliefs with which they work. When discussing a session within the framework of the CCM methodology, it is not part of our method to focus on the ongoing metaphoric processes as such. Despite this not being our objective, by focusing on these processes I will try to pinpoint a perspective to evaluate them. It is important to point out that, even though this is an individual viewpoint, all of the ideas here contained are the product of a rich discussion with the members of our group.

Because I need to create an approach, based on the question asked to us, I am proposing to evaluate the progression of metaphorical processes in terms of how much they cover and how inclusive they are, as part of the evolution of symbolic forms, whether they are part of the analyst's intervention or the patient's narrative.

Due to restrictions of time, I will only focus on some brief sections of the clinical material at our disposal, which will be used as examples of how we might be able to find some common ground among the diverse working groups.

I will try to identify, in each of the categories of either step 1 or 2 of our diagram, the presence of metaphoric processes.

DOI: 10.4324/9780000000002-25

Step 1 is made up of six categories and focuses on the examination of the diverse possibilities of interventions by the analyst.
Step 2 is made up of five categories and strives to unravel the implicit theories with which the analyst is working.

Given this, I could return to our main theme and formulate the following questions: How can one evaluate the areas covered by a metaphor or by a metaphoric process? Can we identify their presence in each of the categories under the headings of steps 1 and 2?

Following Montana Katz (2013) and inspired by Modell (1997), we could say that metaphoric processes may be viewed as systems of mapping out the ongoing symbolic processes in a session or during a certain period of time across many sessions. Inspired by Modell's (1997) ideas, I am thinking of metaphors both as linguistic bridges that connect body to mind and as bridges that connect unconscious affective states to the patient's verbalizations.

When choosing this particular focus, I am assuming that these unconscious affective states, expressed by means of metaphors, are essential for the examination of the transformations occurring in the mental articulation of the patient, whether in their conscious or unconscious manifestations.

But a question then arises. Would we consider everything that transpires in a session (or sessions) a metaphor? But if we do so, the very idea of a metaphor loses all of its heuristic value. Therefore, I will be restricting the use of the word *metaphor* to the expressive aspect of symbolic forms, arising in specific contexts, which I will identify, and I am aware that this sometimes involves arbitrary decisions on my part.

Therefore, how can we evaluate progressions of symbolic forms contained in the metaphors? The answer to this question brings me to a number of papers I have published along with my husband, Elias M. da Rocha Barros (da Rocha Barros, 1999, 2000, 2006; da Rocha Barros & da Rocha Barros, 2016, 2017), on the nature and process of creation of symbolic forms.

The answer we gave to this question takes us back to the work of Donald Meltzer (1984) and Susan Langer (1942). Inspired by these authors, and often following their formulations *ipsis literis*, we suggest that metaphors evolve through 'the progression of symbolic forms' that constitute the vehicle of metaphors.

In order to capture the emotional experiences, included in the unconscious phantasies, we need symbols as mediums. The philosopher Susan Langer (1942), in her theory on how meaning is built, introduces the distinction between two categories of symbols that seem to me useful to understand what occurs in the 'metaphoric process' of reverie.

Langer (1942) distinguishes between *presentational* symbolism and *discursive* symbolism. The first one is associated with expressive forms of emotion, is nondiscursive, and has a fundamentally connotative nature (refers to the subjective meaning and transmits information by *evoking* other realities through associations and sensorial forms). The second is discursive and has mainly only a denotative nature (refers to the objective meaning, the word in its dictionary form).

Words are our most powerful symbols because they provide plasticity to thought when they acquire a connotative character, thus distancing from the concreteness of experience and its representation.

Presentational symbolism is intuitive (many times a form of condensed intuition) and feeds on patterns of our emotional life; it is through this form that affects are evoked. Its aim is not the presentation of ideas as propositions or concepts, such as happens in natural language, but to exemplify a *feel-like* experience. This distinction between symbolic forms allows us to grasp, describe, and reflect on evoked representations.

Langer (1942), commenting on how feelings are grasped and conveyed through symbols, referred to the central role played by presentational symbolism and suggested that it has the property of transmitting what she calls 'likeness'; that is, it 'exemplifies objectively what feelings seem to be subjectively' (Innis, 2009, p. 47). Other authors (Dewey, 1931; Peirce, 1992) refer to this same property of symbols as a quality of *suchness*; that is, of exemplifying a situation or a character through a set of distinctive qualities. By 'suchness', these authors understand something very close to 'similitude' or, rather, the capacity to suggest *types of experience*. Let us look now at the specific qualities of each of these two types of symbolism. Presentational symbolism does not name but exemplifies that about which we are speaking (Innis, 2009). Innis (2009) wrote: 'Feeling itself, the perceived suchness of things is a form of meaning-making, and forms of feeling can be expressed in material media [images for example], which give us true knowledge, although it cannot be put into words' (pp. 47–48).

In this context, we are considering that symbols captured by the means of evocation are the crystallization of intuitions. These may or may not assume an expressive form of an emotional experience.

This term, as we are using it, derives from Collingwood (1938) and Benedetto Croce (1925/2002) and refers to an aspect in art that aims not only to describe or represent emotions but centrally to both transmit and produce them in the other or in one's own self through an evocation, a mental representation colored by emotion. Expression precedes the communicative capacity through words. Within our present context we can say that it is a representation directed to someone. This would be the characteristic feature of communicative projective identification. From the psychoanalytic standpoint, expressiveness is one of the essential components of projective identification.

Meltzer (1984, pp. 28–29) wrote:

> But if we [were] to allow that 'meaning' goes beyond the perception of the gestalten and that mental life goes beyond anything that one could [see] as a property of computers. ... We would need to take this concept as implying the possibility that mentation is non sensuous in its inception, that it is concerned with objects for which forms need to be invented or borrowed from external reality, that emotion as its central phenomenon and laws, are not those of logic or mathematics, but of 'progression' in formal qualities (Langer) or 'transformations' (Bion).

Meltzer (1978) said that the visual images used in dream work, as the result of working through (transformation), increase their complexity, sophistication, and level of abstraction, and it is in this way that the transformation or growth broadens the generality of the mental formulation and, likewise, increases the specificity of its use. To the extent that new emotional networks are open, new memories that were split before or repressed become available through evocation to be integrated in the river of meanings that constitute the mental life of the patient.

The analyst, through their reverie based on the feelings, images, and experiences evoked in their mind by the patient's material, can access what the symbols *represent* in their broader denotative and connotative nuances.

These images evoked in the analyst's mind by the patient's projections are developed in *affective pictograms* [1] (da Rocha Barros, 2000), which include all the expressiveness of mental representation and become something that exists between pure experience and the abstractions of these experiences.

We are suggesting that meanings are broadened as they become related to other parts of the self, due to the breakdown of barriers that prevent contact with other emotional experiences.

***

Within our methodological framework, I believe that step 1 seems to make more sense to examine, taking into consideration the richness of the metaphors in the clinical material.

Zoe's case is especially suited for a more detailed examination with regards to the communication between patient and analyst in terms of the nature of metaphors used, by both analyst and patient. The analyst transpires to be a reliable, serene, and available person. This attitude seems to have allowed an emotional development in Zoe. The analyst uses models and images in her interpretations. We could even call them affective pictograms.

The patient also uses very lively metaphors in her verbalizations, and those seem to gain in complexity as the analysis progresses in a very touching way.

Reasons for the consultation

I am not going to repeat all of the vignettes of the clinical material, because they are available to everybody. I will only refer to some images that seem to me to condense the communication of the patient or of the analyst.

From the very start, we could already consider the manner in which Zoe refers to the reason that brought her to analysis to be a metaphorical communication. Zoe describes very promptly her experience in the first interview. She describes it as a feeling of being 'completely out of my body, with the sense of being far away, as if I was looking at life from behind a glass'.

This image comes to me as a powerful description of a feeling of depersonalization and of estrangement in relation to herself. Additionally, 6 months into analysis, she adds: 'It's a feeling that goes beyond what people talk about, beyond literature, beyond Borges's poetry with the mirrors. … I needed to identify with something. … It happened to me with *The Scream* by Munch. …'

ZOE: I woke up and I felt weird, I thought it was a hangover. … It was as if I had an eternal hangover.

ANALYST: A hangover from your mother's death. You didn't suffer when she died.

Thus, in the first representation of her problem and as the center of her anxiety, Zoe defines herself as depersonalized, as someone who is not a subject, owner of her own feelings, but instead is lived by or through them.

This feeling is expressive of an acute anxiety, but it does bring elements to an understanding of the deep nature of her anxiety.

After 1½ years of analysis, Zoe refers to the image of a hamster going around indefinitely in a wheel to describe the feeling of living her life going around in circles, without any progress, and she illustrates this when she speaks about her life with her boyfriend. It is interesting to note that this same image of the hamster occurred to the analyst some minutes before Zoe made reference to it.

Z: [Pauses for a few seconds. The image of a hamster (8) comes to my mind. For a second, I think to tell her about it, but I don't, and she keeps talking.]

We can see here a metaphorical communication that associates the feeling of paralysis (partly conscious and partly unconscious) that dominates her life projected in the interpersonal relation. It is a metaphor of the pair.

The analyst interprets:

Z: In autopilot, the hamster wheel, being glued to the computer after your mom died. Everything flows but nothing happens.

The interpretation emphasises the depersonalised character that dominated Zoe's mind since the death of her mother, suggesting that it is a defensive maneuver.

These three metaphors would primordially indicate the way that the analyst conceives what is not well with Zoe (one of the categories of our step 2), and Zoe's material suggests a freezing in a given state of mind that impedes the working through of her mourning process.

The metaphors employed both by the analyst and the patient we would tend to see a *standstill* kind of situation, probably associated with the strong defensive structure of the patient insofar as these metaphors do not indicate a progression in formal qualities; that is, an increase of the encompassing of the affective nets involved.

These metaphors would only indicate that the way the analyst sees Zoe's difficulties did not change much in its content. This remark does not imply any judgment of the quality of the analysis, whether from the point of view of the interpretive angle of the analyst or from the point of view of Zoe's availability to cooperate so that the analysis could go on.

Three and a half years later, the analyst, in her interpretation, employs a very rich metaphorical image, suggesting that Zoe maintains an existence between the world of the living and of the dead: 'As if Zoe ceased to be a person, as if she became depersonalized and were trapped in a different world, in a bubble, between the world of the living and the world of the dead'.

Here, having in mind the perspective of our method about identifying what is not well with the patient, we can see a significant change: The patient stops being depersonalized and lives in a transitional space between the living and the dead. The metaphor is richer, more encompassing, and, at the same time, it points to a situation of a very specific space, that is, 'between the living and the dead'. This is a transitional territory (Green, 1986).

Later on, in another session, the metaphors employed by the patient and by the analyst point to a deepening with regards to how the analyst metaphorizes Zoe's internal world, which is now more alive and richer. This indicates, as one would expect, that Zoe is more alive and, for that matter, suffering more.

It is interesting to follow these metaphors. Zoe speaks about her experience of horror of seeing herself facing very painful experiences that were hidden from her before: her mother's depression followed by a fatal car accident and Fred (her fiancé) cancer. None of these were told to her by anyone in her family. She had to find out by herself and she uses metaphoric images to express how she has experienced this tragedy. She then associates this with what is going on in Syria and Aleppo, using a very strong metaphor:

Z: Today I looked at the news from Aleppo and Syria on my cellphone. … There's something, like, horrible in that, like a death, a war. … People want to run away, they hope they'll survive, and then a bomb explodes on them. … And I don't know why this affects me. … Even if I can be happy. … This thought lurks in me, like something impossible to avoid, like what those people go through. …The analyst in a sensitive way points out the following:

A: As if the monster were lying in wait for you, increasingly bigger and meaner, capable of making a bomb explode on you and destroy you, like the terrorists who sacrifice themselves.

Here, from the perspective of our method, we would see, through this metaphor, that the analyst's view of what is not well with Zoe evolves into something richer. This is more general but, at the same time, more specific, when she indicates that there is a monster in Zoe's internal world just about to explode, capable of expelling the equivalent to a missile. The metaphor here accounts for a monstrous internal reality – no longer external – that attacks her from the inside.

This is followed by a very expressive dream of Zoe's dilemma that allows the analyst to deepen her understanding of what is going on. Here the metaphors used by both become much richer and elaborate.

As she mentions the terrorists that immolate themselves, Zoe remembers a terrifying dream:

Z: I had a dream, always with a macabre touch. I related it to Aleppo. … An image I don't want to see, I don't want to know, but. … It was at my place [where she lived alone], and I don't know if it was me or a real estate agent that was going to show the apartment for rent. I started to show it, and there was a dog in the inner courtyard that had fallen, and its head had gone one way and its body the other way. But, since it wasn't dead, it barked and barked, as if it didn't realise that it had no body. … And I said to the people, 'Oh, I'm sorry about this, come this way', and I opened the closet and the drawers where I stored my underwear, my panties, … and the dog kept barking and its body was somewhere else, … as if it didn't realise it was dead. …Then the analyst comments:

A: Thinking all the time, brooding about things, like spinning in the hamster's wheel, could be a way of not getting in touch with that feeling of having something crazy, macabre, and disturbing that is about to explode any minute.

We can see, from the point of view of what we would emphasize in our method, that the analyst employs a metaphor still more encompassing than the previous ones. At the same time, this metaphor is very specific with regards to the existence of an unconscious phantasy of incorporating something monstrous inside herself, very crazy, macabre, and to the point of exploding.

This evolution in the type of metaphors employed by the analyst illustrates what we consider *progression in formal qualities of the symbolic forms* (here, the metaphors). This is precisely the point where we see a possibility of cooperating with the other groups, through the identification of the method employed by each one of us to approach the material of a session, irrespective of the specificity of each method. This is a possible bridge that would not interfere with our specific approach, characteristic of the CCM, and that integrates us in the world of the working parties through the possibility of doing a kind of investigation that would find a common ground between the various working parties.

Interventions and/or interpretation of type 1: Maintaining the basic setting

At this level, we consider both the contractual aspects and mainly the analyst's comments and the patient's responses that have implications in the maintenance or alteration of the setting. What are the implications at this initial level to the question of how we work with metaphors?

It is essential that we examine the analyst's and the patient's interventions that, somehow, affect the essential nature of the function of the setting. This is its condition of becoming an *incubator of symbolic forms* inside which, remembering Socrates (Hartke, 2007, 2017), the analyst searches to voice the *logos spermatikos* – 'the word that fertilises'.

In brief, I would say that the function of the analyst is to maintain the setting as an efficient metaphor that allows the unconscious to express/manifest itself.

Interventions and/or interpretation of type 2: Adding an element to facilitate unconscious process

This refers to interventions that aim to encourage more associations or links at an unconscious level even though, by now, the patient's metaphors reveal more superficial unconscious material, closer to consciousness and, therefore, at the border of verbal formulations.

From my perspective, we here include material that may be linked to the symbols called 'presentational' by Langer (1942, p. 79). They are experiences that are about to bloom into consciousness but still in the form of visual images with a more limited expressive capacity.

Due to time limitations, I will only mention one example of what I would consider a metaphor that would characterize an intervention of this category.

In the session chosen we see Zoe saying:

Z: Yesterday I blew up because I was hearing, 'Dad, Dad, Dad.' I tried to understand but I couldn't. ... I thought, how unfair! I did everything, and I can't even talk with Fred. I pretended to be asleep, and he says to me, 'Are you really tired, are you going to sleep?' And sometimes an enemy appears inside me that says, 'Okay, you know what? You can stay by yourself!' And I fell asleep.This leads the analyst to interpret:

A: It was as if you felt pushed out and unacknowledged. You got mad, you turned around and left, you fell asleep.

From the perspective of our method, this is a metaphoric comment that introduces an element to facilitate the unconscious communication. It is a metaphor that is not very encompassing but rather specific.

Interventions and/or interpretation of type 3: Questions, clarifications, reformulations, aimed at making matters conscious

Because these interventions are mostly in the form of questions, they produce material closer to consciousness. They may be amplified insofar as they connect with more unconscious material. For example, when the question generates an affect that opens a connection with new affective nets.

From my perspective, the degree of expressiveness tends to be larger when compared with material that is mobilized by type 2 interventions. It is likely that, in their responses, the patient will use metaphors that mobilize affects not yet expressed, more encompassing memories in feelings derived from more complex and more stable representations. But this material would still be contaminated by the focus suggested by the question and, therefore, much closer to consciousness and not the result of a genuine free association.

Even if it is in the form of questions, the analyst may be in that moment using metaphors that evoke in the patient situations that are a little more primitive and/or closer to memory. Questions always mobilize situations that are closer to consciousness but that may produce in the future new free associations.

Examples taken from Zoe's material in response to one of the analyst's interventions:

A: And your home? Which one is your home?The presence of an encompassing metaphor is clear here. This is a rich metaphor that may include many experiences and that helps Zoe to unblock a subject that, at this point, becomes conscious.

Z: [Gets very anxious, holds back her tears]. It's like, on the one hand, I want to have more opportunities to talk to Fred about that. What we're going to do, what's going to happen. ... I want to live with him, create something with him. ... I hadn't thought about it until now, but this thing of being on autopilot. ... I don't know if we don't talk about it because he doesn't talk about these things, or we don't talk about it because I don't let us talk about it. ... Now you ask me which one is my home, and I feel shaken, because I don't know which one is my home. ... I spend a lot of time at Fred's. ... My current place doesn't seem like a home, and the spirit of home is gone. I'm not. ... My place has no spirit. ... I like to have the protection of having my own place. ... I'm scared of talking about the future, of getting married, and having a life together. ... On the one hand, I really want to, and on the other, I don't. I had never thought I didn't want to. I'm thinking of it only now that you asked me which one is my home. [She's distressed.]

Interventions and/or interpretation of type 4: Designating here-and-now emotional and phantasy meaning of the situation with the analyst

These interventions are specifically oriented to the emotional meaning of the interaction with the analyst or to the meaning of the phantasy that reflects the nature of the relationship with the analyst.

From this point onwards, the analyst gains access to a more unconscious material that, in my formulation, would contain aspects that are more expressive and that would evoke a reverie in the analyst or a more complex countertransference. This would be both in what concerns the difficulty of transforming them into an interpretation and in what concerns the opening of new affective nets for the patient. This type of intervention tends to generate dreams.

At this level, the metaphors are more complex and tend to be associated not so much to metaphors that refer to singular situations but to metaphoric processes that encompass more than one emotional experience. It is likely that the analyst making interventions of this type will produce a larger opening for more connections with affective nets. Here the expressiveness mobilised by symbolic processes will tend to be broader.

After 3½ years of analysis, the analyst makes an interesting interpretation pointing directly to a possible emotion that the patient might be experiencing in the session in relation to how the patient feels the relationship with the analyst in that moment. The analyst says:

A: Perhaps you're scared of not knowing if I'll survive your anger, not knowing if your anger can kill me. And perhaps you need to know that I'll continue to be here, so that you can let what you feel come out as it is.

This type of intervention is more indicative of feelings that are present in the here and now and, therefore, less metaphoric, despite its power to stimulate the contact with unconscious fantasies.

Interventions and/or interpretation of type 5: Constructions directed at providing elaborated meaning

This category involves observations that are made in more than one session.

The word will only become fertile if it generates a piece of knowledge that goes beyond the facts. In other words, that may be transformed into experience; that is, *knowledge as experience* (Bell, 2017). For such a thing to occur, from my point of view, it is necessary for the analyst to pick up the metaphors employed by the patient and transform them into bridges between the representations of unconscious affects and their verbal formulations.

The metaphors are not any casual metaphors and they must never be an attempt to make an interpretation more attractive. Their aim is to enhance an assimilation of the emotional experience that was unveiled by the patient's metaphors.

In this case, the mother/analyst is a metaphor that includes all types of characters that are experienced by the patient as demanding and oppressive and that, in that particular moment, are synthetised in the maternal figure.

The reference to the mother may mobilise metaphors (or a group of metaphors associated to a metaphoric process) that are very expressive, referring to various temporalities, not only chronological but logical as well.

The phantasies contained in the metaphors evoked in the patient and by the patient may include not only her mother as an ancestor but all the figures that exert a maternal role in her life.

The following intervention by the analyst is an example of this category:

A: Separation is like death. Now that you start finding your center and the wheel is spinning in a different direction, you're happy. It's not like the hamster wheel, which spun in the same place without moving forwards.

Here we have an interpretation that involves a rather complex encompassing metaphor that opens up space for the hope of a meaningful leap in Zoe's analysis.

The analyst uses the previous metaphor of the hamster wheel and gives to it a new meaning in the here and now of the session. In this process, the previous metaphor is expanded and resignified. This opens up new affective associations that are relevant for Zoe's future emotional development.

Interventions and/or interpretation of type 6: Sudden and apparently glaring reactions not easy to relate to the analyst's normal method

Here we are talking about *acting outs* or *acting in(s)* of the analyst and we are immediately reminded of what Cassorla (2013, p. 327) called 'acute and chronic enactments'. For instance (as it is in our diagram), this happens when the analyst comments that the noise the patient complains about is quite normal and immediately realizes that her comment, apart from being unusual, may block the patient's free association.

At this level, we are dealing with unconscious phantasies that may have never been formulated verbally by the analyst or evoked in the mind of the patient by the analyst's *enactment*.

The enactment may be very expressive and, thereby, may contain a very complex metaphor transmitted mostly in action, even when this is a result of a verbal formulation that may be equivalent to an action. These reactions may occur in more than one session.

In view of the limited time that each one of us has to present a complex method, I come to an end, hoping that I was able to exemplify how the CCM could contribute to the exercise proposed by the organizers of this event.

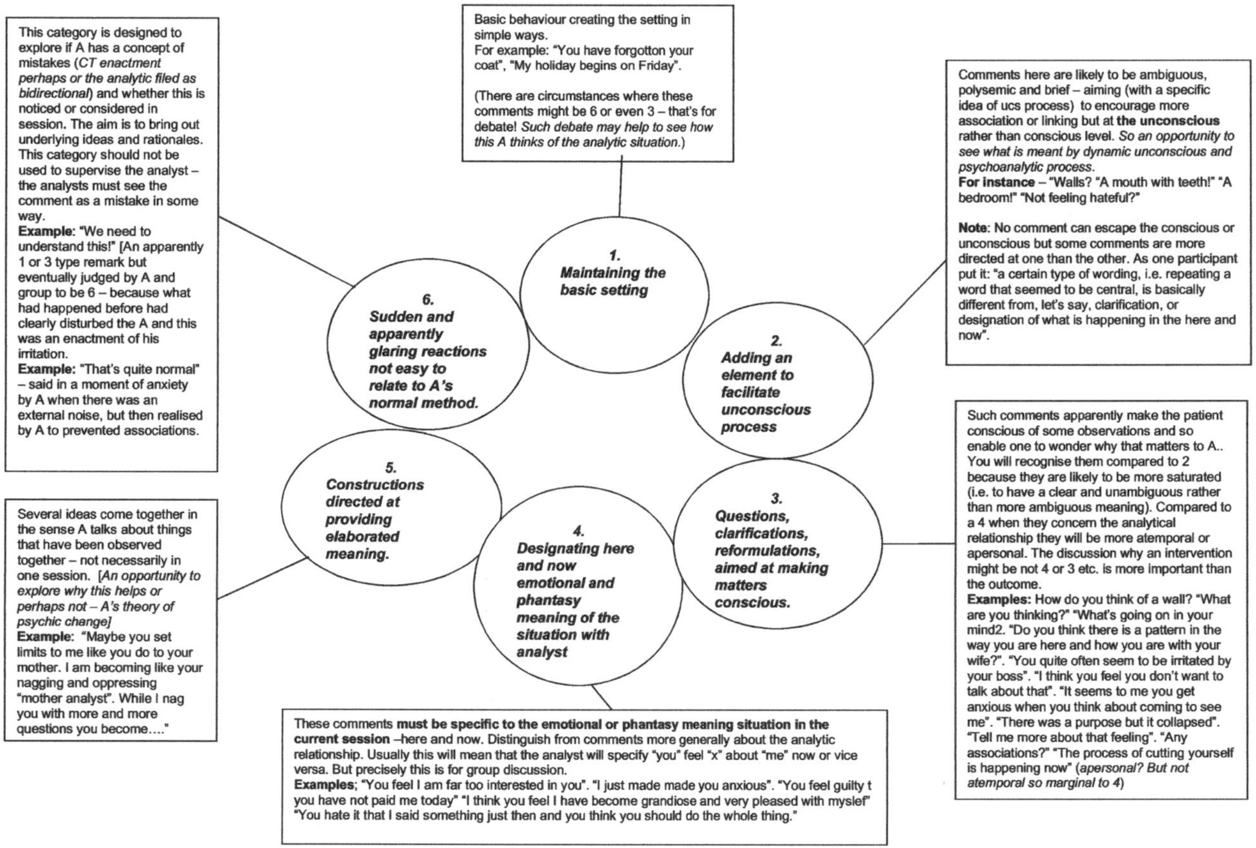

Step 1 appendix diagram

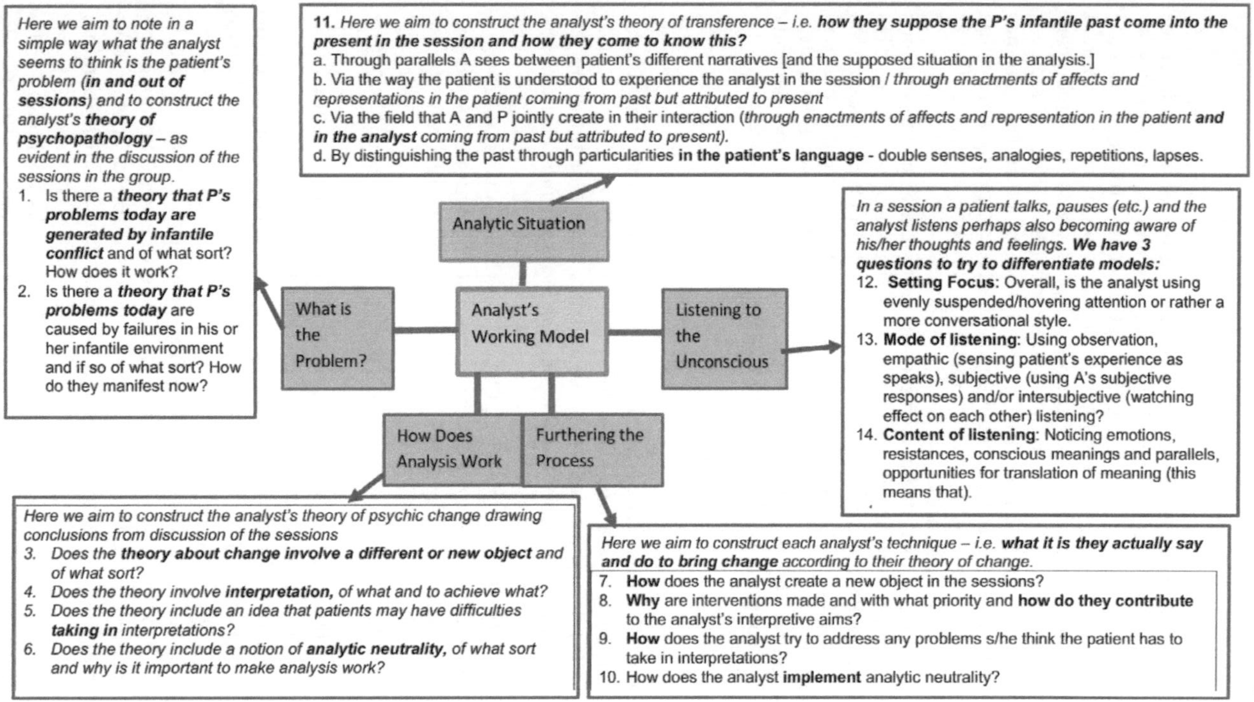

Step 2 appendix diagram

Note

1 The term *pictogram* is defined in Paul Robert's dictionary (1984) as a translation of ideas into figurative and symbolic scenes. I use 'pictogram' in a similar way, to refer to a very early form of mental representation of emotional experiences, fruit of the alpha function that creates symbols by means of figurations for dream thought, as the foundation for and first step toward thought processes. Strictly speaking, however, pictograms are not yet thought processes, because they are expressed in images, rather than in verbal discourse, and contain powerful expressive–evocative elements proper of presentational symbolism. Nevertheless, they are very different from beta elements (Bion, 1963), which are raw elements due to be expelled from the mental apparatus when they are not transformed by alpha function in alpha elements. An affective pictogram has the property of becoming an abstract variable capable of containing several similar (in meaning) emotional experiences.

In the process of being constituted and in their figuration, affective pictograms potentially contain hidden and absent meanings, kept in a suspended state. This absence of meaning is not reduced to the concealment of a presence. It consists more of a state of suspension, a reference to an absence, a discontinuity that will never be overcome and that constantly compels the psyche to broaden its instruments of representation. Representation constitutes a response to a permanently present absence and consists of a discontinuity that will never be overcome.

References

Bell, D. (2017). Unconscious phantasy: Some historical and conceptual dimensions. *International Journal of Psychoanalysis*, 98(3), 785–798.

Cassorla, R. M. S. (2013). When the analyst becomes stupid: An attempt to understand enactment using Bion's theory of thinking. *The Psychoanalytic Quarterly*, 82 (2), 323–360.

Collingwood, R. G. (1938). *The principle of art*. Oxford: Oxford University Press.

Croce, B. (2002). *The aesthetic as science of expression and of linguistics in general*. Cambridge, England, and New York, NY: Cambridge University Press. (Original work published 1925)

da Rocha Barros, E. (1999). Constituição de significados na vida mental. *Psicologia USP*, 10(1), 97–117.

da Rocha Barros, E. (2000). Affect and pictographic image: The constitution of meaning in mental life. *International Journal of Psychoanalysis*, 81, 1087–1099.

da Rocha Barros, E. (2006). Contratransferência e interpretação das relações de objeto. In J. Zaslavsky & M. J. P. dos Santos (Eds.), *Contratransferência: teoria e prática clínica*. São Paulo, Brazil: Artmed.

da Rocha Barros, E., & da Rocha Barros, E. L. (2016). The function of evocation in the working-through of the countertransference: Projective identification, reverie, and the expressive function of the mind-reflections inspired in W. Bion's work. In H. Levine & G. Citivarese (Eds.), *The W. R. Bion tradition*. London, England: Karnac.

da Rocha Barros, E., & da Rocha Barros, E. L. (2017). 'Attacks on linking': The Transformation of emotional experiences and its obstacles. In C. E.

O'Shaugnessy & C. Bronstein (Eds.), *Attacks on linking revisited: A new look at Bion's classic work*. London, England: Routledge.

Dewey, J. (1931). *Philosophy and civilization*. New York, NY: Putnam.

Green, A. (1986). *On private madness*. London, England: Hogarth Press.

Hartke, R. (2007). *Repetir, simbolizar e recordar*. Paper presented at '¿El psicoanalisis cura aun mediante la rememoración?', 45th Conference of the International Psychoanalytical Association, Berlin, Germany.

Hartke, R. (2017). *Lecture in Porto Alegre*. Unpublished manuscript.

Innis, R. E. (2009). *Susanne Langer in focus: The symbolic mind*. Bloomington: Indiana University Press.

Katz, S. M. (2013). Metaphoric processes. In S. M. Katz (Ed.), *Metaphor and fields: Common ground, common language, and the future of psychoanalysis*. New York, NY, and London, England: Routledge.

Langer, S. K. (1942). *Philosophy in a new key: A study in the symbolism of reason, rite and art*. Cambridge: Harvard University Press.

Meltzer, D. (1978). *The clinical significance of the work of Bion*. Perthshire, Scotland: Clunie Press.

Meltzer, D. (1984). *Dream-life*. Strachclyde, Scotland: Clunie Press.

Modell, A. (1997). Reflections on metaphor and affects. *Annual of Psychoanalysis*, 25, 219–233.

Peirce, C. (1992). *The essential Peirce: Selected philosophical writings* (Vol. I) (N. Houser & C. Kloesel, Eds.). Bloomington: Indiana University Press.

Robert, P. (1984). *Le petit Roberto dictionnaire*. Paris, France: Le Robert.

Chapter 21

A clinical illustration on the Working Party on the Specificity of Psychoanalytic Treatment Today – Latin American Group

César Luís de Souza Brito and Ana María Chabalgoity

Introduction

The Working Party on Specificity of Psychoanalytic Treatment Today (WPSPTT) is a permanent working and research group under the auspices of the International Psychoanalytical Association (IPA). With a psychoanalytic methodology, the WPSPTT conducts research on what is specific to psychoanalysis, the process of transformations that are set in motion in the minds of psychoanalysts, when they treat and transform a patient's clinical material. It uses as a device the work that occurs in the clinical groups of psychoanalysts gathered for this purpose, stimulated by the reading of three or four sessions of a psychoanalytic treatment made by an experienced analyst (Bleger, 2011).

The WPSPTT was created in 2006 by Evelyne Séchaud, then president of the European Psychoanalytic Federation. From there it extended to North America. Since the Chicago IPA congress in 2009, a group of Latin American colleagues, encouraged by the founders, have begun its inclusion on our continent. Currently the group consists of colleagues from Argentina: Abel Fainstein (Argentine Psychoanalytic Association, APA), Agustina Fernández (APA), Claudia Roqueta (APA), Elizabeth Chapuy (Córdoba Psychoanalytic Society); Brazil: Cesar Luis de Souza Brito (Porto Alegre Psychoanalytical Society, SPPA), Magda Khouri (Brazilian Psychoanalytic Society of São Paulo), Ruggero Levy (SPPA), Zelig Libermann (SPPA); Peru: Maria Luisa Silva (Peruvian Psychoanalytic Society); and Uruguay: Ana Chabalgoity (Uruguayan Psychoanalytical Association, APU), Ema Ponce de León (APU).

The Latin American group has been conducting its activities in different countries and congresses in South America. It has also proved to be an excellent practice for the development of the psychoanalytic functions of the participants and the interaction between analysts from different psychoanalytic cultures. We have been working with activities of two consecutive work shifts of 4 hours, with a night break between them, which allows a space of dream elaboration by the participants.

We have been very active and have done activities in various cities of the continent, as well as in the Psychoanalytic Federation of Latin America

DOI: 10.4324/9780000000002-26

and in IPA congresses. We have also conducted activities geared specifically towards candidates in various psychoanalytic training institutes. About 5 years ago, we offered our WPSPTT as a curriculum seminar in the analytical training of the APA.

The theoretical assumptions of the methods used by the WPSPTT

We have already described our method of operation in Chapter 16 in this book. Therefore, in this chapter we will make some reflections and expose the model that underlies our work.

The device constructed by the WPSPTT method is essentially based on the application and exploration of the fundamental rules of psychoanalytic treatment: the free association rule and its corollary, the floating attention, and the abstinence rule.

Thus, the device is set by bringing together from 8 to 15 psychoanalysts to free-associate after a stimulus of three or four psychoanalytic sessions. These sessions are obtained from a patient in a psychoanalytic process and reported by the conducting psychoanalyst. As part of the device, we have one reporter/observer and two moderators to conduct the group's free association work. The sessions are read as reported by the case-conducting analyst, without any other objective data about the patient or the history of that psychoanalytic process.

This device triggers the participants to operate the psychoanalytic functions of their personalities at the service of an interanalytic dynamic. This enables the development of an associative tissue, the weaving thoughts (Norman & Salomonsson, 2005), as the result of the immersive experience in the dynamic field provided. Unconscious fragments of the transferential dynamics of the patient's mental life and the dual patient–analyst process are diffracted in the group dynamics. This triggers unconscious, preconscious, and conscious elements in the interplay between individual subject and the *group's subject* (Kaës, 2007/2011) on this psychoanalytic field generated.

This device allows the extraction of certain elements specific to the development of a psychoanalytic treatment and serves as an instrument for research and assessment of the evolution of a treatment and its effects (Séchaud, Frish, & Bleger, 2010).

This work method is inspired by Norman and Salomonsson (2005) and also by Donnet (2005). Norman and Salomonsson (2005) brought inspiration from the model presented by Camargo et al. (1997) at the Bion Centenary held in Turin 1997 and applied it to supervisory groups.

According to Séchaud et al. (2010), the model is based on an analogy between the analytic session and its narrative to a group of analysts that responds to what they listen. The core of the research is to analyse the interanalytical exchanges in the clinical groups, from the discussion of a clinical material.

The WPSPTT is an *action research* (Frish, 2010) aiming to be as open as possible to the listening of what will emerge in the conjunction between the report of clinical material and the group's listening. We can retrace, a posteriori, the path of a research that uses the psychoanalytic technical instrument (Frish, 2010).

From the listened report, the material progressively becomes an associative tissue to which the participants bring their impressions, intuitions (Bion, 1962/1963, 1963/2004a), reflections, ideas, and hypotheses. The associative tissue, the thought work, is closer to a dream thinking, rather than a secondary-process reflection work (Séchaud et al., 2010).

The work material progressively ceases to be the narrative made by the presenter and increasingly becomes the narrative plus its effects on the group. In this immersive experience, the participants begin to explore their experiences from the read material and from the expressions of participants on the interanalytical exchange. All of that, with the load of emotions and symbols that it carries, triggers the participants to think and work with their own reactions to this (Bleger, 2009).

The case's narrative serves to stimulate the exchange of interpersonal experience of different approach styles, theoretical models, and psychoanalytic cultures. In this way, it constitutes a trace between the session and the interanalytic exchange.

The result of this associative tissue is neither a copy nor a duplication of the read session, nor is it intended to collect factual elements of the case. The interanalytic group performs a capture of unconscious and conscious elements of the ongoing treatment. That is, it characterises a replication of certain transferential configurations that are updated in the group's scope. It is also possible to observe the expression of specific processes of the analyst's work.

The associative manifestations of the participants are like resonance boxes and operate a work of transformations and displacements through the work on the transferential field. According to Y. Dorey, they seek to appreciate the conditions of the treatment and what it conveys, discovering and rediscovering the succession of *replicas*, disagreements, and remains that escape saying (cited in Séchaud et al., 2010).

In the group, the transference's elements are diffracted among the participants. A double associative chain is drawn: the one that the group releases in relation to the narrative considered a latent dream. And, at the same time, another in which each participant associates, leaning on what another said, and whose saying was not available to themselves (Séchaud et al., 2010).

The *replica*, the new folding over of clinical material engendered in the group's work, creates a unique potential space, irreproducible, that allows the trespassing of original *invariants* (Bion, 1965/2004b) of the case to penetrate in the group's associative tissue, updated by the analyst's embodied reading.

In the group discourse, multiple associative fragments are produced. These are expressed in speech, action, and emotion. Some of these associative fragments fertilise each other into a consistent narrative. Others move away or get lost in the associative tissue. There are still those that collide with others, oppose them, or even follow divergent or fragmented directions. There are different possible courses that potentially carry the fragmentation of intrapsychic conflicts of the case.

It is in a posteriori reflections, either on the course of the group work with subsequent reading sessions on new work shifts or in the late reflections or research on the reporter/observer reports or on the recorded transcriptions of the group work that it is possible to retrieve the traces of the *invariants* of the case left in the associative trails made by the participants. In this way we potentially have access to some degree of awareness of the latent elements of the patient's inner world and the analytical process.

The Latin American group also began a second design of research using content analysis (Bardin, 1977/2011) in its variant of discursive textual analysis (Moraes & Galiazzi, 2007) as research method as well as the main *action research* design, in a naturalistic and exploratory investigation of the material collected.

The focus of this research group is to analyse the emerging processes during these interanalytical exchanges. We aim to reflect on how psychoanalysis is practised today, after so many changes in the psychoanalytic theory and technique.

It is always surprising that participants in WPSPTT clinical groups, though unaware of the factual elements of the patient or of the process of analysis, retrieve various elements of the patient's factual life and personal and psychopathological history (Levy, Fernández, & Silva, 2015).

It seems to us that a group of analysts that listens to a fragment of clinical material is able to do a decondensation of the many facets and investments of a session by the communion among the participants of the resonances of the analysis presented.

Comments on the group's associations

The following is a partial illustration of this content analysis research using the verbatim of our WPSPTT activity at the international symposium of the IPA Subcommittee on Clinical Research and the APU: Working From the Clinic, Metaphor and Interpretation, held in Montevideo in 2017 (Brito, Chabalgoity, & Ponce de León, 2017).

Due to confidentiality and space constraints of this text, we will illustrate a fragment from the beginning of the patient's speech provided by the analyst, as a stimulus to the reader.

During the activity, the full reading of the session is given by the analyst of the case without interruption. At the end of the reading, the group begins its associations. Although we do not include the reading of the complete session here, we will present some quotations of the participants' associative chain that will allow the reader to get a rough idea of our group's interanalytic work. The associations allow some inference about the material reported in the session. Here, what interests us is the exploration of the group's associative chain as stimulated by the reading of the session.

We chose an initial fragment from the first dialogue that uses the expression *papa* repeatedly. The content was retrieved from an audio recording and from remarks made by the reporter/observer and adapted for this text.

In the associative interanalytic work performed by the group of participants, the utterance *papa* slides from semantics senses (father and meal) into an onomatopoeic form (*pa, pa, pa, pa*). This reveals an array of the emotional experiences potentially present in the patient's life and their personal history. Thus, it is possible to follow the rich development of the group's associations revolving around a potential *invariant*.

The associations described below were grouped into categories. We maintain the temporal linearity of their appearances in the associative work. We think that the associations are, to some extent, shaped by the force of invariants. These invariants allow the group to construct a supposed understanding of the patient's emotional experiences, from simple vestiges to hole theoretical anchorings.

PATIENT: Yesterday I blew up because I was hearing, 'Papa, Papa, Papa.'

I tried to understand but I couldn't. …

I thought, how unfair! I did everything, and I can't even talk with Fred.

I pretended to be asleep, and he says to me, 'Are you really tired, are you going to sleep?'

And sometimes an enemy appears inside me that says, 'Okay, you know what? You can stay by yourself!'

And I fell asleep.

We take the lines of speech as a group production and not as an expression of each individual. We understand the group associative chain as a potential expression of transferential elements, invariants of the emotional experience of the patient and the pair patient–analyst, which are diffracted in the different sayings and actions of the participants.

So, we take the reading of the session as a point of departure, the very first stimulus, which works as a trigger to the associative chain of the group. It is important to highlight that the focus of the work in the WPSPTT is the exercise of the mind of the participants itself, an *action research*.

Therefore, we are not searching the transformations done by the patient or their personal analysis in order to understand their psychic development. Instead, our focus lies on offering the participants a shared immersive experience with their own analytical listening skills and their technical attitudes of free-floating attention and free association, as well as with their own negative capability (Bion, 1970/2006). The intention here is to broaden the participants' mind availability and their capability of reverie (Bion, 1970/2006) in the group's dynamic field (Baranger & Baranger, 1961/2008; Bion, 1961/1975; Ferro, 2005; Freud, 1921/1969; Kaës, 2002, 2007/2011) and to observe the process that took place.

We aim to encourage participants to realise the possibility of using the technical instruments of psychoanalysis as a specific research instrument and enable us to explore what is specific to psychoanalysis today.

We have, as a result of the group activity, a *replica* as Bleger referred to it (as cited in Séchaud et al., 2010) of the case arising from imaginative and rational conjectures of the interanalytic group. This replica is an abstract construction that potentially contains significant inferred elements in the group's associative chain, similar to those presented by the clinical case. The associative disagreements, deviant remains, elements that emerge of group interaction itself and/or from the very own personalities and circumstances of the participants, approach or move away from those present in the case.

However, we have observed in several groups the emergence of replicas that closely resemble the case, including factual approaches not described in the reading of the case that are later revealed by the analyst in the latter part of the activity.

These facts lead us to think that there may be certain *invariant* elements (Bion, 1965/2004b) of the case, which are brought into the group activity by the presence of the analyst, even if unconsciously, or of the associative chain itself of the presented dialogue. Thus, these traces present in the psychoanalytic group field, when captured by the listening of the participants, fruit of the technical attitude of free-floating attention and free association, trigger the dream-thinking processes rather than the rational ones. This is a group condition similar of *reverie* (Bion, 1962/1963), in which the associative chains formed in the group are triggered and somehow modelled by these invariants, allowing the thought processes until reaching the rational pole of participants and researchers. It is this structuring of the group's associative material that enables our potential inference on the similarities and dissimilarities between the themes of the replica constructed by the group and the unconscious elements present in the case.

The methodology applied to treat this material

For the purposes of this symposium we restricted the treatment of material obtained in WPSPTT work to the stimulus provoked in the first segment of the activity after the reading of the first session of the clinical case. So, we got the verbatim of the work done at this stage and the observer's comments on it.

Here we present the design of research developed by the Latin American group WPSPTT using content analysis. The treatment of the interanalytic exchange was done by the first author due to the limited time we had between the group work and the presentation at the symposium. Our methodology comprises the treatment of the material by a pair of external psychoanalysts and two external psychoanalyst judges to confirm categorisation and a later discussion by the WPSPTT Latin American group. We approach the material with an a posteriori categorisation process. Thus, the categorisations emerge from the proper material.

Despite these limitations, the reader will be able to see the general model used by us to collect and to treat the material, as well as to have the scope of the richness and complexity of the interanalytic weaving.

The process to treat the material begins with a free-floating attention reading, as many times as necessary, so that the researcher feels immersed on it. It is similar to psychoanalytic free-floating attention and reverie. The objective of this stage is to permit the researcher to get in touch with the documents and to open themselves to be invaded by the impressions and signs evoked.

Then, the material is explored in order to select *registration units* (RUs). The RUs are units of a text clipping (segments of a sentence or even complete sentences or paragraphs) that are able of express a well-defined meaning by itself.

Next, the categorisation process takes place. The categorisation is a process through which the raw text data are transformed by clipping, with new additions and enumerations, allowing a synthetic representation of a content. The RUs are grouped into *beginning categories*, which are in their turn grouped into *intermediate categories*, and these are finally grouped into *final categories*.

With the categorisation process of content analysis, we retrieve 15 themes that we had taken as initial categories. They are (a) blast, (b) spirit of the empty house, (c) routine, (d) movement/shaking, (e) child trauma, (f) confusion/indeterminism, (g) house/place, (h) papa-papa-papa, (i) translation, (j) abandonment, (k) childhood, (l) support, (m) little quarrel, (n) disorganisation/depersonalisation, and (o) child sexuality/Oedipus.

In this text we regrouped the *intermediate categories* into *contingent categories* (CCs), based on psychoanalytic listening. So, we formulate the following CCs:

(I) Based on the form of emergence:

a From semantics to phonetics – 'papa, papa, papa'.
b Action and circulation: association in act.

(II) II.Based on thematic content:

a The blast and the routine.
b Confusion and delimitations: who is who?
c The house, the support and the abandonment.
d The support fails and a disintegrated self.

Below, we present some CCs followed through the quotations that compose them. The number preceding the quotations refers to the order in which the speeches of participants appear along the work. Thus, the number between brackets, as in (1), refers to the first speech that appears, and so on. We had 88 quotations in this first part of the work.

In the following CC, we can see how the quotes can emerge at different times and thematic contexts. These create a web with comings and goings of contents throughout the work. The themes emerge into a complex system that is organised from what is latent in the material, the trace of the invariants of the clinical situation.

Qualities present in the associative process

The resources used by the group to weave their associative tissue are interesting and varied. The use of semantics in its metaphorical and metonymic senses weaves a richness of material. Also, the sound of words, as well as the rhythm differences of their expressions, are explored, as we will see below.

The evocation of individual experiences and cultural forms, such as memories of novels and movies, weave potential replicas of the emotional and psychic senses of the case. The participants' speeches stimulate and afford material for the associations of others, providing material for them to think and express themselves. But they can also be a factor of inhibition, conflict, or repression.

The silences, the omitted thoughts, and the words that are left without reverberation in the third-party associative chain form residues that sometimes constitute a negative tissue. At some point, this negative tissue is similar to the one in the sense of Green's negative (1993/2010) and may even establish a negative field in the task. The body and the emotional movements of the group provide a background for associations and sometimes become prominent figures in their qualities as *actings*, as we will illustrate in sequence.

a. From semantics to phonetics – 'Papa, papa, papa'

We are struck by how strongly the speech of the patient about the repeated shouting to the father surprises the group: 'papa, papa, papa'.

The emerged movements of associations are of recognition and classification of the material heard. Firstly, there is a theoretical demarcation such as talking about the infantile and the Oedipal triangulation and linking it to the potential feeling of jealousy. A logical understanding of a metonymic process in speech and action follows. It is a process of appropriation of the material in a rational and theoretical way, as if the group were looking for some ground demarcation. The thematic category child sexuality/Oedipus also emerges. Then, child sexuality is directly inferred by taking the manifesto of dialogue in rational conjectures.

(8): And I was very hooked on this 'papa, papa, papa'; then she appears to be jealous.

(28): The routine calms the blast that can have with the sexual, clearly.

(42): And it seems that gathers several things, daddy, mommy, and I thought it is a defence against sexuality and also to the daddy that runs; that the father is the father is very metonymic.A memory of a film shifts the theoretical axis to an experience of emotional dimension with the evocation of a psychic disorganisation of the protagonist.

(11): I feel she said she couldn't talk. But when she said 'papa, papa, papa', I had a memory of an Argentine movie where the main character was a translator for a psychoanalysis congress and there was a clinical material that said, 'mamma, mamma, mamma', and she feels ill and can't keep working.A semantic slip that keeps the sound of the repeated word 'papa, papa, papa' to that one of a meal senses the food, evoking the hunger, the need to be fed.

(41): As well we can hear like a child talk for food: papa.[1]

Another use arises using the sonority of the word papa repeatedly. However, this is done with a modification in the metric of syllable pronunciation, isolated and rhythmically distinct from the original, giving it a sense of an operative, monotonous, soulless, and joyless way of living. It is monotonous and repetitive rhythm that calls for translation of its underlying emotional condition, a condition of childish need.

Here, we see that the analyst's description of an adult scene described by his patient is filled with childish noises that make us think about the analysis, as we listen to the child within the adult. There is a demand from the child that is repeated in the transference but that remains as a background noise of the adult dialogue.

(40): You can also hear the 'pa, pa, pa, pa' ... somehow.[2]

(59): I thought about something that, at first, has to do with the sound 'papa, papa, papa', so often. And I think about the autopilot scene, 'pa-pa-pa-pa'. The translation issue caught my attention in two circumstances: how can I see something from the patient? And, I am asking, what is asking for translation? In the order of what is not listened to, what is not understood. The language that she speaks is a dialect where the talking is something of a child talk.

b. Action and circulation: Association in act

A very interesting associative core arises because it falls short of a verbal sense and semantic slip. The group embodies the thematic of the emotional state of agitation, by its abnormal movement, an acting in.

On the reporter/observer's note, it is written that the group seemed restless, agitated, with many participants rising from their chairs and leaving the group circle. They were going to the bathroom or they were looking for a coffee or a glass of water to drink or to serve others, disturbing the participants' listening and attention.

At the same time, there were many associations within the group. These associations form a CC formed by intercategorical associative chains, such as those in action and those referring to metaphors of circular motions. Based on this, the group takes those metaphors in order to express the sense of obsessive defences. These defences are used to protect the patient from the feelings of despair and abandonment on the face of a psychotic mother and unsupportive father.

The group not only associates but also acts. Potentially, it reacts to a transferential invariant of the case. As will be seen, the group builds a replica of the case where the young patient must deal with an agitated or psychotic mother, while the father becomes absent and silent. The sense of a request for listening and support and the routine defence trying to control their despair and emotional outburst are merging within the group.

(10): In certain situations, it is the only way to confront it [the emotional situation]. This is to lock herself up, and this is the way she says, that there is a carousel, the hamster wheel, and so on.

(25): It is interesting because there is an image of the translation as something mechanical; the little routine.

(54): She is afraid of opening up to Fred. She is ambivalent about him and she has her speech in circular ways. There is a wheel, there is a distaff, there are games. There is a difficulty in letting others permeate her ...

(86): This group movement is not so common ['the group was restless', someone said with surprise].

There are other operational modes of the associative links to form the associative texture, such as the thematic connections.

The thematic tissue

There are associative chains that unfold around thematic axes. The quotations expressed during the activity are taken by the participants as metaphors describing unconscious conflicts, emotional states, and modes of object relations. Based on these, the constructed replica can be used to infer a mode of unconscious conflict of the case. The conducting analyst may or may not talk explicitly about these conflicts to the group in the latter part of the activity.

The following is an illustration of some of the thematic axes of the associations gathered in this group.

c. *The blast and the routine*

The first association that occurs within the group is about the explosion referred to by the patient and her complaint to Fred. The children's repetitive call, 'papa, papa, papa', becomes an annoying noise in the background. These are appeals from unseen, unheard children; there is only the 'badly timed' demand from them.

The theme of routine and circular action is seen to contain and discharge the failure in elaboration and the paternal and the maternal support. The circular action does not move in one direction; there is only movement, discharge in a nonoperative action. There is a demand to fill an empty house – a house without a soul – and a relationship between the patient and Fred; no exchange, no soul, and no sense appear.

(1): I am struck by her exploding and intervening with Fred.
(2): There are references to a house, thought it has to do with her, talking about home and the spirit of the house. What does she want to ask? What is her dream about? What does she want?
(3): Who is she? And the diminutives struck me. She claims there are differences between her routine and the little routine.
(4): I add, 'there is such a traumatic situation that requires such an automatic unfolding, that it implies a displacement on the hamster wheel, that there is no displacement'.
(5): To me came an image of a carousel, which rotates, a certain children's space, of children's games.
(6): It occurred to me that it has to do with a call to her father to run, run, run. Yes, the childish things of circle motion. And there also appears the little routine of the little girl.

We see in this associative chain how the quotations express a web of connections that provide a picture of the patient's emotional conditions and inner world. Distinct initial categories such as blast, spirit of the empty house, routine, movement/shaking, and child trauma intertwine and stimulate associations in an interanalytical way.

d. Confusion and delimitations: Who is who?

The categories movement/agitation, house/place, abandonment, childhood, and disorganisation/depersonalisation intertwine, enabling the understanding that there is a lack of boundary demarcation between child and adult and the roles of man and woman. So, the confusion about who is who that arises among participants expresses a potential conflictive invariant of the case.

(7): At first, I got totally lost because I didn't know who Fred was. And it took me a long time to realise if it was a man or a woman. Secondly, I did not know who this gentleman was. It seemed to me that he was a son. And it was slowly that a man began to appear. Because Fred could be a son. And as you define later Fred and the children. ... Evidently the case is not explained, but how it appears makes me think that the place of woman and the man are not very clearly marked. The place of a child appears well; it is the first thing that I felt.

(9): It also caused me a lot of confusion, it came to me a fantasy that Fred was a child, and that

(10): in certain situations the only way for her to cope was to close up, and the way she says it is a carousel, the hamster wheel.

(27): What about Fred? Why a name that is ambiguous, male or female? And the association with the wheel – that is to pass to a dream with the encircling of sexuality ...

(79): And thinking about it, it completely blurs me; it is really hard for me to put it all together. I listened; I didn't listen. I find it very hard to see it, to apprehend it, to give it a shape.

(80): There is a depersonalisation.Thus, a quotation appears in the group in an attempt to organise the understanding of the distinct fragmented elements.

(13): There are a lot of things happening to me: an explosion, of course, a demand for the father to be supportive. Then this is displaced by her running to the bedroom, the autopilot, the horse, and then the appearance on a wheel. Everything has to do with how it circulates. Then, it has to do with the hamster wheel. And finally, it is linked with the feeling of depersonalisation, a clinical fact, as she is saying. Then comes the interpretation of the analyst – who needs a body? What is the room?

e. The house, the support, and the abandonment

While the group comments on how difficult it is to know the features of the characters present in the session, the participants' sense of confusion and ignorance, and their needs to have positive and clear data, the sense of an abandoned child object that routinely seeks to defend herself against this emotional neglect it also emerges in the quotations.

The thematic categories abandonment, childhood, support, little quarrel, and disorganisation/depersonalisation express an excess of the mother, potentially representing an invasive object (a psychotic or narcissistic mother) with a consequent devitalisation referred by one participant. Meanwhile, another one diverges, perceiving the phenomenon as disorganised agitation. This occurs in the failure of a supportive father.

(16): It came to me that Fred was her partner, her man, and I remembered a wonderful series; the series has been cancelled. I associated this with one of the women of this series in which there was a group of teenagers that was marginalised. They lived on the street and they were abandoned. They were a family and ended up prostituting themselves and using drugs. Boys and girls. And one of them was more masculine than feminine; she seemed homosexual or lesbian, but she was the smartest of all, and the healthiest. At least because she didn't use drugs; her body was her sanctuary.

(17): I think that the film is called *Pubis Angelical*. I don't know. It's a book by Puig. And the 'papa, papa, papa' and their little routine comes back to me. She has a childish way of talking. And in this film, there is something about a relationship between a baby, her father, and a woman.

(18): To me this evocation, 'papa, papa, papa' has, in the bond, an excess of 'mamma'. I thought of the fairy tales, the distaff and the spinning wheel, and now it seems to me that I was giving up and feeling tired. This is what this patient awakens in me.

(19): Look at this feeling of tiredness. It does not give me the feeling of tiredness, but of a disorganised agitation. It seems like a moment of intolerable panic for her that is organised by the little routine. It gives me a bad feeling of 'papa, papa'. Maybe it would be an association of an evocation to get her organised, and maybe the little routine is a way of organising herself, understanding that there are things to do.

(20): A support.

(21): A support for agitation.

(22): In the movie there is a cancer, and a circular situation. Of course, for the cancer in the movie, it's hidden. This is closed.

(23): The film comes back to me because in the movie she is disorganised. She isn't prepared to listen to an analysis session. What I remember about this movie is just this image. And I was thinking about this patient's disorganisation, and I was thinking of the house. She is trying to organise it. I don't know, but she goes on describing all this with the house.

(29): I am thinking about the house, or the house and the routine. And when the analyst asks her, and she starts to think of her house, she thinks of an empty and chaotic house, and this makes me think of her relationship with her father. I wonder, what would this void correspond with? In a couple there is often one that enters the other's world and becomes empty of their own history and their life. And then, I don't know if it is for reasons of clinical complexity, but it is precisely in the house that she is talking about herself. And even this routine does not appear as something of her own self.

(31): When talking about the movie I thought about *The House of the Spirits*, the book by Isabel Allende. It is about a strange house, which has to do with the disappearance of the groom. It was written during Pinochet's times. There is a very beautiful house, and a young girl falls in love with a boy.

(32): Her father is a soldier, and she dates a boy. And in the movie her father saves him, and he puts him in the car. On countertransference, I feel a young woman who is suffering a lot – she is very distressed. She is trying to look for a path in analysis that she cannot find. That 'papa' is a desperate cry, and as she is suffering.

(33): She keeps confusing the house with herself. In her language, what does it mean to say 'no' to a routine? Is it to say 'no' to being strong? Does it mean having no soul?

Here we understand that the two quotes, although contradictory, do not exclude each other because they are diffracted aspects of invariant elements captured and represented in each one of the quotations.

f. The support fails and a disintegrated self

The thematic categories house/place, translation, support, and disorganisation/depersonalisation are also woven into a patient's request for the father to translate this agitated condition, as a good support, and provide the patient with a proper place, the development of a safe self. Faced with the failure of paternal support, as well as her own defensive routine, she disorganises herself and presents symptoms of depersonalisation.

(24): You know what you are talking about. It reminded me of this congress where they asked me for translate the papers. And millions of translation requests came. I like this work. It helps me to be inside. I have a friend, and she is a translator, and a very good translator.

(25): It is interesting because there is an image of the translation as something mechanical, the little routine.

(26): But, in reality, translation is the opposite, because you have to work intensively with you. Each signifier is one thing. It is a very creative thing, and sometimes it goes to places that disorganise you. Shall I explain myself? And this, it goes there; it goes here, and that's how it is. But there is something about this routine that takes you away and puts you in touch with the work of translating the unconscious. And you said that, right now, that disrupts her. I don't know if in this session the mamma disrupts herself.

(34): And such a request, this strong, a 'papa, papa', is for her. She is trying to get some home. And the attempt is to move to Fred's house, and there is something there. I was thinking that she is entirely defended, and I kept myself thinking about the wheel image. In a sense, all that routine stuff means defence, defence, defence.

(35): But in the face of unbearable anguish.

(36): Yes, near the disorganisation …

(37): And when the children call this 'papa', I believe so. It's like begging.

(38): She calls 'daddy, daddy'. And another situation: she doesn't know what she wants, and nobody knows when she closes up either. This is what Lacanians call a no place. However, that demands a place. It seems to me that there is a calling, what place do you want?

(39): We would have to think about why she makes this kind of demand. I was thinking of a mom or dad who didn't pay attention on her.It is very interesting to see the group's movements oscillate from moments when associative work is more rational to moments of loosening of rationality in which participants express themselves with emotions, personal memories, intuitions, and imaginative conjectures that may not be so clear at first to the group.

(70): This persecutory anxiety also appears in each of us. Each one of us speaks from their own experience. For example, I was delighted with the introduction of the film. But the word 'terrorist' struck me, as well as the mistress in *The House of the Spirits*. There is a difference, and these things impact how everyone listens to each of us. If each one of us listens as if she were our patient, we can see how the signifier of each one comes in.

(76): When I said 'terrorist', it didn't occur to me another word. And as I put myself in Pinochet's times, this word came out. I don't think I got myself into this. This word came out. I would rather talk about what we say about the group. Persecuting anxieties appear,

(77): and also this demanding thing, once we have to associate freely. And how can we associate freely, with free-floating attention, with fifteen people here? It is very pertinent what you said.

(78): I believe that, with the patient, we see how each one is responsible for their own voice. What the patient seems not be able to do. She goes on talking a little about her mother, using her mother's voice. How can she get this place from her own subject, from her own desire, by herself?

The replica: The patient built in the group

Thus, along the trail of the associations, an imaginary character was built among the participants. The replica created was a woman with children, who defends herself from the relationship with her partner, obsessively isolating herself with motor discharges in her routine (circular metaphors and action to nowhere like the hamster wheel) and attacking her love link in an ambivalence towards her partner, approaching or disinvesting in him.

She comes from a family with a mother, who supposedly had psychotic crises, possibly with periods of turmoil (such as acting in the group), and a fragile, nonsupportive father. Her fantasy of destroying her links with her childish parents and their current affections, as well as driving her mother crazy, emerges in the group's representation of the association with the words *terrorist, explosion*, and *disinvestment*. The patient breakdowns face strong emotions of love and hate. She misses a paternal support that organises her emotional experience of sexuality and tenderness in face of the terror of a psychotic mother, so she has fantasies of explosion and shattering. In the family there is a feeling of a hidden secret, of something misunderstood about the mother, and there is a feeling of helplessness and abandonment. The father, fragile in his capacity for paternal function and support, leaves her with a feeling of abandonment; thus she has to deal with her agitated and psychotic mother while still young.

Comments from the lead analyst of the case

The presenter analyst briefly wrote us his most general impressions for the purpose of the presentation at the symposium:

The way the work took place was very interesting, they were very respectful.

The group was building a patient who is very similar to my patient.

In a way, the things being built in the group have a lot to do with the patient's conflict.

It's amazing where the word 'terrorist' comes from.

For me, it was also the development of a series of hypotheses that coincide with the patient's family that is surprising and impressive in terms of production.

We see that interanalytic production in some way retrieves and points out the invariants present in the dynamic field. It arises in group work and somehow shapes the metaphorical associations that closely resemble a sort of elements such as the patient's clinical material.

Final comments

We emphasise that the focus of our work is not to verify the objective facts of the patient's life story but rather to encourage the participants to use free association and fluctuating attention, demonstrating its usefulness in capturing unconscious elements.

To the extent that we use a group device that enables the emergence of elements closely linked to psychoanalytic objects, we create conditions for validation and recognition of the scientific and technical value of these essential instruments to psychoanalysis.

The richness of our working party lies precisely in exploring these psychoanalytic instruments that reinforce and expand the capacity for intimate perception of psychic phenomena in contact with narrative elements of a dialogue, often preverbal or arising from interanalytical exchanges and group phenomena. This reinforces everyone's experience with the apprehension of the unconscious elements and the psychoanalytic dynamic field.

We understand that we have shown in this chapter that our hypothesis that free association and fluctuating attention in a group of psychoanalysts immersed in psychoanalytic listening to clinical material is a scientific valid way of grasping unconscious processes.

The recording of the activity also makes it possible to trace specific characteristics of current psychoanalytic listening, which was not the objective of this chapter.

Notes

1 In Spanish and Portuguese, the word *papa* also is a word an adult can use when speaking to a baby or small child to refer to food.

2 The participant refers to the repetitive sound representing a repetitive, monotonous, and routine way of doing things.

References

Baranger, W., & Baranger, M. (2008). The analytic situation as a dynamic field. *The International Journal of Psychoanalysis*, 89, 795–826. (Reprinted from *Revista Uruguaya de Psicoanálisis*, 4(1), 3–54, 1961–1962).

Bardin, L. (2011). *Análise de conteúdo*. São Paulo, Brazil: Edições 70. (Original work published 1977).

Bion, W. R. (1963). *Aprendiendo de la experiencia*. Buenos Aires, Argentina: Paidós.

Bion, W. R. (1975). *Experiências com grupos. Os fundamentos da psicoterapia de grupo* (2nd ed.). Rio de Janeiro, Brazil: Imago. (Original work published 1961)

Bion, W. R. (2000). *Cogitações*. Rio de Janeiro, Brazil: Imago. (Original work Cogitations, published 1992, London, UK: Routledge.)

Bion, W. R. (2004a). *Elementos de psicanálise* (2nd ed.). Rio de Janeiro, Brazil: Imago. (Original work published 1963)

Bion, W. R. (2004b). *Transformações*. Rio de Janeiro, Brazil: Imago. (Original work published 1965)

Bion, W. R. (2006). *Atenção e interpretação* (2nd ed.). Rio de Janeiro, Brazil: Imago. (Original work published 1970)

Bleger, L. (2011). A few postulates and hypotheses: Report of the Working Party on the 'Specificity of Psychoanalytic Treatment Today' (WPSPTT). *European Psychoanalytical Federation*, 65, 45–49.

Brito, C. L. S., Chabalgoity, A. M., & Ponce de León, E. (2017). *Trabajando desde la clínica, metáfora e interpretación: grupos clínicos sobre la especificidad del psicoanálisis hoy*. Paper presented at the Jornada Internacional de la Asociación Psicoanalítica Internacional (IPA), Montevideo, Uruguay.

Camargo, C. A. V., Sandler, E. H., Botelho, E. Z. F., Serebrenic, F. T., Cesar, G. L. M. S., Mattos, L. T. L., ... Wetzel, S. G. (1997). Nine psychoanalysts in search of a myth. Retrieved from http://www.sicap.it/merciai/bion/papers/camar.htm

Donnet, J. L. (2005). *La situation analysante* [*The analyzing situation*]. Paris, France: PUF..

Ferro, A. (2005). Commentary to Madeleine Baranger, field theory. In S. Lewkowicz & S. Flechner (Eds.), *Truth, reality and the psychoanalyst*. London, England: The International Psychoanalysis Library.

Freud, S. (1969). Psicologia de grupo e a análise do Ego (J. Salomão, Trans.). In J. Strachey (Ed.), *Edição standard Brasileira das Obras Completas de Sigmund Freud* (Vol. XVIII). Rio de Janeiro, Brazil: Imago. (Original work published 1921)

Frish, S. (2010). The specificity of psychoanalytic treatment today. *European Psychoanalytical Federation*, 64(Suppl.).

Green, A. (2010). *O trabalho do negativo*. Porto Alegre, Brazil: Artmed.

Kaës, R. (2002). *La consistance du travail psychanalytique en situation de groupe*. Paper presented at the GERCPEA, Luxembourg.

Kaës, R. (2011). *Um singular plural. A psicanálise à prova do grupo*. (São Paulo, Brazil: Loyola. (Original work published 2007)

Levy, R., Fernández, A., & Silva, M. L. (2015, July). *¿Cuál es la especificidad del psicoanálisis?* Paper presented at IPA Congress, Boston, MA.

Moraes, R., & Galiazzi, M. C. (2007). *Análise textual discursiva* (Vol. I). Ijuí, Brazil: Unijuí.

Norman, J., & Salomonsson, B. (2005). 'Weaving thoughts': A method for presenting and commenting psychoanalytic case material in a peer group. *The International Journal of Psychoanalysis*, 86, 1281–1298.

Séchaud, E., Frish, S., & Bleger, L. A. (2010). Especificidade do tratamento psicanalítico hoje. *Revista Brasileira de Psicanálise*, 44(3), 53–64.

Chapter 22

Metaphor transformations in the 3-LM

A systematic clinical exercise with Zoe's case

Andrea Rodríguez Quiroga de Pereira, Bruno Salesio and Adela Leibovich de Duarte

Aims and structure of the chapter

The first purpose of this chapter is to show how metaphors change at different moments in Zoe's treatment, using the Three-Level Model (3-LM).

In a broad sense, this chapter aims to contribute to a knowledge of the phenomenology of practice in psychoanalysis as proposed by Jiménez (2009). This author considers the contribution of the working parties to be a useful methodology for collective investigation into an important part of the field of the implicit in the practice of psychoanalysis.

The study of analytic practice is motivated fundamentally by the aim to process the therapeutic relationship for the benefit of the patient (Hill & Knox, 2009; Jiménez, 2009). Today, it is known that the therapeutic relationship is responsible for 30% of the efficacy of a treatment (Lambert, 2013), but investigation into the therapist's difficulty in recognizing the deterioration of a patient (Macdonald, 2013), as well as into their lack of training for dealing with this, has also been carried out. As a way of reverting this, the systematic observation of empirical data has been proposed as a resource to complement and enhance the reach of our clinical observation (Bernardi, 2018; Rodríguez Quiroga de Pereira, Borensztein, Corbella, & Marengo, 2018), although the same authors highlighted the fact that this requires training that is not always easily obtained.

In our view, analysts and researchers should implement bridging actions between themselves. For this purpose, a second objective of this chapter is the exploration of the metaphors that arise between the patient and the analyst and the observation of the patient's evolution through the operationalisation of the scenes/metaphors proposed. It is presented as a tool that permits the development of a systematic exercise for practice. We consider this an attempt to make a contribution towards the development of different clinical abilities.

DOI: 10.4324/9780000000002-27

In line with these proposed objectives and, given that the specific model of the 3-LM has already been described in previous chapters, here we will only develop (a) the importance of the operationalisation of metaphors in order to perceive the patient's evolution and (b) the utility that the systematic investigation into how the patient and analyst use these metaphors may have for the psychoanalytic clinical practice.

Taking into account these two axes of analysis, this chapter has been structured into three sections. The first section develops possible ways to conceptualise and operationalise metaphors. The second section analyses the use of *ourselves* and *significant others* as indicators to clinically describe the transformations of metaphors within the 3-LM. The third section integrates a description of how the scenes/metaphors evolve in the case of Zoe, according to the 3-LM. This includes the incorporation of the presence–absence of the categories *ourselves* and *significant others* in the metaphors as a criterion for analysis. Finally, we will discuss implications for clinical practice and for empirical research in psychoanalysis.

It is important to clarify that Zoe's case has been provided by the treating analyst, who has defined the ethical considerations regarding confidentiality and the protection of the patient's rights.

Part 1: How do we conceptualize and operationalise metaphors?

The conceptual framework

In a very general sense, metaphors arise in psychoanalytic dialogues and, due to their specificity, become part of the private language of each psychoanalytic pairing. In this sense, we can consider (a) the patient's metaphors, (b) the analyst's metaphors, and (c) the metaphors that are shared by the patient and the analyst.

Historically, in psychoanalysis, the theory of the metaphor appears framed within the theory of creating new symbols. In our clinical practice, we often refer to a patient's capacity to symbolise or to failures in their symbolisation.

There are different ways to conceptualise metaphors according to diverse theoretical perspectives, with no consensus on their definition or on how they function. In a broad sense, we can conceptualise metaphors as figures of speech that are present in the patient's free associations and in the analyst's interventions. They reveal a relationship in the similarity between two terms, a creation of meanings through comparisons. When we compare both terms, there is an implicit duality, or 'twoness'.

Kopp and Eckstein (2004) explained that metaphors present themselves when one wishes to express emotionally charged content in everyday language. Metaphors often employ images and produce and imply a movement, a transfer of meaning. But though the figurative, logical expression is misleading, they express the subjectivity and emotional experience of the person using the metaphor.

Here we will mention only some theoretical positions that we believe support the proposed clinical perspective, because the historical and conceptual trajectory of the topic far exceeds the proposed purpose of this work.

It is worth noting that Freud (1925/1958) characterized thought as the development of a motor action. The authors presented below argue that bodily configurations are the basic categories that give shape to external reality and that the same process applies for internal reality (Enckell, 2002; Rizzuto, 2001). Lakoff and Johnson (1980) and Lakoff (1993), from a different perspective, revealed that our conceptual system is founded on our experiences of the world as mediated by the body and that it structures our thoughts and our actions. They understood the functionality of metaphors, considering that metaphors structure our thoughts and actions (Lakoff & Johnson, 1980). In this sense, metaphors can be understood as matrices for the elaboration of affective and cognitive content, as well as for the creation of mental representations.

Ana-María Rizzuto (2001), a psychoanalyst whose developments we will work with later in this chapter, was interested in the advances in the conceptual metaphor theory (Lakoff, 1993; Lakoff & Johnson, 1980) that were developed in connection with the contexts of psycholinguistics and psychoneurology (Lakoff & Johnson, 1999). Enckell (2002) considered the metaphorical process a fundamental principle of mental functioning, aligning it with a broad application of the theory of the metaphor. The process of transformation in a treatment, meanwhile, was explored by some authors through the construction of connections between different parts of the metaphor (Enckell, 2002).

Rizzuto (2009, p. 20) later indicated that 'contemporary analysts of all convictions agree that analysis is a metaphoric process, and that the patient's and the analyst's metaphoric processes and verbalized metaphors are essential for the transformations the analysand must undergo'.

Towards the operationalisation of metaphors

A second different approach we wish to introduce here is one based on an empirical investigation. Schachter and Kächele (2017) developed a collaborative approach between conversation analysis and psychotherapy process research. Metaphors, in this approach, are part of conversation and, at the same time, create a reflective stance for conversation. In this sense, conversation or 'talking' is the superior concept. It is important to note the fact that characteristics of the primary process appear on the conversational surface and that we can direct our attention to them (Schachter & Kächele, 2017).

The findings of Buchholz, Spiekermann, and Kächele (2015, p. 877, emphasis added) show:

> a) how analyst and patient co-create their common conversational object called psychoanalysis; b) how a lot of up-to-now not described analytical tools are applied, that can be described as 'practices'; c) how a 'dance of insight' is enacted by both participants in a common creation making patterns of interaction visible from 'both sides'; d) *how participants create metaphors as conversational and cognitive tools to reduce the enormous complexity of the analytic exchange and for other purposes*; e) that prosodic rhythmicity and other prosodic features are best integrated in a threefold model for analytic conversation consisting of 'interaction engine', 'talking to' and 'talking about' the patient.

In these terms, the psychoanalytic relationship is a kind of metaphor that co-creates a psychoanalytic process.

The 3-LM proposes a second look, to identify significant clinical patterns that can be expressed as metaphors, the sense of which will be discovered and interpreted at different moments during the analytic process. The model specifically considers that

> they are usually found in the clinical material and are metaphors or scenes that transmit in a vivid and unsaturated form the core of the patient's problems. Some of them appear from the beginning and become the focus of therapeutic work and can be considered as 'anchor points' that serve as a background on which it is possible to identify subsequent changes. (Bernardi, 2015, p. 14)

Taking this into account, metaphors can be operationalized moving from a theoretical concept to an empirical concept, which allows the identification of a unit of analysis. An operational definition articulates a concept's processes or actions that are necessary to identify examples (MacGregor, 2006). Finally, we can say that operationalisation expresses or defines something in terms of the operations used to determine or prove them.

Ourselves **and** ***significant others*****: A useful aspect of metaphors to clinically describe their transformations**

Rizzuto (2001) considered that four dimensions must be present in every metaphor in the psychoanalytical situation. When they are not present in a direct way, their absence awakens our interest, as analysts, to reveal them. In her work, the author developed how these dimensions appear in metaphors throughout the length of the therapeutic process.

In a similar way to other authors (see, for example, Kopp, 1998; Kopp & Eckstein, 2004), Rizzuto (2001) proposed that

> metaphors we create to talk about what is ineffable about ourselves refer directly or indirectly to scenes with four elements: 1) *ourselves*, directly or in disguised form; 2) *significant others*; 3) a particular type of psychic event; and 4) the depiction of an interpersonal experience. (p. 555)

Though we consider that these elements can be operationalised, Rizzuto (2001) does not advance in this direction.

However, some empirical studies suggest the clinical importance of considering the presence–absence of *significant others* in the use of metaphors within the psychoanalytic process. The research work by Fabregat (2004), *Metaphors in Psychotherapy. From Affect to Mental Representations*, shows the role of affect and language in psychotherapy sessions and their possible unconscious integration into speech and cognitive processes.

The author worked with a sample of 39 coded sessions from ten psychoanalytically oriented treatments in 'analytic focus treatment', according to the definition of the treating therapists. Among many of his results, Fabregat (2004, p. 252) observed that 'a higher production of metaphors was related to a greater production of significant objects of reference and associations. When free association functions adequately, according to theory, more objects of reference will be associated'. Under 'objects of reference', the author coded 'all relationships with persons that were mentioned by the patient, the therapist or both in a combined formed; i.e. proper names or important relationships like father, mother, husband, friend, etc.' (Fabregat 2004, p. 269). The results indicate that the patient's *object-of-reference* naming and combined object naming (patient and analyst) advance in the same direction. Also, patients with good outcomes name more objects or have more associations. She also described how patients and therapists that interact with higher levels of metaphor coefficients also name more objects of reference, and that higher metaphor production is related to more associations (Fabregat, 2004).

How do we make this research information useful for an analyst?

The 3-LM and its questions help the analyst in the understanding of the problems of a patient. Let us see three examples: (a) Do changes exist, over the analytic process, about how the patient uses their own mind and body? Is it possible to identify, in the texts of the sessions, when the patient or the therapist speaks of themselves? Can we attempt to connect this question with one of the four dimensions described by Rizzuto (2001)? Can we describe *ourselves directly* or in *disguised form* as one of the elements that are supposed to be part of the scenes to which the metaphors refer us? (b) How does the patient experience others and how do they experience themselves in relation to others? Is it possible to identify in the text of the sessions when the patient and the analyst speak about a *significant other*? Can we describe a *significant other* as one of the elements that are supposed to be part of the scenes to which the metaphors refer us? (d) Are there changes that may be noticed through time, between different sessions? Can we describe any changes from these elements that we can considerer a transformation?

Criteria of exclusion: the analyst's self-reflections to herself that had not been communicated to the patient.

We will attempt, therefore, to describe how the direct or indirect presence of indicators of *ourselves* and *significant others* develop through Zoe's psychoanalytic process, as a clinical tool.

To this end, we will operationalise, as an exercise, the elements *ourselves* and *significant others*. As mentioned previously, these concepts will be defined in terms of the operations used to determine or prove it. That is, we will define them to see whether they are present or not as elements of the scenes to which the metaphors refer.

1 This will then mean that we will operationalise *ourselves* (OU) as all references about how the patient and the analyst use their own minds and bodies, as expressed in the session text that refers scenes in the metaphorical text or in the context where metaphor is included. We will define *ourselves as direct* (OUD) when the reference is expressed in the metaphorical text. We will define *ourselves as indirect* (OUI) when the reference is expressed in the context where the metaphor is included.
2 This will then mean that we will operationalise a *significant other* as all the relationships mentioned by the patient and/or the analyst in the metaphorical texts and in the context where this metaphor is included (links that the patient and/or therapist identify as important).

We will define a *significant other as direct* (SOD) when the reference is expressed in the metaphorical text. We will define a *significant other as indirect* (SOI) when the reference is expressed in the context where the metaphor is included.

We will define as *other nonspecific* (ONS) ones when directly (ONSD) or indirectly (ONSI) alluded to others not categorised as other significant ones in metaphorical texts or in the context where this metaphor is included (e.g., others, them).

3 The results of this exercise will be the answer to this question in Zoe's case.

Evolution of metaphors in Zoe's case according to the 3-LM, incorporating the presence of *ourselves* and *significant others* as analytic criteria

Level 1. Phenomenological description of transformations

This first level adopts a phenomenological perspective and sets out to describe the changes as they appear to the observer, whose observation is informed by their previous analytic experience (Altmann de Litvan, 2015).

We have chosen to work with the following moments in the process – in which we have identified 22 metaphors: the beginning of the treatment (scene A and scene B); 6 months into the treatment; 1½ years into the treatment; 2½ years into the treatment; and 3½ years into the treatment (sessions 1, 2, and 3). We have also included tables to illustrate the presence of *ourselves* and *significant others* for each of the 22 metaphors identified in Zoe's case.

Beginning of treatment: Scene A

The analyst introduces the case, saying that, when she met Zoe, she described that the patient felt the following:

> ... a feeling of being completely out of my body, with the sense of being far away, as if I was not connected to them. ... I'm scared of existing ... of being here, alive, not knowing what I am. ... Sometimes I feel I'm in something unknown, and that's what concerns me ... *looking at life from behind a glass* (1). ... This causes me to have panic attacks that go from fear to madness. ... I see the others living their lives, and. ... (see Table 22.1)

Tables presented throughout the text refer to the presence or not of elements of the scenes to which the metaphors refer. In relation to *ourselves* (OUD or OUI), in relation to a *significant other* (SOD or SOI), and in relation to *other nonspecific* (ONS, ONSD, or ONSI). Metaphors are numbered according to their appearance.

Is she communicating her feelings through this metaphor? The image allows us to specify the way she feels being out of her body, described in that image.

Table 22.1. Categorisation of patient's metaphor: (1).

OURSELVES/SIGNIFICANT OTHER	
(1) Patient OUI (mind and body)	ONSI (others)

OUI: ourselves as indirect
ONSI: other nonspecific indirect

But when she places the glass as an element of separation, she means that the separation is physical, not only visual. Her full visual/perceptual ability generates the anxiety of someone who can see but not touch, who can/could be seen but can/could not be touched (in her primitive experiences and in the transference). At the beginning of the treatment, her relationship with others is almost impossible; she mentions others in an unspecific way, as *they live their lives*, and with whom it seems difficult to connect.

Beginning of treatment: Scene B

> The last day I saw Mom she couldn't insert the key in the keyhole because her hand was shaking. ... I have episodes ... feeling really bad, ... *as if something, a monster, had woken up inside me that started to attack me; it simply woke up* (2). I felt I could die. It was my first personal contact with death, because I'd snorted a lot of cocaine. I felt I was going to die, and perhaps that day I came close to what happened to Mom. (see Table 22.2)

The monster metaphor expresses some part of herself that has become available to her consciousness and has brought her closer to what happened to her mother. What does this monster mean? Is the identification with her mother what scares her so much? Why is it happening now? May the experience with cocaine have been a trigger for the current symptomatology? What does it mean to the patient to '... come closer to what happened to Mom?' How serious is the patient's mental state? What is the intensity and modality of affection present in her metaphors? It seems to oscillate between mental states in which affection feels like an inhibition and another in which it becomes disruptive (a monster that grows). In this second scene we can observe the lack of discrimination regarding herself and her mother.

Table 22.2. Categorisation of Patient's Metaphors: (2).

OURSELVES/SIGNIFICANT OTHER	
(2) Patient OUD (monster)	SOI (Mom)

OUD: ourselves as direct
SOI: significant other as indirect

Six months into treatment

Let us observe a vignette from a session at this moment in the treatment:

ZOE: I've been thinking of what we talked about, ... of connecting what's happening to Mom, or with the things I went through. ... I had a new sensation, something I'd never felt before; I was putting myself on a different level from what I was used to, as if *I had opened an invisible door toward another dimension, as if I was displayed on a window*. I can connect with the world, but I'm very scared, because I'm alone, and the others are on the other side (3), and it's as if I'm dreaming, and I thought how it could be related to Mom or to death. … I don't know if it's a way. … I never thought of death. … It happened to me when I was 17, and my birthday is on the 17th; it was right after I turned 17. I woke up and I felt weird, I thought it was a hangover. …

ANALYST: A hangover from your mother's death. You didn't suffer when she died.

ZOE: I did suffer, but I only realized what it meant to really suffer at 17. Sinister suffering and horror, real horror, I felt at 17. I don't say I was forced to, but I was told to block everything out. My father would say to me, 'turn the page' (4) all the time. (see Table 22.3)

Six months into treatment, the initial scene A seems to have changed. Spatially, Zoe has ceased to look from behind the glass to, instead, be exhibited in a window, perhaps referring to her situation in analysis. She makes associations this with the death of her mother (3). Her mother was killed in a car accident . The mother appears as a *significant other* indirectly and the *others* as nonspecific indirectly, but she is still alone, unable to relate to any of them. In scene 4, a different *significant other* indirect appears: her father. Zoe seems to realise how she and her feelings were not taken into account by him.

Table 22.3. Categorisation of Patient's Metaphors: (3, 4).

OURSELVES/SIGNIFICANT OTHER		
(3) Patient OUD (I)	SOI (Mom)	ONSI (others)
(4) Patient OUI (I)	SOI (Father)	

OUD: ourselves as direct
ONSI: other nonspecific indirect
OUI: ourselves as indirect
SOI: significant other as indirect

One and a half years into treatment

We will present a vignette from a session at this time.

Z: Yesterday *I blew up* (5) because I was hearing, 'Dad, Dad, Dad'. I tried to understand but I couldn't. … I thought, how unfair! I did everything, and I can't even talk with Fred'. I pretended to be asleep, and he says to me, 'Are you really tired, are you going to sleep?' And sometimes *an enemy appears inside me* that says, 'Okay, you know what? You can stay by yourself!' (6). And I fell asleep.

A: It was as if you felt pushed out and unacknowledged. You got mad, you turned around and left; you fell asleep.

Z: I've reacted this way since I was very young. When I got mad, I would run through the hallway, I would run, run to my room and throw myself on the bed until someone came. ... It's odd, because it's a nice feeling, ... and lately, *I'm on autopilot* (7). I'm like that, ... I've always done this thing of being focused on one thing, like horses, who can't see sideways. ...

A: [She pauses for a few seconds. The image of a hamster comes to my mind. For a second, I think to tell her about it, but I don't, and she keeps talking].

Z: And lately I've been very much involved in Fred's routine, taking charge and doing things. *It's like part of the wheel, like spinning yarn on the spinning wheel. ... My mom would say that to me, 'We have to spin on the wheel'. It's as if I had created. ... The image of the hamster wheel comes to mind ...* (8). These things also keep my feet on the ground, creating little routines for myself, creating a small world of things to do. ... It's the exact opposite of the feeling of depersonalization, but it's hard to regulate the intensity, and I'm thinking a lot about his sons, and Fred and me. ...

A: In *autopilot* (9), *the hamster wheel* (10), being glued to the computer after your mom died. Everything flows but nothing happens. (see Table 22.4)

This vignette begins with a metaphor when she says, 'I blew up' (5). It tells us of a request for care that she never received, which happened when the child of her partner calls his father, '... dad, dad, dad', and she hears this sustained complaint, which impedes the attention she seeks from Fred'. It could be considered that a *significant other* appears indirectly here, because it is clear from the context how her impulsiveness stems from Fred's lack of availability to her. However, it is of interest to think, for later associations, that she does not yet manage to distinguish between Fred and Dad in her mind. Faced with them, she reveals the conflicting need for care versus self-sufficiency. Metaphor (6) brings to our understanding the monster that depersonalises her in scene B, converted into an internal enemy that attempts to resolve the conflict posed, and putting a new metaphor into play, 'I'm on autopilot' (7), in a pattern of long-standing defensive behaviour. Then the analyst has an image of a *hamster*, which the patient later verbalises, although she had not told the patient about it.

According to de León de Bernardi (1993), this implies complex dynamics in communication that appears as a game between images, affects and words happens between patient and analyst which are enabled by regression. These moments of the analytic relationship intricately include transferential and countertransferential aspects that, as formations of the unconscious, become established in the field. 'I believe', says de León de Bernardi (1993), 'that these moments constitute true neoformations of the analytic field, "interactive dynamic nuclei" which mark the history of analysis and establish "the shared substratum of interpretation"' (p. 812).

It is interesting to note the presence of a *significant other*, the mother, in the same metaphor (8). Can we think the 'we' is a direct *significant other* as a step towards transformation? This is also interesting in order to distinguish our practices. As the analyst notices again, the patient's metaphors (7), (8), (9), and (10) introduce an indirect *significant other*. The metaphors are more present as a mode of expression at this point of the analysis.

Table 22.4. Categorisation of Patient's Metaphors: (5–10).

OURSELVES/SIGNIFICANT OTHER		
(5). Patient OUD (I)	SOI (Fred)	
(6). Patient OUD (enemy)	SOI (Fred)	
(7). Patient OUD (I)		
(8). Patient OUD (we)	SOD (we)	
(9). Analyst	SOI (patient)	
(10). Analyst	SOD (patient, hamster wheel)	SOI (Mom)

OUD: ourselves as direct
SOI: significant other as indirect
SOD: significant other as direct

Two and a half years into treatment

The relationship with another is now experienced as a pendulum. Could it also be thought of as a metaphor for the mother's bipolarity? For the first time, a complaint appears, with feelings of anger, not only against her father but also against the family from which she was excluded at an early stage.

Z: I don't know what's going on with Fred'. … Things aren't going well. *The relationship is like a pendulum* (11). I can't find stability. … I want to be with him because I like him, because I miss him, because I'm much happier when I'm with him [she becomes anxious]. … I don't know which way to turn. How come no one is taking responsibility for what's happening to me? If I'm suffering, if someone hurts me, that person has to take responsibility. Otherwise, *it's like they throw everything inside me and put a lid on me, like a jar!* (12).

A: [She seems like a very angry little girl, and I feel the need to hug her.] You need someone to hug you. …

Z: [Nods] And to apologise, to say I'm sorry, to empathise with what I'm going through. Perhaps nobody ever said I'm sorry. And on top of that, Fred' is super proud and won't apologise ever in his fucking life. I waited and waited for my father to apologise, for Alicia to apologise, for my sisters to apologise. …

It is interesting to note that the entrenchment in the relationship highlighted in metaphor 11 precedes the possibility of showing her anger towards a nonspecific direct other (ONSD) that appears in metaphor 12, so that she could finally quote them in the subsequent text. Is this second indicator of transformation in the patient?

Table 22.5. Categorisation of Patient's Metaphors: (11, 12).

OURSELVES/SIGNIFICANT OTHER	
(11). Patient OUI (relationship)	SOI (relationship)
(12). Patient OUD (me)	ONSD (they)

OUI: ourselves as indirect
SOI: significant other as indirect
OUD: ourselves as direct
ONSD: other nonspecific direct

Three and a half years into treatment

Extracts from three sessions are presented to consider the evolution of the metaphors that arise at this point of the treatment.

SESSION 1Z: … I FELT A LOT OF HORROR, A LOT OF ANGER. … ABOVE ALL, A LOT OF ANGUISH AND SADNESS. … AND, IF THERE'S *SOMETHING BLOCKED OUT, IT MUST BE THAT. … IT'S AS IF SOMETHING INSIDE ME HAD TRANSFORMED INTO A MONSTER. … IT'S LIKE HAVING A MONSTER ASLEEP INSIDE THAT WOKE UP MUCH BIGGER AND MUCH NASTIER* (13). … BECAUSE IT'S FULL OF THINGS. … IT'S VERY INTENSE. … SO MUCH SO THAT I FEEL LIKE THAT REGARDING FRED' AND THE KIDS. … AND IF I GO ON LIKE THIS, … I'LL HAVE TO SPLIT UP WITH FRED'. …

A: *A monster* (14) that destroys and splits the monstrous aspects of death. And perhaps you need to separate from the monster, the monstrous aspects that killed your mother and that you feel may have remained inside you.

Z: And I'm scared, ... because I identify with my mother, and why does *the monster* (15) appear like that?

A: It could be a way of keeping her inside you, of not separating from her or letting her go so that you can start again.

Z: Maybe my fear, the fact that I don't know who I am, that I don't know who I look like, and that separating from that past. ... Maybe I don't know very well who Zoe is without a mom. ...

A: As if Zoe ceased to be a person, as if she became depersonalized and were trapped in a different world, in *a bubble, between the world of the living and the world of the dead* (16).

Z: That's why I was so multifaceted as a teenager. ... I need to identify with something in order to exist. ... It's so hard! Maybe, ... yes, ... I think I hold back because there are things that I think before I say them. I search for the right way to say them. ... I vent my anger. ... Here I vent things in a very intense way. ... What I don't know is. ... [She remains silent.]

A: Perhaps you're scared of not knowing *if I'll survive your anger, not knowing if your anger can kill me* (17). And perhaps you need to know that I'll continue to be here, so that you can let what you feel come out as it is.Z: It's the only place where I feel I can talk freely. ... Sometimes I'm scared that ... so much of what I feel has no shape. ... I need time to graphically [she makes the gesture of opening her abdomen] *open myself and get everything out* (18). ...

In metaphor (13) we again find the monster. This time it indirectly refers to *significant others* Fred' and the children. The danger it subjects her to has also changed. No longer does she feel depersonalised but rather that she must separate from Fred' if she continues to feel this way. The analyst takes this metaphor (14) but brings it back to the centre, to what at this juncture could perhaps be considered a focus of her work, the patient's conflict of identity connected to the mourning of her mother's death. The patient continues conversing with the analyst and returns to the metaphor of the monster (15) but in a way seems to show a difference with the analyst in the moment of wondering why the monster appears that way. Perhaps this can be thought in relation to how a past conflict appears in her current life. Later, the analyst produces a metaphor (16), in which the living and the dead are nonspecific directs ones, and Zoe is mentioned in an indirect way. She precedes her next transferential intervention (17) directly mentioning a nonspecific other and only indirectly mentions Zoe. We have also noted this in the way the patient addresses the feelings of aggression. Perhaps this can be an observation to follow on how the analytic pair work together through strong feelings. Metaphor (18), connected to the body, shows the intensity of the work between the patient and the analyst and is the first one in which the patient refers indirectly to the analyst.

Table 22.6. Categorisation of Patient's Metaphors: (13–18).

OURSELVES/SIGNIFICANT OTHER		
(13). Patient OUD (monster)	SOI (Fred and the kids)	
(14). Analyst	SOD (patient, monster)	SOI (Mom)
(15). Patient OUD (monster)	SOI (Mother)	
(16). Analyst	ONSD (world of the living and of the death)	SOI (Zoe)
(17). Analyst OUD (I)	SOD (patient, you)	
(18). Patient OUD (myself)	SOI (analyst, it's the only place)	

OUD: ourselves as direct
SOI: significant other as indirect
SOD: significant other as direct
ONSD: other nonspecific direct

Session 2

Z: *I think I have like an iceberg* (19), and maybe I don't, … but I don't know. … But it has to do with what I told you about having something inside and not knowing what it is, … but there's something inside me that I don't want to face. …

A: Speaking and exposing yourself here also upsets you, and you're being careful about showing, about showing yourself.

Z: … When I feel that I want to leave, … that I'm unhappy, … I feel I need to leave. … That's what I don't want to face. … the children … Burdens! Burdens appear, become burdens. … Then, removing those burdens, leaving them behind is a relief, … *as if being in a relationship was a burden. … Taking responsibility is a burden* (20). …

A: What was it like to live with the burden of your mother's illness? A mother who exposed you to situations that embarrassed you, who couldn't think of you during those moments. Her was the one who broke up, who withdrew.

Zoe has to give a presentation at university. Faced with this new risk of exposing herself, the metaphor of the iceberg (19) appears, and freezing is a defence the patient no longer uses. It is interesting to see the turn in this vignette

Table 22.7. Categorisation of Patient's Metaphors: (19, 20).

OURSELVES/SIGNIFICANT OTHER	
(19). Patient OUD (I)	
(20). Patient OUD (being in a relationship)	SOI (the children)

OUD: ourselves as direct
SOI: significant other as indirect

regarding the responsibility of being part of a link. It is also interesting to see how the analyst intervenes to jointly reformulate the problems presented by the patient.

Session 3

Z: I was very nervous all weekend because of today's presentation. … Horrible, horrible nerves. … I can't get like that because of an oral presentation in class. But when I started talking, I felt super confident and calm. I was speaking about a subject I had studied thoroughly. We all did well. … *I'm in a wheel that is spinning and is going somewhere* (21). … I had two feelings yesterday that struck me. I remembered that you talked about the holidays or asked me if I would feel bad when they start, if I would miss you. … I never think about that, the holidays are the holidays and that's it, nothing else, … and yet yesterday I thought how upset I'd be if I never came here again! I want to come always! I never realized. I also felt that I love Fred' so much that it's scary. … I'm really anxious that something may happen to him. … It makes me so anxious and it's so painful to think that I can lose him. …

A: There's also more inside you, not only death and destruction.

Z: Yes, especially today, when I had the presentation and I was so nervous, but when my turn was coming, I started feeling happy … because it was my turn!

A: [I think, 'She's spinning yarn on the wheel; she's starting to spin in a certain direction'.]

Z: I'm experimenting with other things. *It's as if I had found my center* (22). …

This session, the last one presented by the analyst, clearly shows an evolution on the patient's part. Metaphor (21) allows us to observe the sense of agency that the patient has acquired for her life. The analyst does not verbalise the metaphor through which he shares what his patient says. We understand that the last one, a bodily metaphor (22), refers to the patient's identity conflict and her new way of experiencing herself.

Table 22.8. Categorisation of Patient's Metaphors: (21, 22).

OURSELVES/SIGNIFICANT OTHER	
(21). Patient OUD (I)	SOI (we, you-the analyst, Fred)
(22). Patient OUD (I)	

OUD: ourselves as direct

SOI: significant other as indirect

The results of the categorisation of *ourselves* and *significant others* are displayed together in Table 22.9, in order to understand the complete picture. As an initial result we can observe that the element *ourselves* (sometimes direct and others indirect) is present in every metaphoric context. The *significant others* are present in most metaphorical texts or in their contexts (in 17 out of 22). Out of the 5 that do not denote a significant one, 2 of them are linked to other nonspecific ones.

Up to this point we are able to identify *ourselves* and *significant others* as two of the elements that, according to Rizzuto (2001), are part of the scenes to which the metaphors refer us in the selected texts of Zoe´s case.

But is it possible to identify changes in the analytic process about how the patient uses their own mind and body? Or in how the patient experiences others and how they experience themselves in relation to others?

Some specific links between us and *significant others* show transformations from the studied elements.

Studied transformations

At 1½ years into treatment, it is possible to identify the use of the pronoun *we* (8), ('We have to spin on the wheel') for the first time. It is also the first time that an element related to *ourselves* is linked to a direct *significant other*. This could be possibly thought as an initial transformation from the isolated 'I' into an indiscriminate 'we'.

At 2½ years into treatment, the patient is able to express her anger for the first time: linking herself (OUD) to the object of her anger, named as a direct nonspecific other (12) ('Otherwise, it's like they throw everything inside me and put a lid on me, like a jar!'). This could be seen as a second transformation, expressing her anger and linking it to an object. After this, the patient is able to link her anger to herself (OUD) and can think about how this anger can affect her relationships (SOI). Is it possible to think of this as a new transformation?

A last transformation can be detected through metaphor (18), which is connected to her body (OUD) and is the first reference to the analyst (SOI).

Level 2. Can the metaphors and the exercise done with them help to identify the main diagnostic dimensions of change in Zoe's case?

The patient's subjective experience of illness and the contextual factors have changed. Zoe's expectations about her problems and treatment have been radically modified towards a needed intimacy and her recognition of the need of her analyst, not only in the analytic space but also in the fear of losing her *significant others*.

With regard to the patterns of interpersonal relationships, the patient has moved from a freeze defence, 'looking at life from behind a glass' (1) to feeling that being in a relationship was a burden, 'taking responsibility

Table 22.9. Total categorisation of *ourselves* and *significant others* in the 22 metaphors.

Speaker	*Metaphor number*	*Ourselves (OU)*		*Significant others (SO)*		*Nonspecific others (NSO)*	
		OUD	OUI	SOD	SOI	ONSD	ONSI
Patient	(1)		1				1
Patient	(2)	1			1		
Patient	(3)	1			1		1
Patient	(4)		1		1		
Patient	(5)	1			1		
Patient	(6)	1			1		
Patient	(7)	1					
Patient	(8)	1		1			
Analyst	(9)				1		
Analyst	(10)			1	1		
Patient	(11)		1		1		
Patient	(12)	1				1	
Patient	(13)	1			1		
Analyst	(14)			1	1		
Patient	(15)	1			1		
Analyst	(16)				1	1	
Analyst	(17)	1		1			
Patient	(18)	1			1		
Patient	(19)	1					
Patient	(20)	1			1		
Patient	(21)	1			1		
Patient	(22)	1					

OUD: ourselves as direct
OUI: ourselves as indirect
SOD: significant other as direct
SOI: significant other as indirect
ONSD: other nonspecific as direct
ONSI: other nonspecific as indirect

is a burden' (20) and, finally, to being able to speak about the pain produced by the possibility of losing a loved one.

The bonds that imply closeness and intimacy are important for the patient after 3½ years in treatment. The metaphor of the monster and its development clearly show how it has been possible to relate current patterns to childhood experiences.

As main intrapsychic conflicts we can identify an identity conflict and the need for care as opposed to self-sufficiency. The prevailing dysfunctional defences, limiting internal and external experiences, have changed, and the patient has acquired a sense of her own agency.

Regarding the affective regulation, the patient has achieved a better balance between her own interests and those of the others. The patient's symbolisation is rich, full of affective experiences, bodily self, and fantasies. Zoe has certainly improved in differentiated relationship with internal and external objects. It is still an open question how she can tolerate separations.

The metaphors in this case allow us to identify and the elements of the metaphoric text allow us to address (as it has been developed above) several diagnostic dimensions and account for their transformations.

Level 3. Explanatory hypothesis of change

It is possible to identify, in some metaphors, the theory/theories that the analyst uses. The following is an example:

A: *A monster* (14) that destroys and splits the monstrous aspects of death. And perhaps you need to separate from the monster, the monstrous aspects that killed your mother and that you feel may have remained inside you. ... It could be a way of keeping her inside you, of not separating from her or letting her go so that you can start again.

In the example above, we can identify Freudian theories of identification and theories of aggression (Freud, 1915/1957a, 1915–1917/1957b, 1915/1957c, 1920/1955).

In the following intervention by the analyst, we can also clearly perceive her connection with the patient and the support given to her.

A: [She seems like a very angry little girl, and I feel the need to hug her.] You need someone to hug you. ...

Conclusions

This chapter had two main purposes. The first objective of this chapter was to show how metaphors change at different moments in Zoe's treatment, using the 3-LM. It has been seen how the metaphors/scenes A and B have been modified throughout the treatment. At the beginning of treatment, scene 1 showed that Zoe's relationship with others was almost impossible. In the last sessions studied, her links had evolved, and she could recognise her need for intimacy and her fear of losing her *significant others*. The 3-LM group discussion on Zoe's case mentioned that, despite having experienced changes in her interpersonal relationships with the analyst, with Fred' (her partner), with Fred's children, and with her father, Zoe did not develop a great empathy in her life.

Scene 2, the *monster*, as a metaphor for 'herself', has been worked over throughout the treatment and has allowed the patient to face a traumatic situation, the death of her mother and the subsequent abandonment by her family. The work on this metaphor has also helped to perform an internal discrimination between herself and the representation of her dead mother.

A second objective of this chapter was to conduct a thorough study of the metaphors that arise from the patient, the analyst, and the relationship between the patient and the analyst and the observation of the patient's evolution through the operationalisation of the scenes/metaphors proposed. It was presented as a tool that permits the development of a systematic exercise for practice. As a result of this exercise, we were able to identify the two elements selected – *ourselves* and *significant others* – as parts of the scenes to which the metaphors refer us in the selected texts of Zoe's case. Specifics about how their observation allowed us to see transformations are explained throughout the chapter.

As a limitation to this exercise we can indicate that the sessions are reconstructed and not verbatim. We hope that the work done can encourage clinicians to include another perspective through a systematised analysis. Another weakness is that we did not have access to all of the sessions but only those selected by the analyst.

Following that idea, we think that it will be a useful exercise for any analyst-in-training to compare a session's transcripts and reconstructed sessions. A potential new progress of this work would follow that direction.

An interesting path would be to identify how the *dance* between analyst and patient takes place, as we saw in this analytic pair. It is a shared way to introduce themselves through the communication of strong feelings.

It is important to clarify that, though these dimensions have been used to identify metaphoric elements, their reliability or validity has not been examined.

Current studies are intended to contribute to the trustworthiness of the 3-LM (Rodríguez Quiroga de Pereira, Borensztein, Bongiardino, Aufenacker & Juan, 2019).

We thank the patient and the analyst for their generosity in offering this material to attempt to advance towards a better understanding of our work with our patients.

References

Altmann de Litvan, M. (Ed.). (2015). *Time for change: Tracking transformations in psychoanalysis – The Three-Level Model.* London, England: Karnac.

Bernardi, R. (2015). La evaluación de los cambios del paciente. El modelo de los tres niveles (3-LM). *Mentalización. Revista de psicoanálisis y psicoterapia*, 4, 1–16. Retrieved from http://www.revistamentalizacion.com/ultimonumero/abril2015/

Bernardi, R. (2018). Moving from clinical inquiry to clinical research. In *Many faces of psychoanalytic clinical research: From the perspective of different IPA working groups*.

Buchholz, M. B., Spiekermann, J., & Kächele, H. (2015). Rhythm and blues. Amalie's 152nd session. From psychoanalysis to conversation and metaphor analysis – and retour. *The International Journal of Psychoanalysis*, 96, 877–910.

de León de Bernardi, B. (1993). El sustrato compartido de la interpretación. Imágenes, afectos y palabras en la experiencia analítica. *Revista de Psicoanálisis*, 50(4/5), 809–826.

Enckell, H. (2002). *Metaphors and the psychodynamic functions of the mind* (Doctoral dissertation). Retrieved from http://epublications.uef.fi/pub/urn_isbn_951-781865-3/urn_isbn_951-781-865-3.pdf

Fabregat, M. (2004). *From affect to mental representations* (Doctoral dissertation). Retrieved from https://publikationen.sulb.unisaarland.de/bitstream/20.500.11880/23318/1/Fabregat.pdf

Freud, S. (1955). Beyond the pleasure principle. In J. Strachey (Ed.), *The standard edition of the complete psychological works of Sigmund Freud* (Vol. XVIII). London, England: The Hogarth Press. (Original work published 1920)

Freud, S. (1957a). Instincts and their vicissitudes. In J. Strachey (Ed.), *The standard edition of the complete psychological works of Sigmund Freud* (Vol. XIV). London, England: The Hogarth Press. (Original work published 1915)

Freud, S. (1957b). Mourning and melancholia. In J. Strachey (Ed.), *The standard edition of the complete psychological works of Sigmund Freud* (Vol. XIV). London, England: The Hogarth Press. (Original work published 1915–1917)

Freud, S. (1957c). The unconscious. In J. Strachey (Ed.), *The standard edition of the complete psychological works of Sigmund Freud* (Vol. XIV). London, England: The Hogarth Press. (Original work published 1915)

Freud, S. (1958). Formulations regarding the two principles in mental functioning (1925). In J. Strachey (Ed.), *The standard edition of the complete psychological works of Sigmund Freud* (Vol. XII). London, England: The Hogarth Press. (Original work published 1925)Hill, C. E., & Knox, S. (2009). Processing the therapeutic relationship. *Psychotherapy Research* 19, 13–29.

Jiménez, J. P. (2009). Grasping psychoanalysts' practice in its own merits. *The International Journal of Psychoanalysis*, 90(2), 231–248.

Kopp, R. (1998). Early recollections in Adlerian and metaphor therapy. *Journal of Individual Psychology*, 54, 480–486.

Kopp, R., & Eckstein, D. (2004). Using early memory metaphors and client-generated metaphors in Adlerian therapy. *Journal of Individual Psychology*, 60, 163–174.

Lakoff, G. (1993). The contemporary theory of metaphor. In A. Ortony (Ed.), *Metaphor and thought* (2nd ed.). Cambridge, England: Cambridge University Press.

Lakoff, G., & Johnson, M. (1980). *Metaphors we live by*. Chicago, IL: University of Chicago Press.

Lakoff, G., & Johnson, M. (1999). *Philosophy in the flesh: The embodied mind and its challenges to Western thought*. New York, NY: Basic Books.

Lambert, M. J. (Ed.). (2013). *Bergin and Garfield's handbook of psychotherapy and behavior change* (6th ed.). Hoboken, NJ: Wiley.

Macdonald, J. (2013). 'Formal' feedback in psychotherapy as psychoanalytic technique. *Psychodynamic Practice*, 20(2), 154–163. doi:10.1080/14753634.2013.771566.

MacGregor, S. K. (2006). Operational definitions. In *Encyclopedia of educational leadership and administration*. Retrieved from http://sageereference.com/edlea-dership/Article_n408.html

Rizzuto, A. M. (2001). Metaphors of a bodily mind. *Journal of the American Psychoanalytical Association*, 49, 535–556.

Rizzuto, A. M. (2009). Metaphoric process and metaphor: The dialectics of shared analytic experience. *Psychoanalytic Inquiry*, 29(1), 18–29.

Rodríguez Quiroga de Pereira, A., Borensztein, L., Bongiardino, L., Aufenacker, S., & Juan, S. (2019, May). *Testing psychic change hypotheses: A systematic study of a single case of psychoanalytic psychotherapy, using the Three-Level Model (3-LM)*. Paper presented at the 20th Joseph Sandler Conference, Buenos Aires, Argentina.

Rodríguez Quiroga de Pereira, A., Borensztein, L, Corbella, V., & Marengo, J. C. (2018). The Lara case: A group analysis of initial psychoanalytic interviews using systematic clinical observation and empirical tools. *The International Journal of Psychoanalysis*, 99(6), 1327–1352.

Schachter, J., & Kächele, H. (2017). *Nodal points: Critical voices in contemporary psychotherapy/psychoanalysis*. Astoria, NY: International Psychoanalytic Books.

Chapter 23

A descriptive comparison of first interviews under the light of 3-LM and initiating psychoanalysis

Andrea Rodríguez Quiroga de Pereira

I understand that before I start this comparison, I must clarify my context. I have participated in the Working Party on Initiating Psychoanalysis (WPIP) by presenting a case and I have been working with the Three-Level Model (3-LM) for several years, both in its workshops and in research. Beyond what the models describe, I have the experience I have just explained to you.

It is interesting to go back on some points in which the use of both the 3-LM (Altmann de Litvan, 2014) and the WPIP (Reith et al., 2018) contribute to the psychoanalytic community.

The first one I would like to mention is the experience that both working parties share when studying a case and its process, with the presence of the treating analyst and with the view of a third party, the working group. Both working parties have been highly successful throughout the years and their development, and many psychoanalysts in the different regions of the International Psychoanalytical Association have been able to participate in the experience of processing clinical materials. By accepting to participate in these proposals, each working group gets started, based on the clinical practice as well as the different perspectives of its participants. This allows the groups to advance in the production of knowledge about the patient, the analyst, and the process, instead of getting stuck in controversial theoretical discussions.

In this way, both methods allow an approach to a more experienced near-clinical common ground, understanding this as a shared argumentative field (Bernardi, 2003).

By regarding differences and clarity in defining the task, and distinguishing it from a supervision, an 'intervision', these groups generate an emotional state that consents to creating a work field belonging to psychoanalytic thinking.

Curiously, both models use three levels, although only one of them identifies with that name. The 3-LM's three levels are (1) phenomenological description of the transformations, (2) diagnostic dimensions of the change, and (3) explanatory hypotheses of the change. The WPIP's three stages are (1)

DOI: 10.4324/9780000000002-28

first interview(s), processing notes; (2) clinical workshop; and (3) WPIP case study.

It is important to distinguish a difference between the two groups: the 3-LM works with the analyst and the group at each of its levels, whereas the WPIP includes only the workshop moderator and reporter or the group in its third level, not the analyst. Because the third level is a time for investigation into the case, I wonder, why should we exclude the analyst? The reasons for doing so are explained in this way:

> At some point it may be easier to elaborate without the presenting analyst, … just as in stage 2 elaboration is facilitated by the absence of the patient. … [T]hey can also be an opportunity to elaborate the 'sessions residues' of the previous 'stages', leading to a progressively deeper understanding. (Reith et al., 2018, p. 60)

Having passed the experience as a presenter, I would have found it interesting to know the production of the research group regarding my patient and to be able to use it to his benefit, to think together.

In my opinion, both models imply sharing and emphasising the importance of the training of psychoanalysts. Nevertheless, they do so differently. The WPIP guides the discussion through a series of questions to the analyst, in a more traditional way, and still leaving room for free association. As Reith et al. (2018) stated, 'This provides a form of reality testing in which individual group members could come to recognize that their own reading of the process notes wasn't necessarily exhaustive' (p. 42). The emphasis is on the analyst's understanding of their own ideas or associations. As they claimed, the method 'can be thought of as an instrument to "see" unconscious dynamics that are too "blinding" or overpowering for the mind to take in on first contact' (Reith et al., 2018, p. 60). This is the direction of systematic work.

A difference between the models worth noting is that the questions of the 3-LM are aimed at understanding the patient in a systematic way, as a guide or heuristic to observe and describe the patient's changes. This can be considered an essential aspect of analyst training today, because it allows not only for a more complete understanding of what happens to the patient but also for the analyst to engage in dialogue with non-psychoanalysts more clearly.

Having said that, I find that some questions of the 3-LM, such as 'How does the patient use the analyst and his interventions?', could be used to better understand how the analyst selects the material from which they interpret and what they do to arrive at an interpretation. Additionally, this could help to investigate more specifically their countertransference, both before doing the interpretation and in relation to the patient's use of it as well. Other relevant questions are 'What specific conflicts does the analyst have in their mind?' and 'Are they moving towards any of the anchor points selected?' Although this last one is one of the questions in the third level, it could be educational to understand more about their feelings, conflicts, and personal theories from the beginning and throughout the process.

Neither model neglects the analytical situation, the analytical couple, and their vicissitudes. They aim, from different angles, to understand the dynamics of it. Furthermore, both models insist on working with the material as it has been presented by the analyst, thus trying to understand what they are responding to or specifically referring to.

In relation to the aims of each model, the 3-LM is expected to sharpen the clinical observation and description of the transformations that occur during long periods of analysis or in the course of a complete treatment. The first interviews are the starting point, where one must find the anchor points or metaphors that may become focal points to work with throughout the process (Rodríguez Quiroga de Pereira, Borensztein, Corbella, & Marengo, 2018). As for the WPIP, it is interested in seeing whether forms of conscious or unconscious dynamics take place between analyst and patient in the first interviews. Moreover, it observes whether relationships can be found between such dynamics in addition to the decision to begin analysis, also including the process of the analysis. That being said, I must specify that it is difficult for me to understand the emphasis placed by the model on its central objective. As Reith et al. (2018, p. 1) explained, the WPIP 'will try to clarify how analysts actually perform the task resulting in recommendation of analysis, and what goes on that make it possible to initiate an analysis'. Perhaps, partially, this has to do with the different countries where we live and work.

To me, from the first encounter with their analyst, the patient is immersed in an analytical process, not even knowing how far they will be able to move forward as a duo.

Transformations and dynamics, both in the first interviews and over the analysis process, show a mutual interest, from models created in different regions, and reflect a need to promote and share a joint and systematic processing on different issues.

In relation to empirical research, these models have followed different paths. Both have protected the confidentiality of both patient and analyst. From my point of view, as a clinical researcher, I cannot help regretting the destruction of the clinical materials done by the WPIP after investigating them. I say this because I consider that the request for informed consents from both patients and analysts would have provided analysts-in-training with materials of incalculable value through which a patient can be studied from different perspectives. Nonetheless, I still understand the analysts' difficulties in requesting informed consents, and that might have slowed down the sample collection (Rodríguez Quiroga de Pereira, Bongiardino, et al., 2018; Wajnbuch et al., 2017; Rodríguez Quiroga de Pereira, Messina, & Samsalone, 2012).

The WPIP has followed the same predefined procedures in all of the cases they have studied – from the presentation of the clinical material, to the semistructured discussion in the clinic, to the workshops, to the subsequent work of the WPIP with the clinical material. They claim to be conducting an ongoing qualitative investigation and attempting to develop a constructivist grounded theory, taking into consideration the influence of the research process on the results as part of the methodology (Reith et al., 2018).

Upon obtaining their preliminary results, they emphasised that they could not reach any firm conclusions regarding one of their first hypotheses. They could not conclude whether the patient's characteristics could inform, in a useful way, the decision of whether psychoanalysis should be initiated or not or to predict whether psychoanalysis with a given patient would work successfully. With regard to the first point, I have already raised my differences. As for the second point, I understand that the patient is not systematically studied in order to find a relationship between the initial interviews and the outcome of the treatment.

However, the results of these studies have proven that the unconscious dynamics of the initial interviews were much more powerful than anticipated. The authors adopted the term 'unconscious storm', by Bion, to describe the dynamics at play, creating intense transferences and countertransferences. What can be seen is that the result of each session is actually a result of how well the patient and the analyst could adapt to one another unconsciously and also in relation to the emotional situation, the sociocultural context, and the institution. Based on their experience, they believe that an analytical patient–therapist duo is co-created. The role of the analyst is essential at this stage, and it becomes of interest to understand the development dynamics of the duo and how the analyst works in that context (Reith et al., 2018). They specifically allude to the analyst's ability to accept the challenge of opening up emotionally and to how emotions work. Their conclusions give rise to thinking about the coincidences that they have with research studies in psychotherapy about the importance of the first interviews, the attitude of the therapist, and the therapeutic alliance with its ruptures and repairs (Barrett, Chua, Crits-Christoph, Gibbons, & Thompson, 2008; Flückiger, Holtforth, Znoj, Caspar, & Wampold, 2013; Lutz, 2002; Lutz et al., 2006, 2013; Oddli & Rønnestad, 2012).

The 3-LM has chosen a somewhat different path. The 3-LM approaches the process of change undergone by the patient because of the analysis, studying how this is visible in the sessions and a possible hypothesis for why this has occurred. This method gives the professionals a systematic view of the case and an alternative stance on the analysts. From this perspective, to develop a case systematically is essential in order to know the information about the patient the analyst needs to treat them.

The systematisation proposed by the model, specifically at its second level, diagnostic dimensions of change, allows for a knowledge of the patient acquired by being able to think systematically about the patient. The questions posed at this level have been developed based on three diagnostic manuals, the *Diagnostic and Statistical Manual of Mental Disorders*, 5th edition (American Psychiatric Association, 2013), the *Psychodynamic Diagnostic Manual* (PDM Task Force, 2006), and the *Operationalized Psychodynamic Diagnosis OPD-2: Manual of Diagnosis and Treatment Planning* (OPD-2; OPD Task Force, 2007, 2008). The model is a dynamic clinical tool, in the sense that it is open to modifications and developments that may come from its use. Its validity and reliability are being tested, and this growth is done in order to cater to the needs of modern and evolving analysts.

The first study (A. Garbarino, M. Luzardo, & A. Corti, personal communication, 2019) about the degree of agreement between analysts in clinical trials on the unconscious processes of change over prolonged periods of analysis allows us to answer that, from the analyst's perspective, they are very satisfied with the model as a valid instrument for observing and understanding changes in the unconscious processes of long-term analysis. However, the author says that, to obtain a response about the reliability of 3-LM, they must improve the research design and the same team of judges-analysts should evaluate a certain number of patients.

A second study has also been carried out on a single-case study in psychodynamic psychotherapy, working with the 3-LM becoming a possible predictor of treatment results. The changes in the four initial interviews were studied and, in relation to that, the possible changes of the patient were hypothesised after 9 months of treatment. A general convergence was observed between the different perspectives (3-LM, therapist, judges, and patient). These results may be viewed as a small step towards a greater trustworthiness of the 3-LM (Rodríguez Quiroga de Pereira, Borensztein, Bongiardino, Aufenacker, & Juan, 2019).

A third study, an International Psychoanalytic Association Grant, 'Multicentric Qualitative Study: Trustworthiness of the Three Level Model (3-LM)' (Rodriguez Quiroga et al., 2021) that aims to produce empirical evidence regarding the validity and reliability of the 3-LM, is currently being reported. It compares the production of groups of psychoanalysts from different regions with the same clinical cases and then analyses the production with the same structured qualitative methodology. On the one hand, results of the qualitative analysis are going to be compared between sites, analysing whether similar ideas are found in the independent groups, in an equivalent way to inter-judge agreement but at a group level and with a qualitative approach. On the other hand, production results of the 3-LM groups based on their forms are going to be compared to empirical findings from psychoanalytic process measures used in the single case. In that case, we would have partial and preliminary evidence of trustworthiness of the 3-LM method. Consensual qualitative research (Hill et al., 2005; Hill, Thompson, & Williams, 1997) will be used to analyse 3-LM's levels 1 and 3 (phenomenological description of the transformations of the case and the tests of the explanatory hypotheses of such modifications), and the OPD-2 (von der Tann & OPD Task Force, 2008) will be used to analyse the 3-LM's second level (diagnostic dimensions of change).The aim of the analysis and results will be to test the logic and structure of the 3-LM model, in line with the current need for empirical inquiry, both for psychoanalysis and for therapies based on psychoanalytic theory and technique (Barber & Sharpless, 2015; de Maat et al., 2013).

In this way, both projects, the 3-LM and the WPIP, are part of current International Psychoanalytical Association priorities, related to providing evidence on psychoanalytic premises and procedures, both for clinical psychology in general and for psychoanalysis as a discipline in particular.

At the same time, the use of cases of psychoanalysis, along with cases of psychoanalytic therapy (as is done in the 3-LM), generates possibilities for discussion of the results that encompass the clinical practice based on psychoanalysis in a broad sense.

Finally, the multicentric nature of the studies will allow for an analysis of the role of the context in the psychoanalytic conceptualisation of the cases.

The future directions of the 3-LM methodology and its applications, linked to other strategies to evaluate effectiveness in dynamic therapies – such as OPD-2 – will be analysed.

The long-term possibilities of both projects involve, among others, comparing cases of abandonment versus cases of therapeutic completion, or clinical situations centred on conflict versus clinical situations dominated by structural vulnerabilities (see, for example, Juan, Chávez, López Fediuk, Manubens, & Gómez Penedo, 2018).

References

Altmann de Litvan, M. (Ed.). (2014). *Tiempo de cambio: Indagando las transformaciones en psicoanálisis. El modelo de los tres niveles*. London, England: Karnac.

American Psychiatric Association. (2013). *Diagnostic and statistical manual of mental disorders* (5th ed.). Washington, DC: Author.

Barber, J. P., & Sharpless, B. A. (2015). On the future of psychodynamic therapy research. *Psychotherapy Research*, 25(3), 309–320.

Barrett, M. S., Chua, W. J., Crits-Christoph, P., Gibbons, M. B., & Thompson, D. (2008). Early withdrawal from mental health treatment: Implications for psychotherapy practice. *Psychotherapy: Theory, Research, Practice, Training*, 45(2), 247–267.

Bernardi, R. (2003). What kind of evidence makes the analyst change his or her theoretical and technical ideas? In M. Leuzinger-Bohleber, A. U. Dreher, & J. Canestri (Eds.), *Pluralism and unity? Methods of research in psychoanalysis*. London, England: International Psychoanalytical Association.

de Maat, S., de Jonghe, F., de Kraker, R., Lesichering, F., Abbass, A., Luyten, P., … Dekker, J. (2013). The current state of the empirical evidence for psychoanalysis: A meta-analytic approach. *Harvard Review of Psychiatry*, 21(3), 107–137.

Flückiger, C., Holtforth, M. G., Znoj, H., Caspar, F., & Wampold, B. E. (2013). Is the relation between early post-session reports and treatment outcome an epiphenomenon of intake distress and early response? A multi-predictor analysis in outpatient psychotherapy. *Psychotherapy Research*, 23(1), 1–13.

Hill, C. E., Knox, S., Thompson, B. J., Nutt Williams, E., Hess, S. A., & Ladany, N. (2005). Consensual qualitative research: An update. *Journal of Counseling Psychology*, 52(2), 196–205.

Hill, C. E., Thompson, B. J., & Williams, E. N. (1997). A guide to conducting consensual qualitative research. *The Counseling Psychologist*, 25, 517–572.

Juan, S., Chávez, I., López Fediuk, L., Manubens, R., & Gómez Penedo, J. M. (2018, June). *Mecanismos de cambio en un caso único sistematizado de terapia psicoanalítica*. Paper presented at the VI Jornadas de Investigación en Psicología, Instituto de Investigaciones de la Facultad de Psicología y Psicopedagogía, Universidad del Salvador, Buenos Aires, Argentina.

Lutz, W. (2002). Patient-focused psychotherapy research and individual treatment progress as scientific groundwork for an empirical based clinical practice. *Psychotherapy Research*, 12, 251–272.

Lutz, W., Ehrlich, T., Rubel, J., Hallwachs, N., Röttger, M. A., Jorasz, C., … Tschitsaz-Stucki, A. (2013). The ups and downs of psychotherapy: Sudden gains and sudden losses identified with sessions Reports. *Psychotherapy Research*, 23(1), 14–24.

Lutz, W., Lambert, M. J., Harmon, S. C., Tschitsaz, A., Schürch, E., & Stulz, N. (2006). The probability of treatment success, failure and duration. What can be learned from empirical data to support decision making in clinical practice? *Clinical Psychology & Psychotherapy*, 13(4), 223–232.

Oddli, H. W., & Rønnestad, M. H. (2012). How experienced therapists introduce the technical aspects in the initial alliance formation: Powerful decision makers supporting clients' agency. *Psychotherapy Research*, 22(2), 176–193.

OPD Task Force. (2007). *Operationalized psychodynamic diagnosis OPD-2: Manual of diagnosis and treatment planning* (1st ed.). Cambridge, MA: Hogrefe & Huber Publishers.

OPD Task Force. (2008). *Operationalized psychodynamic diagnosis OPD-2: Manual of diagnosis and treatment planning*(E. Ristl, Trans.). Ashland, OH: Hogrefe & Huber.

PDM Task Force. (2006). *Psychodynamic diagnostic manual*. Silver Spring, MD: Alliance of Psychoanalytic Organizations.

Reith, B., Møller, M., Boots, J., Crick, P., Gibeault, A., Jaffe, R., … Vermote, R. (2018). *Beginning analysis. On the process of initiating psychoanalysis*. London, England: Routledge.

Rodríguez Quiroga de Pereira, A., Bongiardino, L., Borensztein, L., Marengo, J., Aufenacker, S., & Mango, C. (2018). Consentimiento informado: Su uso y opinión entre psicoanalistas latinoamericanos. *Revista Caliban*, 16(2), 204–218.

Rodríguez Quiroga de Pereira, A., Borensztein, L., Bongiardino, L., Aufenacker, S. I., & Juan, S. (2019, May). *Testing change hypotheses: a systematic single-case study of psychodynamic psychotherapy using the Three-Level Model (3-LM)*. Dialogue at the 20th Joseph Sandler Conference: Understanding and Psychoanalytic Treatment of Depression: Dialogues Between Clinicians and Researchers, Buenos Aires, Argentina.

Rodríguez Quiroga de Pereira, A., Borensztein, A., Corbella, V., & Marengo, J. C. (2018). The Lara case: A group analysis of initial psychoanalytic interviews using systematic clinical observation and empirical tools. *The International Journal of Psychoanalysis*, 99(6), 1327–1352.

Rodriguez Quiroga de Pereira, A., Juan, S., Bongiardino, L., Aufenacker, S. I., Crawley, A., Botero, M. C., & Borensztein, L. (2021). *Multicentric qualitative study: Trustworthiness of the Three Level Model (3-LM)*. International Psychoanalytic Association Grant.

Rodríguez Quiroga de Pereira, A., Messina, A., & Samsalone, P. (2012). Informed consent calling for debate between analysts and researchers. *The International Journal of Psychoanalysis*, 93, 963–980.

von der Tann, M., & OPD Task Force (Eds.). (2008). *Operationalized psychodynamic diagnosis OPD-2: Manual of diagnosis and treatment planning* (E. Ristl, Trans.). Boston, MA: Hogrefe & Huber.

Wajnbuch, S., Bonifacino, N., Durand, N., González, L. A., Koppittke, C., Nader, V., … Rouilon, G. (2017). Confidencialidad, disfraz y ¿consentimiento informado? *Revista Uruguaya de Psicoanálisis*, 127, 129–151.

Part VI

Final considerations and questions raised

Chapter 24

The impact of clinical investigation on the analyst

Vera Regina Fonseca

Altmann de Litvan (2019) quoted Hinshelwood about the need for triangulation in order to overcome the inherent subjectivity of our task as analysts. Triangulation is considered the 'simultaneous examination of two perspectives' (Hinshelwood, 2013, p. 126) and may refer either to the methodological realm, or a set of data, or to using different investigators, or even different theoretical approaches for analysing data. Nowadays the triangulation is considered part of most clinical work inside the analysis room, because the analyst uses a combination of information coming from her countertransference with the patient's free association and behaviour. A multiple triangulation (of perspectives, methods, and analysts) is of paramount importance in the present investigation.

Thus, clinical research is not only a valid instrument for enlarging general psychoanalytic knowledge but it is also a means to throw light into the dark corners of the psychoanalytic field created by each patient/analyst pair. The multiple triangulation results of the group study (working party) would provide a wider angle to observe clinical phenomena. Indeed, the very process of research is expected to impact on the perspective and attenuate blind spots of the actual analytical pair.

The endeavour of analysis does not count on a protocol; instead, the analyst fumbles to find the way, but one should ask how much of this fumble contains her own bias and collusion in order to avoid hard spots and conflict areas. 'In what concerns the research team, the goal is to look beyond the Ivory tower created by our theories and beliefs. For the analyst, the aim would be to unveil possible 'bastions''' (Ferro, 1993, p. 919).

For all these purposes, we have to rely on triangulation in its varied forms.

I will try to bring proof of the importance of psychoanalytic research not only for psychoanalytic knowledge in general but also for the particular case of the analyst, due to the long-lasting improvement on her ability to widen and deepen her angle of vision.

Let me begin with some background information. When I was the scientific chair of the Brazilian Psychoanalytic Society of São Paulo, under the

DOI: 10.4324/9780000000002-30

presidency of Nilde Franch, Liana Chaves proposed a partnership to me to help organise the conference of the International Psychoanalytical Association Committee on Clinical Research, to which she belongs. After several meetings and exchange of ideas, we decided to propose an exercise: How would different types of working parties (WPs) deal with the same clinical material? Would they arrive at similar conclusions? Despite the differences in methods and aims, would it bring a deeper understanding of the psychoanalytic process?

Notwithstanding an initial mild resistance, the groups accepted the challenge to partly change their methods in order to fit the new proposal. Five kinds of WPs were included:

- Comparative Clinical Method (CCM)
- Specificity of the Analytical Method
- Microscopy of the Analytic Session
- Listening to Listening.

All of these were accomplished using a transversal cut with three sequential sessions during one week of treatment.

- The Three-Level Model (3-LM): a horizontal cut, covering 10 sessions over an 8-year time span.

The core questions were the following: To what extent can the several modalities of WPs be considered clinical research? What results would we get using the same clinical material for the five types considered? What convergences and divergences would be gotten? What are the difficulties and advantages of such a task?

The answers to these questions will be dealt with in another part of the book. The present text concerns the last one, which was not included in the protocol: What would be the impact of the research process on the analyst?

In this presentation I will focus on only two of the WP modalities: the CCM and the 3-LM.

Summary of the patient's history

Helena (H) is 60 years old and is in her seventh year of analysis, with three sessions a week. She is married, has kids and grandkids, and retired about 4 years ago.

She was born in a state up to the North; her parents split for some years when she was 7, and she and her mother had to move to another town, where the two of them had no family or acquaintances. Some years later the couple reunited and settled in a big city.

She looked for analysis because of anxiety and dizziness attacks 2 years after the death of her mother, who she described as a hardworking woman who had professional success but was scarcely sensitive to Helena's needs. Her motto was: 'One has to endure!'

Helena's gait is a bit rigid and she is very conservative in her attire and has short, cropped hair and no makeup.

The clinical case was presented without disclosure of the analyst's identity.

Result of the CCM

I will now transcribe the part of the conclusion that has impacted the analyst most:

> Taking into account the methodological limitations ... it seemed to the group that the analyst, during the sessions considered, works with an implicit model (i.e., not conscious) of deficit, in which the experience of analysis turns out to be an experience with a new object instead of the repair and regeneration of internal objects. It seemed to us the kind of intervention the analyst used is coherent with this implicit model.

This observation implied that in the binomial conflict/deficit, the dimension of conflict has been overlooked; this implication was registered by the analyst, bringing her to a questioning state of mind, sometimes only as a background, other times occupying the forefront. Another striking point was about the reliance on the idea of the analyst as a new object in detriment of the repair of internal objects. This point will be dealt in the next section.

After the investigation

Fresh new material from sessions that took place some months after the seminar are transcribed below:

H begins the session showing the analyst some pictures of her relatives and grandkids, which is a bit unusual. Then she talks about the weekend she spent in X, her hometown. She travelled there with her husband and father to attend her cousin's birthday party; she talked a lot with her relatives until late into the night. Her cousin was moved to see Helena's father, who is quite old.

HELENA: It was quite nice. I decided to bring along my father, and, in the morning, he asked me if I didn't want to go to Y [a small village close to X] to buy some sweaters, as my mother used to do. Then I realised he really wanted to go there. We went and we met other relatives we hadn't seen in ages. It was quite enjoyable. …

ANALYST: Indeed, you seem more relaxed, … you even showed me your pictures, and are enjoying the big family you have. …

HELENA: Yes, … in the past maybe I wouldn't even think of attending the birthday party, but this time I insisted my son about him going too and I decided to bring my father along.At this precise moment the analyst recalled the sentence of the WP report about her implicit theory of deficit and she asked herself if she was avoiding bringing to the field the aggressive and conflicting aspects of Helena. It was such a powerful idea that it made her do the following intervention:

A: Maybe your resistance to visit your relatives in the past meant a kind of protest, of resentful distance. …

H: Yes, I resented the fact that when we went visit the big family everything turned around my mother, and it seemed there was no room for me. I didn't even appear, as I was just an extra. …

Considering this confirmation, the analyst reflected and wrote later: 'I think about the late interpretation of aggressive aspects, which maybe allows for a greater amount of confidence concerning the constructive tendencies: the splitting is attenuated, by virtue of the very analysis, and now can be successfully interpreted'.

In what concerns the part of the CCM report about 'the experience of analysis turns out to be an experience with a new object instead of the repair and regeneration of internal objects, …' it is possible that the analytic process as a whole contributed to a more benevolent relationship with both internal and external parental objects: despite great fluctuation in Helena's disposition towards her parents (in this set of sessions the father is highlighted), she may intuit his father's longing to meet the distant relatives and somehow revive with H his experiences with his late wife. This parallels a movement of repair of internal parental objects, even if this is not explicitly addressed in the considered sessions.

Three-Level Model

Below are the points the analyst considered the most important from the WP report:

- Emotions are cancelled to move on with her life. Why does she cancel them? The intense anxiety, the panic attacks described in the beginning, caused Helena a loss of functions, made her freeze and be prone to a great inhibition. She has many dreams, but scarce associations, revealing some difficulty in thinking about them. Also, her sexuality is excluded to the point that the analyst can't feel free to ask about it.

- Dreams/houses: The different houses and hotels depicted in the dreams are linked to a very important line in the present case, concerning the body. In the beginning it is presented as a rigid one, with a stiff gait, displaying an expressionless facial mask.
- Perplexity, suspension, and disconnection. The analyst brings a comment about the patient: she felt her as perplexed and on the edge of an abyss. This metaphor emerged as a thread uniting different parts of the clinical material.

After the investigation

Some months after the symposium, H tells a dream: Her granddaughter was in a hospital with two other girls. She wanted to find someone to help, but she could not; she got lost and while still searching she walked past beautiful landscapes, as if they were scenes from the holiday trips she enjoys so much. Nevertheless, she was still lost.

The analyst speaks about the three girls, one of which may be H, who is separated from her object of love as if by the wrongdoing of a wicked witch. She keeps searching and may even find beautiful landscapes that maybe compensate for the loss (her long-lasting desire for trips may contain a kind of erotic pleasure). She goes on:

A: The love you have both for beauty and for your granddaughter is like the love an infant has for her mother, a desire to be close, to hug, to be in bodily touch. And the beautiful scenery may, sometimes, be a kind of consolation, of putting together love and beauty.

As soon as the analyst makes this quite long intervention, she recalls a dream she had the previous night: she was sleeping, and H was crawling under her duvet.

After this session, the analyst wrote:

> I think my dream contained a movement of grasping both Helena's longing for intimacy and my fear of being intruded by such powerful love. Indeed, in the dream there was the kind of eroticism an infant may have regarding her mother, first aiming at physical and emotional intimacy before being linked preferentially to sex. For the first time, in all these years, Helena wrote to me during the sessions to unburden her fear of being sick. This signalled an attenuation of her rigidity, a decreasing of the abyss (as in the metaphor). At the other side of the abyss is the Other, now able to be eroticized.

Conclusions

Presenting a case and listening to the comments made by peers is a process of widening the perspective and deepening the understanding about the dynamics of the analytic pair. It goes without saying that just writing down a session offers the analyst the opportunity of seeing beyond what had already been seen during the session. If we take a horizontal perspective, as in the case of 3-LM, we will have a wider perspective of the whole analytic process and its more striking characteristics, including its blind spots kept over time.

The results of the 3-LM highlighted both the metaphor of the analyst (the patient on the edge of an abyss) and the oversight in tackling of the patient's sexuality. Again, several months after the investigation, it has been possible to hypothesise a link between the abyss and the absence of sexual contents, triggered by a dream the analyst had.

In the case of a transversal cut, as in the CCM, the research team will look for the implicit theory of the analyst (and why not of the pair?) about the patient, which may or may not be a constant in the process (i.e., the analyst may bear such implicit theory all the time or only at some moments). Anyway, listening to these descriptions may bring a transformative/questioning impetus to the analytic dynamics, challenging the tendency of immobility and repetition. This is clear in what concerns the idea of conflict that popped in to the analyst's mind during the session that occurred several months after the investigation. The time needed to transform the idea from 'superegoic' into assimilated is noteworthy, in such a way that a fruitful intervention was possible. The balance of a transformative approach versus a more 'familiar' one is never a black-and-white question, of good and bad quality; instead, there is the need for opening alternate avenues little by little for the analytic pair to enjoy a genuine development.

To conclude, investigation in psychoanalysis is a multifaceted enterprise, aimed at making the body of psychoanalytic knowledge more robust and the exchange with other disciplines more feasible; another effect concerns the changes in the analyst's mind and, consequently, the expansion of the analytic field.

Thus, it is worth finishing this text with the following quote by Hinshelwood (2016): 'I think we should not be shy to demand respect for our difficult form of research'.

References

Altmann de Litvan, M. (2019). Los sueños como indicios de algunas transformaciones del paciente. In F. M. Gómez (Ed.), *Percepción y sueño. Perspectivas actuales*. Buenos Aires, Argentina: APA.

Ferro, A. (1993). The impasse within a theory of the analytic field: Possible vertices of observation. *The International Journal of Psychoanalysis*, 74(5), 917–929.

Hinshelwood, R. D. (2013). *Research on the couch*. East Sussex, England, and New York, NY: Routledge.

Hinshelwood, R. D. (2016, November) *What is psychoanalytic knowledge? And how do we get it?* Paper presented at the Brazilian Psychoanalytic Society of São Paulo Symposium 'The Several Faces of Clinical Research', São Paulo, Brazil.

Chapter 25

The analyst's perspective

Commonalities and differences of working parties on a clinical material

Luisa Pérez Suquilvide

The clinical observation models developed through the working parties of the International Psychoanalytical Association are useful instruments to enter the roughness of the psychoanalytic research frontier. This is a border that challenges us to open ourselves to different outlooks and new questions.

It is not an easy task to compare methodologies with such different goals, so I will focus on the contributions of the Three-Level Model (3-LM), the Specificity of Psychoanalysis model (De Souza Brito, Chabalgoity, Ponce de León, & Levy 2018), and Faimberg's 'Listening to Listening' method (Faimberg, 2007; 'Método Faimberg', 2014) for my comprehension of the clinical material.

My first presentation was at the 3-LM working party. I chose an analysis of 4½ years that I was working on to write my final paper to become an associate member of the Uruguayan Psychoanalytic Association. I selected five significant sessions of different moments of the analysis. The affective resonance and the metaphors that emerged at those moments of the transference were the elements that guided my selection.

According to the goals of each model, the group received the clinical material in different ways. In the 3-LM the group receives the material before the discussion, along with a series of questions guiding the description and identification of the transformations and the primary diagnostic dimensions of change. In the Specificity of Psychoanalysis and Faimberg's Listening to Listening models, the group listens for the first time to a cut-out version of the material in the analyst's reading. Although I was aware of these cut-outs, I was slightly surprised when reading the material to the group.

In the model of Specificity of Psychoanalysis, the goal is to place the group in the ambiguity of the analytic field, focusing primarily on the analytical course. According to this method, the context of group associative dynamics co-creates a new transference field and a 'new patient'. Thus, the cut-out conveys the necessary content of the sessions with no biographical or anecdotal data of the patient, nor timeline.

In Faimberg's Listening to Listening method, the cut-out of the sessions into small fragments highlighting analyst's interventions aims to place the

DOI: 10.4324/9780000000002-31

group in the same 'not knowing' situation of the analyst with the patient so that the participants can focus on the listening of each intervention. The hiatus occurring between what the presenter thinks they said and what was heard by the participants opens the space to identify what Faimberg (2007) raised as 'the misunderstanding', allowing for the recognition of the underlying assumptions from which the analyst and each participant listens and intervenes.

These models aim to put the group as if the members were in the analytical session. Although both work over fragments of several sessions, the work centred on the transference–countertransference relationship in the Specificity of Psychoanalysis model and on the interventions in Faimberg's Listening to Listening model blurs the longitudinal perspective, giving the idea of a cross section of the process. The 3-LM observes the transformations in a cross-sectional look at each session, but tracking them throughout the analytic process gives us a longitudinal look.

A common feature of these models is that the group device has an amplifying effect in relation to the phenomena that occur in the analytical field. The group works as a sounding board in which the oral transmission, the reading of the material by the analyst, is central to give life to the analytical scene. This plays a particular role in the case of the 3-LM, because the participants can integrate the emotions transmitted by the analyst's reading to the plain written text they had already worked over.

As in music, the voice of the analyst, with its tone and rhythm, introduces us to the melody co-created with the patient in the different moments of the process, placing us vividly in the affective atmosphere of transference–countertransference. The metaphor of music brings me closer to transmitting the resonances that the different models produced in the presentation of my clinical material.

In the Specificity of Psychoanalysis model, the group worked as a symphonic orchestra playing live, in which each instrument – the participants – enters, giving a different nuance in terms of the music's sound. An intense work of transference–countertransference with the group promoted the updating of other moments of the transference with an intense affective resonance, which led me to acknowledge a different approach to the relational models of the patient. I would describe it as an analytic 'second experience' because it placed me in front of something new from the original sound of the transference with the patient. I think that being a silent but committed observer enhanced the intensity of the affective resonance of the group associative process. Nonetheless, in certain moments the new transference co-created by the group associative dynamics took a turn that, in my view, moved away from my patient. This partially 'new patient', besides making me feel some frustration and anxiety – because I had to remain silent – made me wonder about the risk of this method of creating another patient, away from the real patient.

The resonances in Faimberg's Listening to Listening model led me to the experience of listening to a live jazz band, in which the background rhythm appears interrupted by the surprise of the solo artists. The group interventions highlighted, at some points, the misunderstanding to which Faimberg (2007) referred as 'I did not mean that'. This second look focusing on my interventions made me ask myself 'Did I said that?', 'What did I mean?', or 'Did I mean that?' In retrospect, the group discussion opened up different perspectives that made me think about the possible biases about my interventions linked to the implicit and explicit theories working in my mind.

The 3-LM, like the flatter sound of a musical recording, with an equal richness of nuances but different in terms of its emotional intensity, gives the possibility of going back and forth, to meet the 'anchor points', often expressed as metaphors. It allowed me to refine and resignify the transformations, the aspects that did not change, and those I did not address with the patient. As for tuning an instrument, the different levels enriched the 'second analytic look', with the subtlety of observing the changes in different mental dimensions and interpersonal functioning of the patient.

One interesting fact that surprised me was finding that diverse groups of analysts, working with different methodologies, came up with similar and complementary metaphors on the same clinical material, reinforcing the idea of a common knowledge shared among analysts (common ground). However, in Faimberg's Listening to Listening method, there was a smaller number of metaphors.

Because it was an ongoing analytic process, these three models had an interrelated contribution to my comprehension of the patient and influenced my work. The model of the Specificity of Psychoanalysis, amplifying the emotional aspects of the transference–countertransference relationship, highlighted relational patterns of the patient that helped me to clarify the dynamic of the transference at specific moments. Faimberg's Listening to Listening method drew my attention to the unconscious aspects of the misunderstandings and made me more attentive to question possible biases in my interventions according to the patient responses. The meticulous but panoramic look of the 3-LM, apart from giving me a new and refined understanding of the degree and nature of the changes, helped me think about the reasons behind the aspects left out while working with this patient.

As posed by Altmann de Litvan (2014), understanding is the only way to respond to the questions about what happens to patients in our practice, why it happens, and how we can use our analytic tools to help them. Working parties appear to be useful research tools in the attempt to answer those questions.

References

Altmann de Litvan, M. (2014). *Time for change. Tracking transformations in psychoanalysis – The Three-Level Model*. London, England: Karnac.

De Souza Brito, C. L., Chabalgoity, A. M., Ponce de León, E., & Levy, R. (2018). *Contributions to the research on psychoanalysis Working Party sobre a Especificidade do Tratamento Psicanalítico Hoje*. Paper presented at XXXII Congreso Latinoamericano de Psicoanálisis: Deconstrucciones y transformaciones, Lima, Peru.

Faimberg, H. (2007). *El telescopaje de generaciones: A la escucha de los lazos narcisistas entre generaciones* [*The telescoping of generations: Listening to narcissistic ties between generations*]. Buenos Aires, Argentina: Amorrortu Ed.

Método Faimberg. La escucha de la escucha. (2014). *Diccionario de Psicoanálisis Argentino*. (Vol. 2). Buenos Aires, Argentina: APA Publicaciones.

Chapter 26

Clinical psychoanalytic research with the working party method

State of the Art

Rudi Vermote

Introduction

This book starts with several chapters discussing the research conducted by distinguished psychoanalyst researchers and scientists. It is a clear, diverse, and sophisticated discussion on clinical psychoanalytic research reflecting the focus of the International Psychoanalytical Association (IPA) Clinical Research Committee. Many of the points raised resurface in the subsequent chapters on the working parties (WPs) as research groups. In comparison with the first part of the book, the data of the WPs are complex, making it difficult to see the forest for the trees. Over the years, I have attended several meetings with representatives of the WPs (Prague, 2013; Boston, 2015; São Paulo, 2016). These meetings covered a lot of data, thoughts, commitments, discussions, enthusiasm, and criticism. When faced with such abundance, synthesis becomes complicated. The divergences and similarities in methods and aims of the WPs make it difficult to get an overview. Moreover, the research presented in this book is done in groups and was therefore influenced by group dynamics. Remember Bion's words: The major aim of a group is to go on existing as a group (1961). To facilitate a discussion on these findings, it is necessary to simplify and summarise. This is the aim of this chapter.[1]

The discussion is solely based on what is presented in this book – no further enquiries were made.

Very simple definitions used as a background for this review

Psychoanalysts use both a method (the psychoanalytic device; Donnet, 2005) and a body of theories in dealing with mental processes. Psychoanalysts require training to properly employ this device.

When defined in the broadest way possible, research is a systematic investigation. Although psychoanalysis is a systematic method, this does not necessarily imply that it is a systematic investigation as well.

We can discern three ways of systematic investigation, detailed in the introductory chapters (Chapters 2, 4, 5, 6, 7, 8, and 9):

DOI: 10.4324/9780000000002-32

1 Investigation using an empirical method: a highly structured investigation, employing a hypothesis, validated instruments, and a statistical analysis of the data.
2 Investigation using a qualitative method: a structured systematic investigation but with open questions and no statistical analysis.
3 Investigation using an exploratory method: a very open investigation, unstructured.

The six research groups or WPs featured in this book can be classified into the last two categories. The Comparative Clinical Method WP, the WP on Initiating Psychoanalysis, and the Three-Level Model (3-LM) WP all use a qualitative design and method for all of their activities. The WP on Specificity, the WP on Listening to Listening, and the WP on the Microscopy of a Session, on the other hand, use an exploratory design and method, but qualitative research with content analysis has been done on some material of the WP on Specificity (see Chabalgoity, De Souza Brito, & Ponce de León, Chapter 16) and some material of the WP of Microscopy (see Cassorla, Chapter 18).

The empirical research method is far removed from the psychoanalytic treatment method (this is less the case for behaviour therapy, for example, which takes empirically based data as its starting point). The difficulties in conducting empirical psychoanalytic research are known: multiple variables, a closed and private setting, few validated instruments, a small number of clinical researchers to gather data and to do statistical analysis, and resistance by external researchers. Nevertheless, a large body of empirical research on psychoanalysis with publications and reports exists: Open Door Reviews (Leuzinger-Bohleber, Arnold, & Kächele, 2019) and a research network (from the Society for Psychotherapy Research) and a group of research fellows from the IPA). The IPA even offers a competitive funding scheme and yearly training. The psychoanalytical community is indebted to P. Fonagy, M. Leuzinger-Bohleber, H. Kächele, P. Luyten, S. Blatt, and many others for this training. Empirical research is often conducted by colleagues working in adjacent academic fields, not necessarily by psychoanalysts. Most of the findings are published in non-psychoanalytical journals. Besides its findings, empirical research in the field has played a crucial role in both safeguarding psychoanalysis's position as an academic discipline and acquiring support from health insurances. The qualitative and exploratory research discussed in this book can at some point be combined with empirical research (Bernardi, Chapters 6, 27, this book).

Psychoanalysis as a method of treatment relates much more closely to the exploratory method of research. Many analysts have participated in the clinical research project with WPs for over 20 years, despite the existing resistance to research within psychoanalysis. It is short-sighted to place qualitative and exploratory research in opposition to empirical (see Bernardi, Chapter 6, this book).

The origin of the new approach by working parties

When D. Tuckett was president of the European Federation of Psychoanalysis (1999–2004), he delineated the problems that psychoanalysts would be confronted with in the future: education, initiating psychoanalysis, and the multiple psychoanalytic techniques and theories. He suggested an original method to investigate and facilitate communication about these problems. Tuckett's method consisted of investigating these vital topics through the psychoanalytic method of observing and making links, namely, 'free association on clinical material' (Tuckett et al., 2008). The observation of the clinical material by free association is enhanced by doing this in a group of analysts. When doing this, it is important for the group to adopt a nonjudgemental or nonsupervisory attitude. The group of analysts freely associates on the clinical material and tries to understand why a colleague says or does something instead of judging it. In a second stage, the same procedure on the same material is used by an expert group of analysts familiar with the method and coming from different analytic cultures (countries). This expert group similarly processes the data coming from these groups and makes hypotheses and instruments, organising the project of the WP over the years.

A bottom-up project of 2 decades by now

The European Federation of Psychoanalysis (EFP) started a 10-year program using this new method to better understand the issues psychoanalysts face, aiming to solve them. The WPs began this program in 2001 (see Glover & Reith, Chapter 12, this book). The most notable of these programs were End of Training on training criteria; Comparative Clinical Methods, comparing different techniques and the relationship with implicit theories; and Initiating Psychoanalysis, designed to help understand the relationship between preliminary sessions and the engagement in a psychoanalysis.

For each of these research topics an international expert group was set up, meeting around four times a year generally over a period of 10 years. The case presentations and the working groups that gathered data were organised in preconferences at each yearly EFP conference. This approach consists of three stages[2]: (a) the patient and analyst session; (b) the preconference groups (often up to three groups of the same WP); and (c) the expert group.

While they were presidents of the EFP, E. Séchaud (2004–2008) and S. Frish (2012–2016) added a WP on Specificity with a different methodology.

The already existing Listening to Listening method of H. Faimberg was also added as a WP (Faimberg, 2019).

Over the years, these successful WP preconferences spread to the Federación Psicoanalítica de América Latina (Latin American Psychoanalytic Federation) and were also held at IPA conferences.

A similar approach, the 3-LM by the IPA Latin-American Clinical Observation group of M. Altmann de Litvan and R. Bernardi, was added as a WP in 2014. The WP of Microscopy of the analytic session by Cassorla et al. has been running since 1990 and was added as a WP in 2009. Finally, an IPA Working Parties Committee regrouped the WPs under discussion in this text in 2017 (see Glover & Reith, Chapter 12, this book). As D. Taylor, former chair of the IPA Clinical Research Committee, reports in the Note on the IPA's Committee for Clinical Research in Psychoanalysis earlier in this book, in addition to other projects, the WP methods were discussed in two conferences. These were the 2016 Sao Paulo Conference 'Many Faces of Clinical Research' and the 2017 Montevideo Conference 'Working From the Clinic. Metaphor and Interpretation', mainly organised by Liana Pinto Chaves – member of the IPA Clinical Research Committee – and Marina Altmann de Litvan – member of the IPA Clinical Research Committee and current chair of the IPA Clinical Research Committee, within which the 3-LM became prominent. This book is actually a good reflection of the current work of the IPA Clinical Research Committee: a diverse approach to clinical research in psychoanalysis as exemplified in this book by the diverse theoretical contributions and by putting the research of different WPs together. These WPs have their own IPA Working Parties Committee (chaired by Ruggero Levy).

The aim and importance of this book

1 This book brings six WPs of the project together for the first time to compare and specify the working groups. It paints a picture of where we are and what we can expect in the future.
2 An interesting and promising new approach was first conceived during the 2017 Montevideo conference with different WPs. The idea was to narrow down the wide focus of the WPs to the use of metaphors. The function and importance of metaphors in psychoanalysis is argued in specific chapters of this book (Rizzuto, Chapter 10; de León de Bernardi, Chapter 11; Glover & Reith, Chapter 12; Altmann de Litvan, Introduction; and da Rocha Barros, Chapter 20). Three WPs look at the study of metaphors, each using their own distinct method. Whereas the Specificity WP approaches the study of metaphors on a more theoretical level, the 3-LM WP gives a categorisation of the use of metaphors and applies it to a case. The Clinical Comparative WP, on the other hand, applies it to the same case but uses its own categorisation.

An overview of the methods of the different working parties

Table 26.1. Comparing the six working parties in this book.

	CCM	*WPIP*	*3-LM*	*Listening*	*Specificity*	*Micro-scopy*
Start	2001	2001	2009	2006	2006	2010
Research method design	Qualita-tive	Qualita-tive	Qualita-tive	Explora-tory	Explora-tory One qualita-tive study	Explora-tory One qualita-tive study
Number of analysts involved	500–1,000 ?	500–1,000	2000	>500 ?	500 ?	?
Funding	EFP/ FEPAL ?	EPF	IPA/ FEPAL ?	?	EPF	IPA ?
Preliminary theoretical review	+	+	+	+	– ?	+
Moment or process	Moment	Moment	Long-itudinal	Moment	Moment	Moment
Focus	Analyst	Interac-tion analyst–patient	Patient	Analyst and patient	Patient	Field
Group free association as a method	++	++	+	++	+++	++
Semi-structured questions	+	+	+	–	–	–
Expert group as stage in method	+	+	+ ?	?	–	+
Validated rating scales	–	–	+	–	–	–
Results published	++	++	++	?	–	–
Research value	++	++	++	–	?	+
Training value	+	+	+	++	++	++
Impact on psycho-analytic community	++	+	++	++	++	?

Note. + = affirmative or presence of in a low degree. ++ = affirmative or presence of in a greater degree. +++ = affirmative or presence of in an even greater degree. - = negative or no presence of. ? = no confirmed information.

Qualitative research groups

Comparative Clinical Methods WP

The group begins with a presentation of a session, followed by free association on the interventions of the analyst. After this free associative approach, the group focuses on 'what-the-other-does', 'how-the-other-does-it', and 'how-this-other-think-it-works' (see Calich, Chapter 15, this book). The set of categories used in this method has been refined over the years. The method was demonstrated by da Rocha Barros (Chapter 20).

Step 1 of this method uses six categories, which focus on the examination of the diverse possibilities of interventions by the analyst. Step 2 works with five categories on the implicit theories guiding the analyst's work. In this book, Calich (Chapter 15) presents one set of 17 categories to detect the implicit theories employed by the analyst.

WP on Initiating Psychoanalysis

This group begins with a presentation of one or more preliminary analyst and patient interviews (first stage). Afterwards free association by the group is followed by semistructured questions (second stage). Here, the focus is on detecting the dynamics and unconscious patterns in the analytic couple during the first interviews. The group also seeks to study the relation of the characteristics of the initial interview with the proposal and starting or refusing psychoanalysis. This differs from the existing studies on indication that focus on the characteristics of the patient instead of the dynamics of the analytic meeting. Then the second stage is repeated but this time by an expert group (third stage), which similarly looks for patterns. Based on these patterns, hypotheses that are further tested in a way similar to grounded theory qualitative research are formulated (see Reith, Chapter 13, this book).

Three-Level Model WP

The analyst reads six sessions to the group of analysts. The sessions are based on the beginning, middle, and final or recent phase of the analysis. The presenting analyst is present as a participant-observer. The clinical material is made available to the group beforehand, and they are allowed to study it. Level 1 consists of phenomenological resonance and defining anchor points and changes. In level 2, the group measures change by some dimensions of the *Operationalized Psychodynamic Diagnosis OPD-2. Manual of Diagnosis and Treatment Planning* and *Psychodynamic Diagnostic Manual*. In level 3, the group looks for the effect of interpretations on change and theoretical explanations.

Exploratory research groups

WP on the Specificity of Psychoanalysis

This method starts with a case presentation of one or more sessions to the group. The presenting analyst is present but does not participate during the discussion. The group freely associates about parts (deconstructed) of the material following a 'weaving thoughts' method (Norman & Salomonsson, 2005). This very open method fosters a resonance that makes it possible to relive the session in such a way that a 'replica' of the patient is dreamed and created. At the end, the analyst reveals what new insights they have gained and how far or close the group associations were to their analysis of the patient.

Listening to Listening WP

The presenting analyst reads one or more sessions to the group. The presentation is stopped every time before the analyst intervenes. In the group, each participant is listening to their own and other's 'listening' (which Faimberg calls 'decentred listening'; see Chapter 17). Analysts tend to interpret or 'listen to' the material using a single theory, using their 'basic assumptions'. The group tries to deduce the basic assumptions of both the presenter and each participant (Faimberg, Chapter 17, this book). In this way, any divergences and misunderstandings are exposed. Focusing on these misunderstandings reveals the singularity of the other as well as the unknown. Faimberg calls this 'recognition of otherness' (Chapter 17, this book).

Microscopy of the Session

An analyst presents part of a session, which is stopped before the analyst's interventions. In the group, an analytic field is created consisting of different elements that are to be transformed in symbolisations. (a) The group is open to this process and freely associates and dreams the material. (b) The group makes tentative interpretations. The group's work is then compared with the interpretation of the analyst. (c) The group tries to look for the theories behind the analyst's interpretation. (d) The groups discuss how the interpretation was received by the patient. This is noted, recorded, and then transcribed. In a second step, a researcher looks for patterns and new hypotheses. These patterns and hypotheses can then be presented to the group to be discussed. The work of one session is about 100 to 120 pages. This book presents a nice clinical example of this way of working.

Results

- The WP Comparative Clinical Methods WP worked with both preconference groups and an expert group at an EFP level for 10 years and is now continuing at an IPA level. The categorisation of interventions and implicit theories they use has evolved over time and can be retested time and time again. The method was enriched by analysing sessions from analysts of very different psychoanalytic backgrounds. Six years after the group was founded, they published a book discussing their results (Tuckett et al., 2008). This way of working has proven to be very valuable in situating one's own work, in comparing methods, in linking theory and practice, in communicating about clinical material, and in supervision.
- The WP on Initiating Psychoanalysis worked at an EFP level for 10 years. It began with a review of the literature on initial interviews conducted in different psychoanalytic cultures. The WP has published a book compiling the most relevant papers on this topic, which included comments by the expert group. The data from the preconference groups and from the expert group were processed and patterns were revealed and tested according to a grounded theory approach. These results are presented in a second book by Reith et al. (2018). The book's major findings include the unexpected conscious and unconscious intensity of initial interviews and also the importance of a 'third' (theory, psychoanalytic society, etc.) to deal with this intensity.
- The 3-LM WP developed a multimethod approach, concentrating on longitudinal change in the clinical material of the patient. By analysing the rating of two tests, the *Operationalized Psychodynamic Diagnosis OPD-2. Manual of Diagnosis and Treatment Planning* and the *Psychodynamic Diagnostic Manual*, and then studying links with psychic change, this method seeks to gain a deeper understanding of the psychic transformations of a patient. The focus is on the patient. Two books have been published discussing this method (Altmann de Litvan, 2014; Altmann de Litvan, Fitzpatrick-Hanly, & White, 2021, pp. 34–59). Out of all of the WPs, the 3-LM WP has the strongest link with empirical research, because parts of validated tests are used at the second level. The reliability and validity of the method are currently being tested in three studies: two by comparing groups using the method and one by predicting results in a single case (Rodríguez Quiroga de Pereira, Salesio, & Leibovich de Duarte, Chapter 22, this book).
- WP on the Specificity of Psychoanalysis. The specificity groups have been a great success at psychoanalytic preconferences. The success of this WP's method lies in its ability to help analysts observe and relive the unconscious dynamics of a patient–analyst meeting by freely associating in group, a technique that has been proven to be successful time and time again.

As de Souza Brito and Chabalgoity state in this book, 'We understand that we have shown above that our hypothesis that free association and fluctuating attention in a group of psychoanalysts immersed in psychoanalytic listening to clinical material is a scientific valid way of grasping unconscious processes' (Chapter 21). A research group is now looking at processing material from a group. This research is still in its preliminary phase. It started with a categorisation in units of meaning and themes. This is illustrated in this book.

WP on the Microscopy of the Session

Some WPs have been processed using a qualitative research method, first formulating a hypothesis and then testing its validity. One example in the book illustrates this method (see Chapter 18). It is unclear from the text in this book whether this intensive processing only applies to this one case or whether many other cases have been processed this way. Furthermore, it is unclear whether any other results have been published apart from the example given in this book.

Discussion

General remarks

Although clinical research and exploratory investigation in particular are often used to generate hypotheses, I did not find any new hypotheses in the presentations, except perhaps in the WP on Initiating Psychoanalysis on the emotional storm in preliminary interviews. New concepts are not present but instead happen in the individual mind of the analyst when they process the material of their patient (see also Dreher, Chapter 2, this book). Perhaps the concepts of Faimberg are an exception here. However, many existing concepts are used to understand and elaborate on the clinical data. This deepening of existing concepts is, of course, a welcome result. Psychoanalysis as a discipline is already rich in concepts.

Out of curiosity, I looked into whether my view or implicit theory could find a place in any of these methods. Most categories in the WP refer to understanding, giving meaning, and symbolising. In line with Bion (1965), I think that transformations by experience and intuition are the most important aspects of an analysis, more so than understanding and even 'thinking'. These transformations often stem from a zone outside of representation (Vermote, 2011, 2020). In my reading of this book, I found a link between the Comparative Clinical Methods (CCM) categories of 'interventions that seem to come from nowhere' but also in the WP on Specificity, which makes room for intuition, as well as in the WP on the Microscopy of the Session.

Cost–benefit and impact of the global project

This is, of course, a topic that the IPA Working Parties Committee can better address. The figures in Table 26.1 are approximate and were not checked with the different WPs. I am sure that they are higher in reality. Nevertheless, it would not be fair to talk about the meaning of clinical research for psychoanalysis without mentioning this aspect that illustrates the significance of this clinical research method. I have no clear view on the amount of funding this huge project required, but the members alone must have paid at least US $1,000,000 over the 15 years that these WPs have been taking place (EFP, Latin American Psychoanalytic Federation, and IPA), not including the expenses of the participating analysts at the workshops.

The endurance and motivation of the core/expert groups of the WPs is astonishing. For over a decade, these international events have been taking place, putting a lot of energy in the research of their group. Often members worked for more than four weekends a year together, notwithstanding all of the work they did at home.

The impact of these research groups is overwhelming. Over the years, thousands of analysts from all different regions have participated in the WPs during preconferences. The communicative side of the project should therefore be considered a far-reaching success.

Moreover, all of these groups communicated in a nonjudgemental or nonsupervisory attitude, making this communication qualitatively different and far more open than was previously the case in the psychoanalytic community.

Furthermore – and this is unheard of in the history of psychoanalysis – different schools of psychoanalytic thought were able to discuss clinical case material at a clinical level without getting lost in theoretical discussion.

This general way of working had both an indirect and a direct effect on the training and supervision in many psychoanalytic societies, because colleagues brought the experience they gained at WPs back to their respective societies.

We may conclude that this kind of clinical research so far has had an unexpectedly deep impact on psychoanalysis. I assume that part of its success is based on the fact that most WPs have had charismatic leaders, showing great endurance: Tuckett (CCM), Reith (WP on Initiating Psychoanalysis), Altmann de Litvan (3-LM), Séchaud, Frish, and Abram (Specificity), Faimberg (Listening to Listening), and Cassorla (Microscopy of the Session).

State of the art of the different WPs

Chapter 19 in this book by Luisa Pérez Suquilvide, who presented clinical material at the 3-LM, Specificity, and Listening to Listening WPs, is especially relevant. She describes the comparison of these three methods based on her first-hand experience as a presenter. In summarising her impressions, the 3-LM WP offered new insights on change and transformations in the patient over a longer time, the WP on Specificity served as an amplifier reliving the session, and the WP on Listening to Listening was used to remain attentive to possible biases and misunderstandings.

Vera Regina Fonseca presented the same case to a CCM WP and a 3-LM WP and includes in her report the reactions of the patients months after the seminar, demonstrating the impact of the WP on the patient, which is another important point of view (see Chapter 24).

Qualitative investigations

The CCM WP developed a set of categories that were refined over the years. The questions make it possible to compare the way analysts listen to the clinical material with how they interpret it. Here, the instrument transcends theoretical dogmas and jargon but yet remains open to the specific findings and specificities of each theoretical model. This method offers a way out of the authoritative thinking that has plagued psychoanalysis since its beginnings. This research should continue at an international level; it is most enriching when different models are at stake in the discussions. This method has an impact on both supervision and intervision, making it valuable in training.

From the research side, there are many unexplored possibilities. The categorisation that has become more and more refined and open through its use is a valuable result.

Furthermore, different psychoanalytic schools can be compared. It is also possible to highlight the difference between the way the analyst theoretically believes they work and their actual intervening. The method helps to understand what happens in the mind of the analyst. Many further research options remain to be explored: longitudinal studies, for example, or comparative studies about patient change and its relation to the different types of intervention. Other possibilities include studies that compare intervention types with patient and analyst characteristics. It is similarly possible to use the method in $n = 1$ research. A multiperspective approach in combining it with validated tests in longitudinal studies seems a possibility as well. The possibilities are numerous without losing touch with the core of psychoanalytic practice.

The WP on Initiating Psychoanalysis began with a clear research question about the link between the dynamics in preliminary interviews and initiating analysis. The group conducted an in-depth study of the first interviews structured around a free associative method and semistructured questions, resulting in the delineation of several patterns in the dynamics between patient and analyst. What the results reveal about the link between the dynamics of the first interview and the start of analysis are sobering: The decision to engage in analysis depends only partly on underlying psychodynamic patterns. Availability of the analyst, economic reasons, the analyst's character traits (like narcissism), and the analyst's level of experience and professionalism all play a role as well. One pattern became clear: The intensity of the emotional contact in the preliminary interviews and the condensation of themes in the transferential–countertransferential field is enormous. This is accompanied by a corresponding mobilisation of defences. The three-stage approach (analyst–patient; analyst presenting at a preconference workshop; the expert group without the presenting analyst) further highlighted the intensity of emotional contact. The emotional field extended and was reenacted in the preconference groups. This phenomenon is also experienced in other WPs, especially in the Specificity group. The emotional storm during an initial interview is so strong that it still radiates in the more distant expert group, from which the presenting analyst is absent. It is intriguing that the remoteness of the expert group seemed necessary to be able to see the relational patterns more clearly, because they were less blurred by the emotional storm. It also became clear in reviewing the sessions that analysts who could remain open and observant and stay in contact with the inner world of the patient amidst this emotional storm were characterised by their reliance on a third look (frame, society, set of theories). These hypotheses took shape based on a grounded theory approach, which has all been accurately documented in a book. This WP has since finished its research, and its findings can be implemented in the training of candidates. The WP method can further be used to refine skills in first sessions and further allows for a comparison between the ways in which these first steps are taken in different psychoanalytic societies. It should be noted that this study differs greatly from empirical approaches of indications for psychoanalysis, which focus more on the characteristics of patients. This study is not so much about who receives the indications but about the dynamics in the encounter as indication.

The results can be implemented in training and practice

The 3-LM is an elaborate method to study the change in the patient during analysis. It is probably the WP method that has been most inspired by research. The questions are more focused than in the other methods and take a more reflective, understanding approach to the clinical material. It is also the only method that implies the use of validated tests (second level). The method can be used for proper single-case research.

Even though I did not take part in a 3-LM group, I believe that the method is based on some undiscussed assumptions. For example, it is assumed that there is a clear link between clinical outcome and psychoanalytic process. As Vaughan and Roose (1995) demonstrated in their work, this link is unclear. In their study, they found that, according to their analysts, only 40% of analysands developed a psychoanalytic process during their analysis, yet most analysands who did not develop a psychoanalytic process also felt helped by their analysis. Another assumption is that understanding and giving meaning is the mechanism of change in psychoanalysis. This is different from the CCM WP, which offers several alternative mechanisms of change, derived from different schools of thought.

A promising point is that the 3-LM method has the capacity to integrate findings of other WPs. The first level or analytic observation in the 3-LM could benefit from the findings of the WP on Specificity and be more open, whereas the third level discussing the interventions of the analyst could benefit from the findings of the CCM. Another point is that the 3-LM method is already multimethod and could easily add a multiperspective approach. Currently, its perspective only concentrates on the analyst's point of view on the patient. The patient's view could also be taken into account by using a questionnaire or interview. Similarly, validated tests could be performed and processed by independent (even nonanalytic) interviewers to minimise any bias.

This book suggests making the method less time consuming (12 hours per case discussion), by focusing on the use of metaphors. This is an interesting new approach that will be discussed. The 3-LM is an extensive method that is still developing, and it is structurally open to links with other WPs.

Explorative investigations

The Listening to Listening WP's approach is unique. Its method seeks to be an antidote to the 'knowing' attitude. It allows participants to experience the 'otherness', the singularity of the subject, and the unknown in psychoanalytic experiences. It sensibilises participants to an open presence during the sessions. This method appears to be a wonderful instrument to improve training and increase skills. Its unique approach has influenced the psychoanalytic attitude of many analysts, and the WP should continue taking place at preconferences. Its research focus is not obvious from the chapter in this book (Chapter 17).

The method of the WP on the Specificity of Psychoanalysis most closely resembles the work of an analyst. The group shows time and time again how precious and enriching the instrument of group free association can be. It demonstrates how participants' 'unconscious' can be in contact with each other and experience what happens during the transference–countertransference field of the presented session. The most important result of the WP on Specificity is probably the overwhelming and repeated experience of how sensitive the method is. The processing of data to better understand the specificity of psychoanalysis has just begun. Given the massive amount of data and the fact that this research is not structurally integrated in the method, it is hard to imagine how this can be done. The book, however, offers one example of such a study on content analysis (de Souza Brito & Chabalgoity, Chapter 21). The method of the Specificity WP has served as an excellent training instrument for candidates and members. The method has already had a significant impact on supervision and case discussions.

The WP on the Microscopy of the Session illustrates the wealth of material that can be produced by studying the dynamic unconscious of a group in contact with the recreated field of a session. It shows how interpretations stem from this field and how choices of intervening are made. The method tests whether the choice of intervention is meaningful by looking at the response of the patient. It is a far-reaching but laborious method, resulting in reports counting around 100 to 120 pages per case. An expert group was set up to process the data, of which the book offers an example. This elaboration is then reported to the group, which can work on it again, although it is unclear in how many cases a similar processing of the data has been done as yet. Based on the presentation, it seems to me that there is no research question. This method is very sensitive and useful for both training purposes and improving psychoanalytic skills.

Metaphors

The book offers a rich theoretical background on metaphors. This inclusion was inspired by the 2017 Montevideo conference, which was focused on metaphors. As a trial, the CCM WP also focused on metaphors while analysing the same case (da Rocha Barros, Chapter 20, this book). For the 3-LM, focusing on metaphors seems like a good choice. As far as I am concerned, the 3-LM edges more to the side of understanding than the other WPs. Metaphors, however, stem from another level; they both happen and are the result of a 'thinking' in the way Bion conceived it (Bion, 1965). They exist in between thinking and the body. As Modell stated (as cited by Altmann de Litvan, Introduction, this book), 'Metaphors are detectors of unconscious patterns' and they offer a connection with bodily sensations and feelings. Moreover, by focusing on metaphors, the 3-LM's approach is more focused, shorter, yet, at the same time, deeper and closer to the psychoanalytic method of working. The 3-LM presents a categorisation of metaphors based on the presence of 'others' in metaphors (see Rodríguez Quiroga de Pereira, Salesio, & Leibovich de Duarte, Chapter 22, this book). I do not understand why this categorisation is reduced to the presence of others (objects). This limitation is defended by referring to a research project by Fabregat (2004). Following this newfound approach, I recently reread Fabregat's doctoral thesis. In her study of 18 patients in psychoanalytic psychotherapy, she succeeds in achieving statistically significant results about the use of metaphors. Her approach to metaphors, however, expands beyond just concentrating on the presence of others in metaphors. In fact, in a paper about this research, she does not even mention the relational side (Fabregat & Krause, 2009). Personally, I prefer the approach da Rocha Barros takes to metaphors in this book (Chapter 20), highlighting the level of symbol formation or mentalisation. Moreover, the use of metaphors in the 3-LM seems based on the unproven assumption that richness of metaphors is correlated with the evolution of the psychoanalytic process. This may be partly true, but metaphors also relate to intelligence, educational background, and personality style/pathology. An approach focusing on metaphors is a very promising point of entrance, but the operationalisation could profit from further elaboration.

Conclusion

The project with WPs has spread worldwide and has had a deep impact on psychoanalysis. Firstly, it has improved training and supervision. Secondly, the project has shaped the ways in which we communicate about theory and clinical material. Finally, it also transformed how we understand and link different theories. It has helped psychoanalysts shift their attitude from authoritative and all-knowing to exploring, not-knowing, and learning.

From a research point of view, the three WPs that use a qualitative approach show results that can be implemented as discussed above. The three WPs that use an exploratory approach are rich in methodology but are mostly important in training right now – an aspect that is enhanced in the meeting of international groups.

Notes

1 The personal background from which I make this discussion is that I am a practicing analyst and did empirical process-outcome research for years. Moreover, I was a member of the expert group of the WP on Initiating Psychoanalysis for over 10 years. I also participated in groups working with the specificity method and as part of the Comparative Clinical Method WP. I am also a member of the IPA Clinical Research Committee chaired by M. Altmann de Litvan.

2 The word *stages* is used to avoid confusion with the Three-Level Model research group.

References

Altmann de Litvan, M. (Ed.). (2014). *Time for change: Tracking transformations in psychoanalysis – The Three-Level Model*. London, England: Karnac.

Altmann de Litvan, M., Fitzpatrick-Hanly, M. A., & White, R. (2021). Underlying clinical thinking on change and therapeutic action. In M. A. Fitzpatrick-Hanly, M. Altmann de Litvan, & R. Bernardi (Eds.), *Change through time in psychoanalysis: Transformations and interventions with the Three-Level Model*. pp 34-59. London, England: Routledge.

Bion, W. R.(1961). *Experiences in groups and other papers*. London, England: Tavistock.

Bion, W. R.(1965). *Transformations: Change from learning to growth*. London, England:Tavistock.

Donnet, J. L. (2005). *La situation analysante (Le Fil Rouge)* [*The analyzing situation*]. Paris, France: PUF.

Fabregat, M. (2004). *Metaphors in psychotherapy: From affects to mental representations* (Dissertation, Saerlandische Universitaets und Landesbibliothek). Retrieved from https://publikationen.sulb.uni-saarland.de/handle/20.500.11880/23318

Fabregat, M., & Krause, R. (2009). Metaphors in psychotherapy: From affects to mental representations. In P. Giampieri-Deutsch (Ed.), *Geist, Gehirn, Verhalten, Sigmund Freud und die Modernen Wissenschaften*. Würzburg, Germany: Könishausen und Neumann.

Faimberg, H. (2019). Basic theoretical assumptions underpinning 'Faimberg's method listening to listening'. *The International Journal of Psychoanalysis*, 100(3), 447–462.

Leuzinger-Bohleber, M., Arnold, S. E. A., & Kächele, H. (2019). *An open door review of clinical, conceptual, process and outcome studies*. Retrieved from https://www.opendoorreview.com/

Reith, B., Møller, M., Boots, J., Crick, P., Gibeault, A., Jaffè, R., … Vermote, R. (2018). *Beginning analysis: On the processes of initiating psychoanalysis*. London, England: Routledge.

Norman, J., & Salomonsson, B. (2005). 'Weaving thoughts' A method for presenting and commenting psychoanalytic case material in a peer group. *International Journal of Psycho-Analysis*, 86(5), 1281–1298.

Tuckett, D., Basile, R., Birksted-Breen, D., Böhm, T., Denis, P., Ferro, A., … Schubert, J. (2008). *Psychoanalysis comparable and incomparable. The evolution of a method to describe and compare psychoanalytic approaches*. London, England: Routledge.

Vaughan, S. C., & Roose, S. P. (1995). The analytic process: Clinical and research definitions. *The International Journal of Psychoanalysis*, 76, 343–356.

Vermote, R. (2011). On the value of 'late Bion' to analytic theory and practice. *The International Journal of Psychoanalysis*, 92(5), 1089–1098.

Vermote, R. (2020). Psychic functioning outside of representations. Implications for psychoanalysis. *Japanese Journal of Psychoanalysis*, 2, 3–17.

Chapter 27

Working groups and the search for clinical evidence

Ricardo Bernardi

The chapters in this book highlight the many directions in which clinical discussion groups have developed. I will use the term working groups (WGs) to refer to the original working parties, as well as the Three-Level Model (3-LM) and other experiences with similar characteristics. What all of them have in common is the discussion of clinical material among analysts with different theoretical approaches, according to the specific objectives and procedures of each group. I am interested in reflecting on these groups from a historical perspective first, seeking to understand the reasons for their development, and then to discuss their present importance for psychoanalysis, the challenges they face, and their potential for the future.

The circumstances in which my training and career as a psychoanalyst took place condition this reflection.[1] It led me to appreciate the richness of current pluralism but also to understand the need to go beyond a vision of pluralism as the simple coexistence of different theoretical and technical systems. To go beyond this coexistence, it is necessary to find a common clinical basis that makes a consensual and nonauthoritative comparison of the different approaches based on shared criteria of evidence possible. The theoretical discussion undoubtedly leads to the conceptual enrichment of the discipline, but it has to go together with a peer-to-peer exchange that helps us to keep learning from clinical facts. I think this is the historical role played by the WGs.

The 4 decades that followed Freud's death in 1939 saw the emergence of different psychoanalytic schools, each with original aspects. In my opinion, a significant change occurred in the 1980s, when the most influential authors disappeared (Klein in 1960, Hartmann in 1970, Winnicott in 1971, Bleger in 1972, Pichon Rivière in 1977, Bion in 1979, Lacan and Kohut in 1981, and A. Freud in 1982). They left behind a wealth of valuable teachings that the psychoanalytic community continued to deepen and develop. However, important problems also remained unsolved, namely, the integration of the theoretical differences and the consequences of these differences for clinical practice.

DOI: 10.4324/9780000000002-33

When I finished my psychoanalytic training, it was urgent for me to know to what extent the adoption of one psychoanalytic approach or the other influenced the results of the analysis. At that time, I found R. Wallerstein's presidential address at the 1987 Montreal Congress very illuminating. Wallerstein (1988) asked to what extent was there a common clinical ground among analysts with different theoretical affiliations. In my opinion, this question is at the origin of the WGs as a tool for clinical research.

It could be expected that by becoming aware of the difficulties of theoretical integration the psychoanalytic community would seek ways to compare its diverse theories and determine which hypotheses were of greater value in the presence of which clinical problems. However, this was not a feasible path because of the way in which the dominant psychoanalytic theories were formulated and transmitted and internalised. To the extent that each theory was based on different premises and utilised terms that were conceptually rich but imprecisely defined, psychoanalytic theories behaved as if they were incommensurable paradigms, making the possibility of scientifically useful controversies difficult (Bernardi, 1989, 2002). Consequently, a top-down mode of clinical reasoning was adopted in clinical papers. In these, deductive inferences predominated, seeking to demonstrate the way in which each theoretical system allowed all clinical facts to be satisfactorily explained. It is important to note that this type of clinical reasoning is different from Karl Popper's hypothetical–deductive method, which Hinshelwood defends in this book (Chapter 4). This method requires that experience confirms or falsifies theoretical hypotheses. However, it is very difficult, if not impossible, to find examples of Popperian falsification in the psychoanalytic literature. Usually, if one looks at the psychoanalytic literature, authors always confirm their previous hypotheses. This is because the clinical material is presented in a way that it is not possible to actually test such hypotheses, because only confirmations of the author's hypotheses are highlighted, without their limitations being examined. For this reason, Hanly's discussion in this book (Chapter 5) of the hypothetical–deductive method as the basis of clinical reasoning in psychoanalysis is important. I agree with his proposal that psychoanalytic hypotheses should meet criteria of correspondence, coherence, and pragmatic utility. In the session, as Hanly says, these hypotheses are experienced 'in the analyst's thinking not as hypotheses and predictions as such but as questions, doubts, uncertainties, and hunches' (Chapter 5, this book). I would add that, from my point of view, the answer that the analysts seek consists primarily in finding the best possible explanation for their doubts and uncertainties. This search, which goes primarily from the particular to the particular, resembles abductive processes or Edelson's eliminative inductivism, to which I have already referred in this book (Chapter 6). I believe that this is the kind of reasoning that we find in good clinical examples. However, when narrated, they tend to be presented deductively. But in practice, clinical inferences advance in an ascending manner, 'from the bottom up', moving from concrete clinical experience towards more general statements, whose explanatory scope is examined in terms of their predictive and pragmatic usefulness (Jiménez, 2009). I believe that this is the inferential process that we find in WGs. For that reason, they allow a fruitful dialogue among analysts who adhere to different theoretical approaches.

I would now like to refer to the topics that aroused the interest of the WG, returning to the decade before its emergence, that of 1990. It is interesting to observe the topics highlighted in the international congresses that followed Wallerstein's address. The congress in Rome, in 1989, was titled: 'Common Ground in Psychoanalysis – Clinical Aims and Process', and in the two following congresses the theme was 'Psychic Change' (Buenos Aires, 1991) and 'The Psychoanalyst's Mind – From Listening to Interpretation' (Amsterdam, 1993). We can see that these three topics are still on the agenda of the WGs. In all of them, the observation of what happens in the analyst's mind occupies an important place. The distinction proposed by Sandler in 1983 between official or public theories and private or implicit ones opened the way to the study of the processes that occur between listening and interpretation from a descriptive perspective (how analysts really think) instead of a normative one (how they should think). During his presidency, C. Hanly stimulated the study of the problems of theoretical integration and clinical observation. This last interest led to the emergence of the WG based on the Three-Level Model (3-LM) for the analysis of patient transformation (Bernardi, 2014). The investigation of the effects of interpretation is also present in other WGs, such as Listening to Listening and 'Microscopy of the Session, among others.

As Glover and Reith point out in this book (Chapter 12), 'The Working Parties (WPs) originated in the European Psychoanalytic Federation (EPF) in 2001 as a way to promote an investigative spirit into the fundamentals of our profession, in which all psychoanalysts could take an active part' (p. 000). The fundamental ideas were developed during the 1990s. Although the discussion groups always took place in psychoanalysis (e.g., the 'Wednesday Psychological Society' that took place in Freud's house), the Psychoanalytic Electronic Publishing Archive consigned for the first time the term 'clinical discussion group' in a paper by D. Tuckett (1994). He proposed 'the exploration of alternate hypotheses within the framework of groups of psychoanalysts discussing case material and making independent judgments which can be assessed as to their reliability' (Tuckett, 1994, p. 1178). Therefore, communication between analysts has to be supported by clinical evidence. It is based on 'the psychoanalytically-honored ordinary human conversational capacities (Tuckett, 1994, p. 1178). But for this to be possible, it is necessary to 'allow theory and observation to be at least somewhat separated' (Tuckett, 1994, p. 1178). A decade and a half later, J. P. Jiménez (2009) formulated a similar claim mentioning the experience of the WP: to detach practice from theory, studying the former in its own merits utilising a plurality of methods ranging from systematic investigation to the recent methodology of the WPs.

This path enables analysts coming from different traditions to look for new insights into the clinical material. The WG, as Glover and Reith point out, develops 'a more third-person view of their own preferred theory, with its advantages and limitations' (chapter 12, this book). This last aspect, in my opinion, marks a historical change in psychoanalysis, because it means putting clinical observation and critical comparative reflection back in the foreground, abandoning the pretension of giving an account of all of the problems of the discipline from the exclusive perspective of a single theoretical approach. Pluralism becomes something more than the coexistence of different systems of ideas, to constitute a space of clinical reflection where the contribution of these hypotheses can be examined. The question about the criteria of evidence that supports our theoretical and clinical hypotheses then comes to the fore.

In this book, Marianne Leuzinger-Bohleber (Chapter 8), Ursula Dreher (Chapter 2), and Hinshelwood (Chapter 4) rightly highlight the challenge that evidence-based medicine (EBM) poses to psychoanalysis. As these authors point out, there are clinical research trials and meta-analyses on dynamically oriented psychotherapies that meet the requirements of EBM. To the references that these authors mention we can add authors like Leichsenring et al. (2015) or Shedler (2015), among others. However, it is important to keep in mind that the question of evidence is not limited to the field of systematic empirical research. From the perspective of this book, it is necessary to raise the question of the level of evidence that can emerge from clinical research and, especially, from the work of the WGs. It is important not to separate the clinical evidence from the evidence that comes from systematic empirical research. When EBM emerged, Sackett, Straus, Richardson, and Rosenberg (1997) defined it as 'the integration of best available evidence, clinical expertise and patient preferences and values' (p. 1), giving equal emphasis to the patient's goals, the research evidence, and the clinical expertise of the practitioner. Psychoanalytic clinical research unites scientific tradition with hermeneutics, although it is not always easy to combine both. I would like to highlight some topics in this book related to research that, in my opinion, open paths that still require further exploration. Dreher distinguishes in their work the perspective of first-, second-, and third-person knowledge (Chapter 2). Psychoanalysis is in a privileged position to combine the strengths of second-person knowledge, which is essential in the transferential–countertransferential relationship, with first- and third-person information. I cannot expand on this point here, yet I would like to point out its importance for the current development of the theory of mind.

The WGs discuss the verbatim transcripts of an analyst's interaction with their patient. As Tuckett (1994) pointed out, 'The essence of psychoanalysis is that the analyst, as a receptive human being making sense within a communicative field, unconsciously as well as consciously picks up the data within a framework of meanings' (p. 1160). The type of investigation in the session is, by its therapeutic nature, a form of action research. The clinical material constitutes the record of this action research and the diverse WG proposes various forms of studies of this clinical material, each with its own goals and methods. I believe that this book constitutes a privileged opportunity to reflect on the type of evidence on which each of them intends to rely.

Examining the evidence provided by clinical research requires assessing its strengths and limitations. For this reason, scientific papers, from any discipline, after presenting their objectives, methods, and results, include a discussion section in which the author examines the significance of these results, but also their possible limitations. This discussion is usually absent in psychoanalytic clinical publications – a point that needs to be noticed. The insufficiency of explicit critical reflection on the possible limitations, omissions, and biases of a study was pointed out as a warning sign, because it is one of the causes of the so-called crisis of replicability that exists in many fields of current scientific knowledge (Ioannidis, 2005, 2007). If a clinical psychoanalytic paper does not examine the strengths and limitations of the ideas it proposes in comparison with other existing hypotheses, it will necessarily confirm these ideas based on circular reasoning. Freud critically reviewed many of his findings and was careful to point out when the evidence that supported a hypothesis was inconclusive (*'non liquet'*; Freud, 1918/1955, p. 60).

EBM developed explicit criteria that relate the level of research evidence to the strength of the recommendations that are supported by those studies. In the case of statistical documents or meta-analyses, these criteria are well systematised. On the other hand, in the case of psychoanalytic clinical works, although there are numerous references in the literature, there are no systematised or shared criteria in this regard. However, it is possible to move in that direction (Bernardi & Pérez Suquilvide, 2021, pp. 281–305). In my opinion, it is important for the WGs to explain the evidence criteria that they used in its investigation of the clinical material.

At least three characteristics have to be examined when conclusions are drawn from clinical material (Bernardi & Pérez Suquilvide, 2021, pp. 281–305). First, it is necessary to establish to what extent the author's conclusions are grounded in the unconscious material provided by the material – which means a high level of evidence – or whether they are only based on the author's speculations based on their theoretical assumptions – which means a lower level of evidence. The criteria listed by S. Isaacs (1939) for evaluating the patient's unconscious response to interpretation continue to be a firm reference on this point, to which numerous contributions by other authors were added. Another criterion, related to the previous one, arises from the examination of alternative hypotheses; that is, from comparing the proposed explanation with other possible explanations, examining the strengths and weaknesses of each one. However, to do this, a third condition is necessary: that the author provide sufficient contextual information about the main variables that can influence the phenomenon under study. Boesky (2013) has shown that adequate information about contextual factors is crucial when evaluating the evidence (see Appendix 27.1).

To achieve their role as clinical research tools, WGs need to propose answerable questions, a solid methodology, replicable results, and conclusions based on a traceable inferential process. Complementing with other extraclinical research methods through triangulation procedures of methods, materials, and theoretical frameworks reinforces their conclusions. An issue that requires both conceptual and empirical research is the extent to which the various WGs currently working at the International Psychoanalytical Association can complement each other. The study of the metaphors of a clinical case presented in this book offers a promising example of the convergence of points of view that I cannot examine here.

The documents contained in this book show that some WGs are more oriented towards aspects related to the analytical process and others, especially the 3-LM, towards the relationship process–results in an analysis. In the field of psychotherapy research, the relationship between process and results is a central theme. Therefore, it an increasing complementarity between the different WGs would be fruitful. This path requires, for the reasons that I have just pointed out, advancing the understanding of the potentialities and limitations of each one of them. This task includes problems of different types, both conceptual and methodological. To begin with, both terms, process and results, contain problematic aspects.

There is no consensual definition of 'psychoanalytic process' (Vaughan, Spitzer, Davies, & Roose, 1997). For this reason, it is prudent to adopt Kernberg's (2013) recommendation that the term 'analytical process is a highly complex condensation of variables that need to be studied independently to evaluate their relationship to treatment outcome' (p. 988). The identification of which process variables are relevant is a challenge that each WG must respond to according to its objectives and methodology. I will return to this point.

Regarding psychic change, there is no agreement not only on the key variables but also on the convenience of establishing psychoanalytic aims. However, it is possible to move forward if, instead of looking for a normative answer, we look for a descriptive answer and ask ourselves what the real transformations that take place in patients under analysis are. This is an empirical question whose answer interests not only psychoanalysts but also patients and society. However, systematic descriptions of patients' changes do not abound in the psychoanalytic publications. There are excellent operationalised diagnostic manuals such as the

Operationalized Psychodynamic Diagnosis OPD-2. Manual of Diagnosis and Treatment Planning (OPD-2; OPD Task Force, 2008) and *Psychodynamic Diagnostic Manual* (PDM Task Force, 2006), whose criteria are coincident with the alternative *Diagnostic and Statistical Manual of Mental Disorders*, fifth edition (American Psychiatric Association, 2013), and with the *International Classification of Diseases*, 11th revision (World Health Organization, 2018). These criteria are relevant to psychoanalysis: the functioning of the self and the relationship with others. However, they are seldom used or substituted by any other systematic approach. Consequently, clinical discussions about change become decontextualised and vague. The 3-LM aims to identify what dimensions we are talking about in what type of patient. The same necessity appears if we are discussing emotional storms in the initial interviews of the analysis. These storms are probably not of the same kind in a borderline patient with high emotional instability as in an obsessive patient with rigid defences. This is an empirical question but requires conceptual and contextual information. In the case of the 3-LM, which is the WG with which I am most familiar, the categories of these systems, especially the OPD-2 (OPD Task Force, 2008), are the basis of the questions that guide the group discussion. But, because of the mentioned reasons, reliability of group evaluations is problematic and needs to be further investigated. Probably due to the same reasons, frequently group participants consider patients more severely ill than indicated by these diagnostic systems. Additionally, it is not easy to carry out reliability studies in a traditional way, because the reliability of the evaluations would undoubtedly improve if we selected only analysts trained in one of the diagnostic systems. Then they would no longer reflect what is happening in the psychoanalytic community under usual conditions. This kind of study would only replicate something that is already known; that is, that under appropriate conditions these categories are reliable. In a more general world, these limitations hamper the possibility that psychoanalysis will join current trends for developing clinical practice networks and the growth of 'practice-based evidence'.

Coming back to process variables, each WG selects process variables according to their theoretical approach, research questions, and methodology. Let us take the WG on Comparative Clinical Methods as an example. The theoretical framework is important because the study of interpretations will differ if at the conceptual level we adopt a monadic or a dyadic definition of the analytical process. In the first case, the focus is on studying the process in the analyst's mind. This does not mean ignoring other variables, such as what is wrong with the patient, or the effects of the interpretation, etc., but they are not an essential part of the unit of analysis. Instead, from a dyadic perspective, analyst–patient interaction is a key aspect of the unit of observation, and the effects of the interpretation on the psychopathological dimensions of the patient's personality need careful examination. It is important to bear in mind that the choice of one or another unit of analysis will determine the required methodology and the scope of the conclusions, so it is essential to indicate, in the case of each working group, what its aims and methods are, and therefore its potentialities and limitations.

It is also convenient to clarify the conceptual definition of key terms. Some WGs, like the WP on Specificity of Psychoanalysis, use the concept of free association in a way that it cannot be distinguished from that of free-floating attention. Free association is stated as the fundamental part of the method or device used by specificity groups. However, from my point of view, it would be necessary to clarify the reasons why the term 'free association' is preferred over 'evenly suspended attention'. According to its traditional definition, in an analysis, the analysand is asked to say everything that occurs to them, without selecting anything or omitting anything. This is the fundamental rule, and free association is more than a voluntary decision because its occurrence is related to complex phenomena such as resistances, regression, transference, and the effect of interpretations. The situation in a WG is quite different. Participants are not expected to talk about their personal problems, childhood memories, or any ideas that come to mind unless they think that they are related to the clinical material. For that reason, evenly suspended attention seems to be a more adequate model. Free-floating attention seeks that, by listening to the clinical material, the analyst allows their unconscious activity to operate as freely as possible, suspending the motives that generally direct their attention. There is also another point where further clarification would be helpful. The WG on Specificity states that there is a replication in the discussion group of certain transference configurations of clinical material. This could mean that the group is an excellent magnifying glass to enrich the understanding of the material. However, it is necessary to establish when it is so and when it is not, and this cannot not be an a priori decision because it is an empirical question that needs to be researched. It is necessary to provide criteria to differentiate when there is a parallel process in the group and when we observe other kind of group phenomena, such as Bion's (1961) basic assumptions, groupthink, or other sources of group biases.

The 3-LM stimulates in the first level (phenomenological) an attitude that is very similar to the free-floating attention, seeking the unconscious resonance of the material at the level of the group participants (Bernardi, 2014). At this level, it is possible to observe a clinical common ground among participants (Bernardi, 2017). The chapters in this volume on the metaphor show that at this level there is also a convergence with other WGs. In the case of the 3-LM, later levels of analysis require that this first understanding be accompanied by reflective elaboration processes, as Glover and Reith call them (Chapter 12). Group members are invited to take a 'second look' at the process, evaluating the psychopathological and temporal aspects of patient's change. In addition, there is a 'third look' when a research group studies the experience. There are still many pending issues to be investigated at the second level, in addition to those already mentioned related to the use of the operationalized categories of *Psychodynamic Diagnostic Manual* and OPD-2. Perhaps the categories of the Heidelberg scales (OPD Task Force, 2008) or Stiles' (2001) assimilation of problematic experiences could be a more sensitive tool for studying certain aspects of the change process (Bernardi, 2021, pp. 148–154).

The third level of the 3-LM has an ambitious goal: to formulate hypotheses about the mechanisms of change. This involves identifying mediating and moderating factors, differentiating them from confounding factors, and relating them to the foci of analyst's work during the analysis. This type of analysis is generally carried out by statistical means. However, if the psychoanalytic hypotheses are true, the phenomena of change must be detectable not only through psychometric instruments but also, at least partially, through narrative analysis and resources of a qualitative or hermeneutical nature. The richness of metaphor study is an example in this direction.

As a final reflection, I would like to emphasise that behind this book it is possible to perceive a long road that arises from the need to find an answer to the theoretical and technical fragmentation of psychoanalysis. This path led to the recognition that it is necessary to take the problems posed by clinical practice as a starting point and then humbly accept that we respond better to these questions if we do so through exchange with other colleagues in pluralistic clinical discussion groups. In this way, we all also commit ourselves to the task of finding the best way to put what happens in the analyst's minds at the service of the changes that the patient seeks. To perform this task better, we need to transitorily separate theory and practice and start an inferential path that leads us from the problems posed by clinical experience to the theoretical hypotheses that allow its explanation. This step needs be followed by a next step in which we try to illuminate the answers that we have found in our upward journey with the accumulated knowledge of the discipline. Research becomes more necessary and exciting where these two paths do not meet and we do not find convincing answers available.

Note

1 My society, the Uruguayan Psychoanalytic Association, was strongly pluralistic and open to different theoretical and technical approaches. In the 1980s, I co-chaired with Marta Nieto a research group within the Society that analyses clinical materials from a double perspective. The group compared the interpretation of a clinical material in light of different theoretical approaches and, in parallel, which relevant facts defied theoretical explanations. For many years I have also been a member of the International Psychoanalytical Association Research Committee. My participation in that committee, as well as in the International Psychoanalytical Association Research Training Program, allowed me to learn from important researchers.

References

American Psychiatric Association. (2013). *Diagnostic and statistical manual of mental disorders* (5th ed.). Washington, DC: Author.

Bernardi, R. (1989). The role of paradigmatic determinants in psychoanalytic understanding. *The International Journal of Psychoanalysis*, 70(2), 341–357.

Bernardi, R. (2002). The need for true controversies in psychoanalysis: The debates on Melanie Klein and Jacques Lacan in the Rio de la Plata. *The International Journal of Psychoanalysis*, 83, 851–873.

Bernardi, R. (2014). The Three-Level Model (3-LM) for observing patient transformations. In M. Altmann de Litvan (Ed.), *Time for change: Tracking transformations in psychoanalysis – The Three-Level Model*. London, England: Karnac.

Bernardi, R. (2017). A common ground in clinical discussion groups: Intersubjective resonance and implicit operational theories. *The International Journal of Psychoanalysis*, 98(5), 1291–1309.

Bernardi, R. (2021). Discussion of Bruno Salesio's 'The case of John'. Extent and sequence of changes. In M. A.Fitzpatrick-Hanly, M.Altmann de Litvan, & R. Bernardi (Eds.), *Change through time in psychoanalysis: Transformations and interventions with the Three-Level Model*, pp. 148–154. London, England: Routledge.

Bernardi, R., & Pérez Suquilvide, L. (2021). Assessing the strengths and limitations of clinical evidence in a psychoanalytic clinical material. In M. A. Fitzpatrick-Hanly, M. Altman de Litvan, & R. Bernardi (Eds.), *Change through time in psychoanalysis: Transformations and interventions with the Three-Level Model*, pp. 281–305. London, England: Routledge.

Bion, W. R. (1961). *Experiences in groups*. London, England: Tavistock.

Boesky, D. (2013). What does the presentation of case material tell us about what actually happened in an analysis and how does it do this? *The International Journal of Psychoanalysis*, 94(6), 1135–1143.

Freud, S. (1955). From the history of an infantile neurosis. In J. Strachey (Ed.), *The standard edition of the complete psychological works of Sigmund Freud* (Vol. XVII). London, England: The Hogarth Press. (Original work published 1918)

Ioannidis, J. P. A. (2005). Why most published research findings are false. *PLOS Medicine*, 2(8), e124.

Ioannidis, J. P. A. (2007). Limitations are not properly acknowledged in the scientific literature. *Journal of Clinical Epidemiology*, 60, 324–329.

Isaacs, S. (1939). Criteria for interpretation. *The International Journal of Psychoanalysis*, 20, 148–160.

Jiménez, J. P. (2009). Grasping psychoanalysts' practice in its own merits. *The International Journal of Psychoanalysis*, 90(2), 231–248.

Kernberg, O. F. (2013). Response to Zepf and Gerlach. *Journal of the American Psychoanalytic Association*, 61(5), 985–991.

Leichsenring, F., Luyten, P., Hilsenroth, M. J., Abbass, A., Barber, J. B., Keefe, J. R., … Steinert, C. (2015). Psychodynamic therapy meets evidence-based medicine: A systematic review using updated criteria. *Lancet Psychiatry*, 2, 648–660.

OPD Task Force. (2008). *Operationalized psychodynamic diagnosis OPD-2. Manual of diagnosis and treatment planning*. Cambridge, MA: Hogrefe & Huber Publishers.

PDM Task Force. (2006). *Psychodynamic diagnostic manual*. Silver Spring, MD: Alliance of Psychoanalytic Organizations.

Sackett, D. L., Straus, S. E., Richardson, W. S., & Rosenberg, W. (1997). *Evidence-based medicine: How to practice & teach EBM*. New York, NY: Churchill Livingstone.
Sandler, J. (1983). Reflections on some relations between psychoanalytic concepts and psychoanalytic practice. *International Journal of Psycho-Analysis*, 64, 35–45.
Shedler, J. (2015). Where is the evidence for 'evidence-based' therapy? *Journal of Psychological Therapies in Primary Care*, 4, 47–59.
Stiles, W. B. (2001). Assimilation of problematic experiences. *Psychotherapy*, 38, 462–465.
Tuckett, D. (1994). Developing a grounded hypothesis to understand a clinical process: The role of conceptualization in validation. *The International Journal of Psychoanalysis*, 75, 1159–1180.
Vaughan, S. C., Spitzer, R., Davies M., & Roose, S. (1997). The definition and assessment of analytic process: Can analysts agree? *The International Journal of Psychoanalysis*, 78, 959–973.
Wallerstein, R. S. (1988). One psychoanalysis or many? *International Journal of Psychoanalysis*, 69, 5–21.
World Health Organization. (2018). *International classification of diseases for mortality and morbidity statistics* (11th Revision). Retrieved from https://icd.who.int/browse11/l-m/en

Appendix 27.1. Assessment of the Weight of Evidence Provided by the Clinical Material for Answering 3-Lm Third-Level Questions

	High evidence	*Moderate or low evidence*	*Very low evidence*
1. Clinical information about treatment foci	Initial Interviews combine associative and exploratory aspects There is contextual information about the experience of illness, stressful events, trait/state, conflict/structure, and severity markers	The patient's subjective suffering is clearly described at level 1 of the 3-LM, but there are omissions and insufficient information about level 2 dimensions	Clinical descriptions are insufficient at both levels 1 and 2 Clear bias (availability, confirmatory, selection, etc.)
2. Relationship between analyst's interventions and patient's change process	There is clear evidence of an interactive dialectical process and its progress during the sessions, and it is linked to long-term changes Hypotheses are a coherent and plausible explanation of the process	Weak relationship between interpretations and change process	Changes cannot be linked to interpretations (without evidence in favour of a nonlinear system model)

	High evidence	*Moderate or low evidence*	*Very low evidence*
3. Inferential processes Consideration of alternative hypotheses	Hypotheses are clearly linked to the clinical material and reasonable alternative hypotheses are discussedClinical reasoning and arguments or thought experiments are carefully described	Hypotheses are theory-driven and insufficiently grounded in the clinical material Alternative hypotheses are discarded on the basis of theoretical preferences An insufficient conceptual analysis. Alternative hypotheses are deemed complementary	Strong confirmation bias. One-sided or authoritative arguments

Source: From *Change Through Time: Relating Interventions and Transformations in Psychoanalysis – The Three-Level Model*, edited by M. A. Fitzpatrick-Hanly, M. Altmann, & R. Bernardi, 2021. London, England: Routledge. Reproduced with permission.

Chapter 28

Clinical research in working parties through metaphors

Marina Altmann de Litvan

The general spirit of this book is the search for an improvement to our clinical work for the benefit of our patients. We know that, as authors, we have differences in our worldviews, aims, methods, and scientific backgrounds, for we belong to different regions. Therefore, it is important to be aware of our own positions and pre-assumptions and to formulate them explicitly. Such transparency may facilitate a critical and productive dialogue between researchers of different scientific beliefs and between researchers and clinicians.

In this final part we share the perspectives of authors who give their impressions on different aspects after having studied all the chapters of this book. Firstly, we present Luisa Pérez Suquilvide's and Vera Regina Fonseca's comments on their experiences as presenters of clinical material in the working groups, followed by Rudi Vermote's and Ricardo Bernardi's discussions about the working parties (WPs) and clinical research.

Let us remember that the works collected in this book were the result of the invitation to observe metaphors in one common clinical material. We expected to open new paths of exploration and reflections, aware that more systematisation was needed. The originality of this proposal lies on this experience of gathering different International Psychoanalytical Association working groups to observe meaningful clinical facts from the perspective of each method.

We have done an important collaborative exercise with the different WPs, studying the same clinical material. The three WPs that I will refer to in this work (Comparative Clinical Methods [CCM], Specificity, and the Three-Level Model [3-LM]) did a thorough analysis, and Faimberg's Listening to Listening method, Microscopy of the Analytic Session, and Initiating Psychoanalysis WPs participated by presenting their models and reflections about the topic in the conferences organised in São Paulo and Montevideo.

What have we learned from this experience? What critical reflection can we make? Answers to these questions will be found in Ricardo Bernardi's (Chapter 27) and Rudi Vermote's (Chapter 26) accounts.

Here I would like to share some reflections on the work that the different WPs have done with metaphors.

Strictly speaking, a metaphor is a rhetorical figure or trope in which the meaning is transferred from one concept to another, establishing a relationship of similarity or analogy between the two terms. The word, as such, comes from the Latin *metaph⊠ra*, which derives from the Greek (*metaphorá*), which means 'translation', 'displacement'. Metaphors are images, concepts, or ideas that have a subtle relationship between them that is summoned or suggested when they are associated in a text and that produce impressive relationships that resize the literal meaning of words.

Psychoanalysis has extensively widened this meaning, introducing the concept of metaphoric processes (Modell, 1997), as the analytic method for addressing memories that unconsciously guide action and as the way of unconsciously processing emotional experiences originated in bodily sensations and feelings (Modell, 2009). The concept was further developed as embodied metaphors and behavioural metaphors were introduced (Rizzuto, 2009).

The relevance of metaphors as a salient clinical factor to explore transference is underlined by analysts from different theoretical perspectives and, as Barnett and Katz explained,

> provides a possible theoretical base for interacting features of treatment (the intrapsychic and the intersubjective), as well as change. The potential synthesis of analytic perspectives around the ingredient of metaphor suggested that close attention to its workings in treatment could clarify and advance theories of psychoanalytic practice, expanding the common ground among them. (2009, p. 1)

Systematically observing clinical material with analysts from different theoretical backgrounds, cultures, and languages for several years in clinical observation groups using the 3-LM, we have experienced and evidenced this particular feature of metaphors (Altmann de Litvan, 2021; Bernardi, 2021; de León de Bernardi & Altmann de Litvan, 2014). These observations made us wonder whether it was a shared view with other International Psychoanalytical Association working groups.

The complete path of our work with metaphors was explained in detail in the Introduction. We thought that the analysis of the same clinical material with the different group methods could give us meaningful clues. I will briefly share my understandings of the work done by each group with metaphors, focusing on the three groups that made the complete experience with their model and documented it in a written production.

The CCM provides a framework for a group of psychoanalysts from different traditions, languages, and cultures to discuss and compare how different psychoanalysts work (Calich, Chapter 15, this book; Tuckett et al., 2008).

Although the CCM usually does not focus on metaphors, for the proposal of these conferences and this book the CCM observed the metaphorical processes. The group identified three main metaphors/images in the clinical material:

1 'Looking at life from behind a glass'. Description brought by the patient in the first interview. She describes it as a feeling of being 'completely out of my body, with the sense of being far away'.
2 *The Scream* by Munch. After 6 months of analysis, the patient says she identifies herself with it. This image leads to other images: the existence of a monster in Zoe's internal world just about to explode, capable of expelling the equivalent to a missile.
3 A hamster going around indefinitely in a wheel. After 1½ years of analysis, the patient uses this image to describe the feeling of living her life going around in circles, without any progress. This same image of the hamster occurred to the analyst some minutes before Zoe referred to it.

The group observed that these three metaphors 'indicate the way that the analyst conceives what is not well' with the patient – her feeling of depersonalisation and estrangement of herself, freezing in a given state of mind that makes it impossible to work through her mourning process.

The group underlines that at the beginning of the treatment metaphors do not show amplification of the affective networks involved. It is only 3½ years later that the analyst articulates what is wrong with the patient with the presented metaphors, employing a rich metaphorical image, 'an existence between the world of the living and of the dead' that indicates that the patient stops being depersonalised and lives in a transitional space between the living and the dead. At this moment, the analyst metaphorises more the internal world of the patient, who shows herself more alive but at the same time suffering more.

Later, the metaphors employed by the patient and by the analyst point to a deepening metaphorisation of the patient's inner world, which is more alive and richer, by the analyst. The patient uses metaphoric images to express how she has experienced tragedies not spoken by her family. She then associates this using a powerful metaphor – with what is going on in Aleppo, Syria. This evolution in the type of metaphors illustrates what we consider progression in formal qualities of the symbolic forms.

The analysis of the interventions and/or interpretations of the CCM helps to get deeper into how metaphors expand and acquire a new meaning, at a verbal level, displaying the presence of acute and chronic enactments (Cassorla, 2013), where the analyst realises how there is an element (noise) that could block the patient's free association. 'The enactment may be very expressive and, thereby, may contain a very complex metaphor transmitted mostly in action, even when this is a result of a verbal formulation that may be equivalent to an action' (da Rocha Barros, Chapter 20, this book).

The different metaphors that appear in the clinical material are seen in the context of the analytical situation, so the CCM helps us to understand more clearly what the patient brings, what the analyst interprets, and how the patient answers. By focusing on the analyst's interpretations, this method helps us to observe more precisely than others how the analyst uses the metaphor. In this case the analyst uses the metaphor as a technical tool to bring back to the patient the depersonalised aspects that have dominated her mind since the death of her mother. The group work denotes the idea that there are metaphorical processes and that metaphors can indicate changes in the patient.

The aim of the 3-LM is to observe the changes or no changes in the patient during the course of an analysis. The presence or absence of changes are analysed at each of the three levels, as presented in Altmann de Litvan, Bernardi, and Fitpatrick-Hanly (Chapter 14, this book). In this working group, there is an initial assumption that through metaphors we can approach the core of the patient's problems.

Through the metaphors that gradually emerge in the different stages of the analysis, the group observes the evolution of mental processing. For example, this patient at the beginning of analysis states 'to be fully out of my body, as if I saw life "from behind a glass", as if I was "in a hamster wheel"'. Six months later the patient states, 'I woke up and I felt weird; I thought it was the hangover'. And 3½ years later, experiences of 'monster', 'bomb', 'terrorism', and 'destruction' appear. Through these metaphors, we can observe how the patient did not connect with her emotions at the beginning of the treatment and she starts feeling herself (feeling weird) 6 months later. As the analytical process advances, she is able to face her conflicts. This group found that metaphors are a key access to approach the unconscious problems and to understand changes in the patient.

The 3-LM shows that metaphorical expressions have the characteristic of condensing more information than nonmetaphorical ones. Sometimes one word or expression conveys an amount of affective and associative information that otherwise does not emerge.

To the analyst who presented the clinical material, metaphors can be 'anchor points' and they allowed to refine the patient's understanding and follow the transformations as well as the aspects that did not change and those not addressed with the patient. Metaphors addressed in the different dimensions of the 3-LM were indicators of the changes and no changes in different mental dimensions and interpersonal functioning of the patient.

There is an interesting consistency in the findings of the clinical work with the 3-LM and the exercise done by Rodríguez Quiroga de Pereira, Leibovich de Duarte, and Salesio (Chapter 22). More metaphors emerge, and some metaphors indicated modifications in the treatment concerning how the patient saw herself in the bond with the others and where she could acknowledge her intimacy and the fear to lose meaningful people. In the discussion group with the 3-LM, participants also observed that she had not developed an empathic capacity in her life. The patient brings a metaphor for herself (the monster) that, through this method used by these authors, showed to have helped her perform an internal discrimination between herself and the representation of her dead mother. This metaphor was worked throughout her treatment. This systematised exercise confirms that the monster is a representation of herself and the representation of her dead mother.

Here I would like to briefly refer to Rudi Vermote's comments on the lack of reliability and validity studies of the 3-LM (Chapter 26). This model is a dynamic clinical tool, in the sense that it is open to modifications and developments that may come from its use. Its validity and reliability are being tested, and this growth is done in order to cater to the needs of the modern and evolving analyst. Different studies have been done regarding this issue (Garbarino, Luzardo, & Corti, 2019; Rodríguez Quiroga de Pereira, Borensztein, Bongiardino, Aufenacker, & Juan, 2019; Rodríguez Quiroga de Pereira, Borensztein, Corbella, & Marengo, 2018).

The aim pursued by the Specificity WP is for participants in the group to become more sensitive to their own analytical skills, especially free association, free-floating attention, and attentive listening. When they finish their work, they compare the 'replica' of the patient generated during the work sessions with the analyst's presentation of the patient. There is a subsequent reflective process, based on the reports or transcriptions of the group work, in which the invariants of the case that result in the associative chains of the participants are sought. This allows access to elements of the patient's internal world and the analytical process (Chabalgoity, De Souza Brito, & Ponce de León, Chapter 16, this book).[1]

The group worked with free-floating attention and listened to the analyst who read the clinical material aloud. Then, they did an exercise of free association, constructing different metaphors to account for a work of metaphorical deconstruction, unveiling the invariants of the patient's sessions. The material was derived from the patient's conflicts and modes of psychic functioning and the transferential modulations of the patient–analyst pair. This deconstruction work took the group closer to the metonymic form of expression and to emotional experiences and their transformations in the analyst's mind.

They worked with the image of the carousel, the hamster wheel. It was translated into something mechanical; the little routine was seen as the only way the patient had to confront her emotional situation, by locking herself up. They associated it with her speech, which also had circles. 'There is a wheel, there is a distaff, and there are games. There is a difficulty in letting others permeate her' (de Souza Brito & Chabalgoity, Chapter 21, this book). The replica built by the group construction included a description of the patient that took some of the metaphors involved in the other groups (hamster wheel), especially underlining her circular routines.

The group made an association with and 'reacted' to a transferential invariant of the patient. Based on this, the group took this 'circular motions' metaphor to express the sense of obsessive defences used to protect the patient from her feelings of despair and abandonment to cope with a psychotic mother and an unsupportive father. 'The sense of a request for listening and support and the routine defence trying to control their despair and emotional outburst are merging within the group' (de Souza Brito & Chabalgoity, Chapter 21, this book).

Although it is not strictly a metaphor, I found a discovery in the clinical material that allows to capture something of the transferential relationship very interesting, 'And I think about the autopilot scene, "pa-pa-pa-pa"' (de Souza Brito & Chabalgoity, Chapter 21, this book). The sonority of the word *papá* ('father' in Spanish), said repeatedly, monotonously, allowed the group to see an underlying emotional condition of a childish need. This refers to the transmodal concept of metaphor linked with archaic experiences that are repeated in the transferential situation. In the substratum shared with the group, the underlining, preverbal, subsymbolic metaphors emerge.

These phenomena have a verbal expression, with an emotional charge but not accompanied by the process of symbolisation. They sometimes help finding meaning throughout the process. They are expressions of the patient that emerge and may become bridges to their unconscious conflicts.

What we call metaphor in the other groups appeared through associative chains in this group. From these associative chains, the analysts made inferences and hypotheses about what happened to the patient. Some issues such as the autopilot, the hamster wheel, child abandonment, and depersonalisation arose. They describe unconscious conflicts, emotional states, and ways of object relations. These give the analyst input to rethink the patient from the replica built by the group.

This working group shows how, through their methodology, they capture the unconscious processes linked to the presented clinical material, including aspects that were not included in it but were later confirmed by the analyst.

The presenting analyst states that the group discussion was centred on the transference–countertransference relationship, and the context of the group associative dynamics co-creates a new transference field and a 'new patient' (the replica).

The process by which the group arrived at the inferences was based on certain premises of the mental functioning of patient and analyst and the group functioning. It remains a question to what extent both can be equivalent.

The main contribution of this group, in my opinion, is to help develop the analyst's listening skills and to amplify the capacity to perceive psychic phenomena. It also helps the permeability among unconscious, conscious, and preconscious processes, as the work of the group facilitates different and regressive states of the mind, enabling a creative potential in the analysts through a more irrational, imaginative way, having an amplifying effect on the phenomena that occur in the analytic field.

Discussion

I consider that the most important achievement of the WPs is to address clinical observations that are specific to each patient and each analytic dyad. This contrasts with the works and observations of analysts in previous years, which were deeply impregnated with psychoanalytic theories. As Jiménez (2021) pointed out, the methodology of the WPs has innovative features concerning the discussion of clinical material because

> it does not start from a theory or a framework (frequency of sessions, couch, etc.); it does not start from a hypothesis but from an open investigation, and it starts from the observation of what happens in practice when a psychoanalyst 'is doing psychoanalysis' (p. 156).

They have enabled a significant advance in analytical knowledge because they all start from listening to clinical experience. However, there is still a long way to go before they become reliable methods to answer to precise questions and to be replicable beyond their important value in enhancing the plural dialogue, as developed by Bernardi (Chapter 6, this book).

Regarding this experience, the three groups were able to work with metaphors, each in a different way, even though we did not propose a single definition of the concept of metaphor. The concept itself is not considered in the methods as such – although the proposal has its origins in the experience of 3-LM. The Specificity group speaks of the metaphorical process as a metonymic deconstruction. As for the CCM, it identified and analysed metaphors that arise from the clinical material, from the analytical field, brought by the patient as they are in the mind of the analyst and structured in the analytical field, in the transferential relationship. The 3-LM finds anchor points in the clinical material as

> metaphors or scenes that transmit in a vivid and unsaturated form the core of the patient's problems. Some of them appear from the beginning and become the focus of therapeutic work and serve as a background on which it is possible to identify subsequent changes. (Bernardi, 2015, p. 14)

The analyst who presented the clinical material also found that the different groups 'came up with similar and complementary metaphors reinforcing the idea of a common knowledge shared among analysts' (Pérez Suquilvide, Chapter 25, this book).

The CCM and the 3-LM underline that the patient has achieved a better balance between her own interests and those of the others. The patient's symbolisation is rich, full of affective experiences, bodily self, and fantasies, improving in differentiated relationships with internal and external objects (Pérez Suquilvide, Chapter 25, this book). Both the 3-LM and the CCM show that the interventions made by the analyst through metaphors lead to processes of change in the patient.

The three groups found that metaphors or metaphorical processes are significant for the understanding of clinical material. Do these underlined metaphors lead to an explanatory theory of what happens to the patient? All of the groups referred to the traumatic situation in relation to the mother, the patient's depersonalisation, and her inner monster. They came to observe the same aspects through different working methods.

Barnett and Katz (2009) stated that there is a 'clear accord on the use and value of metaphor as a clinical tool' (p. 2), meaning by this that psychoanalytic treatment aims to nurture the capacity for using and understanding metaphoric processes and articulate the present at many intersecting and interrelated levels of metaphor (Gargiulo, 2006). We tried to go beyond this notion in our work, and now we should reflect on the following question: Are metaphors *research tools* that contribute to a research process; that is, to help better understand phenomena in the field of study? In this book, metaphors were displayed as clinical research tools. Still, we also have their use as research tools, which aim to complement with extraclinical research methods and triangulation procedures.

The use of triangulation procedures, such as those developed with the specificity (Brito & Chabalgoity, Chapter 21, this book) method and the 3-LM (Rodriguez Quiroga de Pereira, Salesio, & Leibovich de Duarte, Chapter 22, this book), with empirical methods, specifically for the study of metaphors in the same clinical material, constitutes an advancement.

The unit of analysis in each of these groups was different. In the Specificity method, it is about thematic units and, in the 3-LM, the operationally defined metaphors about ourselves and significant others. Despite this, the results of both groups corresponded with those presented with the CCM, in the sense that metaphors used were all the same, as well as the assessments made from them about the patient. This reaffirms metaphors as a tool that is close to the clinic and they allow a common clinical field.

Empirical work introduces more metaphors that complement or extend previous ones. There is agreement between the findings of the clinical working group and those of the empirical research with 3-LM.

Expressions with a strong impact, determined by emotions, sensations, and bodily representations, emerged in all groups, even if they were not referred to as key metaphors. The three groups underline certain expressions that gain especially metaphorical meaning in the analytical communication and can be considered key metaphors in different ways and levels of abstraction or symbolisation (de León de Bernardi, Chapter 11, this book).

Even though we have to be aware of the difficulties in comparing methodologies with such different aims as the WPs, in this book the metaphor was used as a research tool, complementing the field of analytical study. New knowledge about the patient could be built from metaphors.

The richness of metaphors as indicators of the evolution of the psychoanalytic process was discussed by Vermote[2] in Chapter 26. Two WPs (CCM and 3-LM) refer to this notion. I believe that this richness is seen as the development of different kinds of images that indicate a change in the patient's view of their conflict, the relationship with themselves, and the emotional connection they express with that metaphor/image, instead of a richness of cognitive elaboration or the emergence of more complex images.

This experience contributes to Bernardi's (Chapter 27, this book) concern over finding 'a common clinical basis with a consensual and non-authoritative comparison of the different approaches based on shared criteria of evidence' (p. 000), forcing us to describe more rigorously and accurately what we observe and 'to draw out precisely both the viewpoint of observation and the inferential processes that follow' (Tuckett, 1995, p. 660). Therefore, it seems to me that the metaphor should continue to be considered an important bridge between the clinic and the different analysts who have different approaches and methods to analyse the clinical material. It can trigger an improvement in our conceptualisation, categorisation, and understanding of the different uses that analysts make of metaphors.

Notes

1 For this book, the group applied a systematic methodology of content analysis and its variety of discursive textual analysis to the material (de Souza Brito & Chabalgoity, Chapter 21, this book).

2 The table he presents in his chapter 'Clinical Psychoanalytic Research With the Working Party Method: State of the Art' is based on the information contained in this book.

References

Altmann de Litvan, M. (2021). Changes and no change in the representation of self and others through images and metaphors. In M. A.Fitzpatrick-Hanly, M.Altmann de Litvan, & R. Bernardi (Eds.), *Change through time in psychoanalysis: Transformations and interventions with the Three-Level Model*. London, England: Routledge.

Barnett, A. J., & Katz, S. M. (2009). Prologue. *Psychoanalytic Inquiry*, 29(1), 1–5.

Bernardi, R. (2015). La evaluación de los cambios del paciente. El modelo de los tres niveles (3-LM). *Mentalización. Revista de psicoanálisis y psicoterapia*, 4, 1–16. Retrieved from http://www.revistamentalizacion.com/ultimonumero/abril2015/bernardi.pdf

Bernardi, R. (2021). A common ground in clinical discussion groups: Intersubjective resonance and implicit operational theories. In M. A. Fiztpatrick-Hanly, M. Altmann de Litvan, & R. Bernardi (Eds.), *Change through time in psychoanalysis: Transformations and interventions with the Three-Level Model*. London, England: Routledge.

Cassorla, R. M. (2013). When the analyst becomes stupid: An attempt to understand enactment using Bion's theory of thinking. *Psychoanalytic Quarterly*, 82(2), 323–360.

de León de Bernardi, B., & Altmann de Litvan, M. (2014). The Three-Level Model in psychoanalytic training. In M. Altmann de Litvan (Ed.), *Time for change. Tracking transformations in psychoanalysis – The Three-Level Model*. London, England: Karnac.

Garbarino, A., Luzardo, M., & Corti, A. (2019). *Agreement among clinical judgments of psychoanalysts regarding the effects of unconscious mental processes of change during long periods of psychoanalysis*. Research granted through an IPA Research Grant, International Psychoanalytical Association.

Gargiulo, G. J. (2006). Ontology and metaphor: Reflections on the unconscious and the 'I' in the therapeutic setting. *Psychoanalytic Psychology*, 23(3), 461–474.

Jimenez, J. P. (2021). Discussion of Bruno Salesio's paper 'Sequence of Changes and Interventions in the Analysis of a Violent Patient'. In M. A. Fitzpatrick-Hanly, M. Altmann de Litvan, & R. Bernardi (Eds.), *Change through time in psychoanalysis: Transformations and interventions with the Three-Level Model*. London, England: Routledge.

Modell, A. H. (1997). Reflections on metaphor and affects. *The Annual of Psychoanalysis*, 25, 219–233.

Modell, A. H. (2009). Metaphor – The bridge between feelings and knowledge. *Psychoanalytic Inquiry*, 29, 6–11.

Rizzuto, A. M. (2009). Metaphoric process and metaphor: The dialectics of shared analytic experience. *Psychoanalytic Inquiry*, 29, 18–29.

Rodríguez Quiroga de Pereira, A., Borensztein, L., Bongiardino, L., Aufenacker, S. I., & Juan, S. (2019, May). *Probando hipótesis de cambio psíquico: Un estudio sistemático de un caso de psicoterapia psicoanalítica, utilizando el modelo de tres niveles (3-LM)*. Paper presented at the 20th Joseph Sandler Conference, Buenos Aires, Argentina.

Rodríguez Quiroga de Pereira, A., Borensztein, A., Corbella, V., & Marengo, J. C. (2018). The Lara case: A group analysis of initial psychoanalytic interviews using systematic clinical observation and empirical tools. *The International Journal of Psychoanalysis*, 99(6), 1327–1352.

Tuckett, D. (1995). The conceptualization and communication of clinical facts in psychoanalysis. *The International Journal of Psychoanalysis*, 76, 653–662.

Tuckett, D., Basile, R., Birksted-Breen, D., Bohm, T., Ferro, A., Hinz, H., … Schubert, J. (2008). *Psychoanalysis comparable and incomparable*. New York, NY: Routledge.

Index

Page numbers in *italics* denote illustrative material.